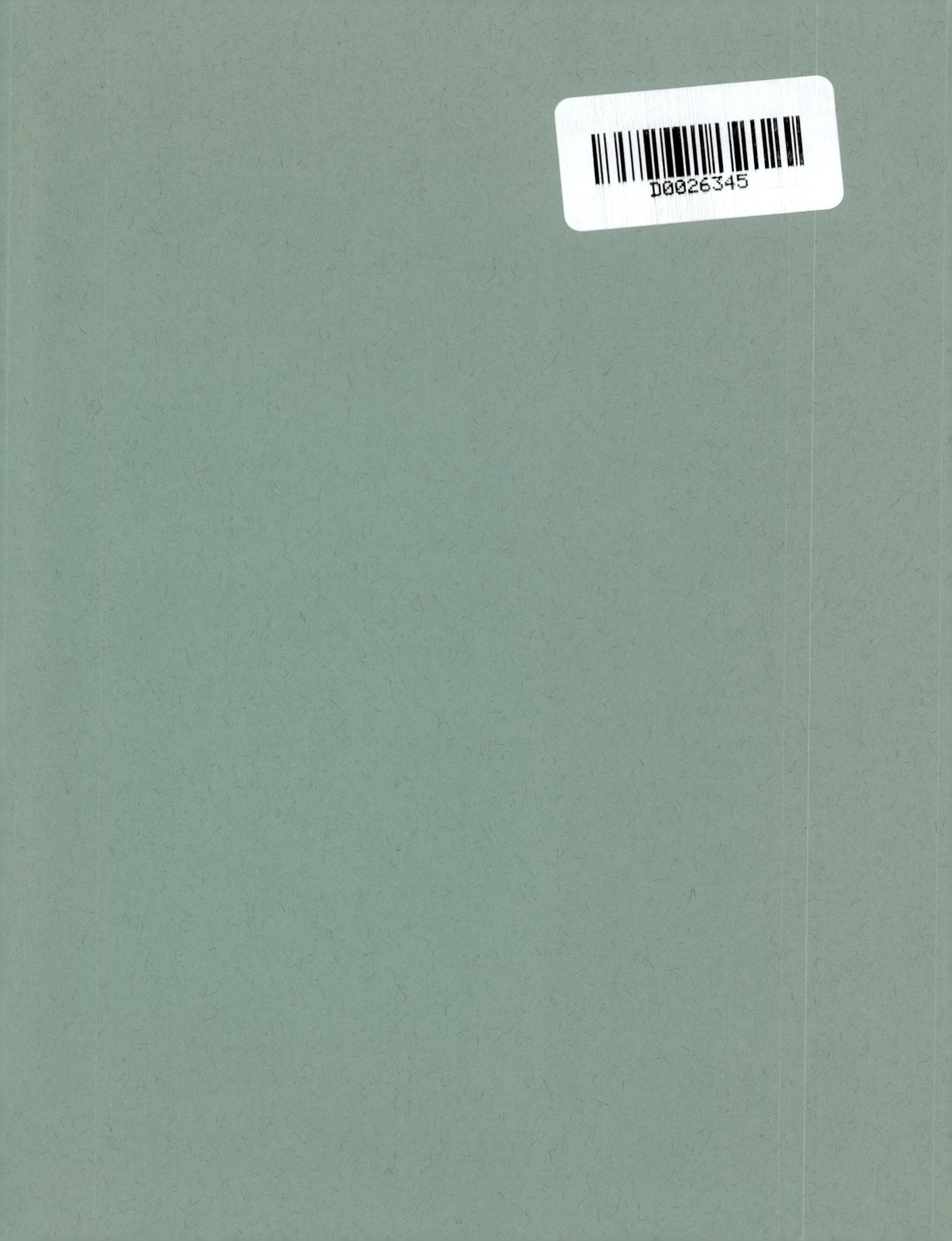
D0026345

CLINICAL DECISION MAKING IN PHYSICAL THERAPY

CLINICAL DECISION MAKING IN PHYSICAL THERAPY

STEVEN L. WOLF, Ph.D., R.P.T.
ASSOCIATE PROFESSOR
DEPARTMENT OF REHABILITATION MEDICINE
ASSISTANT PROFESSOR
DEPARTMENTS OF ANATOMY AND SURGERY
EMORY UNIVERSITY SCHOOL OF MEDICINE
ATLANTA, GEORGIA

F. A. DAVIS COMPANY 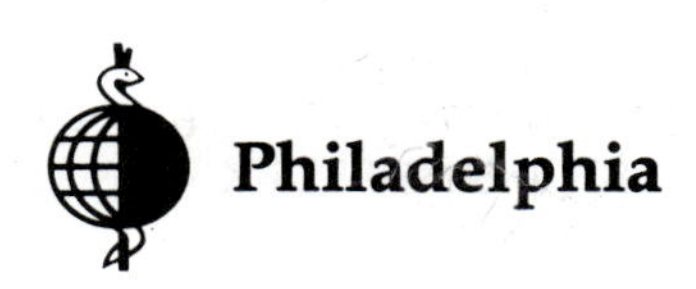 Philadelphia

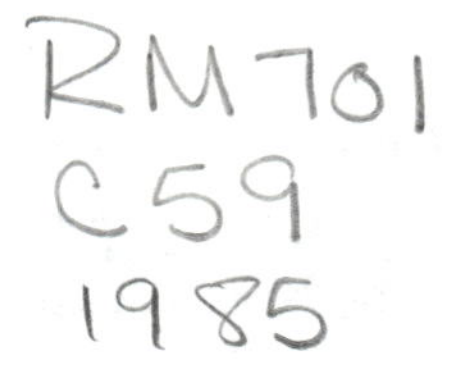

Second printing 1986

Printed in the United States of America

Library of Congress Cataloging in Publication Data
Main entry under title:

Clinical decision making in physical therapy.

Based on a conference held in Atlanta, Ga., Sept. 22-26, 1982.
Includes bibliographical references and index.
1. Physical therapy—Decision making—Congresses. I. Wolf, Steven L.
[DNLM: 1. Decision Making—congresses. 2. Physical Therapy—congresses.
WB 460 C641 1982]
RM701.C59 1985 615.8′2 84-9631
ISBN 0-8036-9525-X

DEDICATION

To the physical therapists in the State of Georgia, without whose financial support, personal involvement, and tireless efforts this text would not be possible.

To all physical therapists, present and future, who believe that to best serve their patients, the bases for clinical competence and professional excellence must reside within the processes of unending inquiry and reasoning.

A NOTE TO EDUCATORS

Clinical decision making is a process that is usually enacted within the context of patient treatment. Clearly, the genesis for this essential phase of effective intervention begins well before professional responsibilities are finally handed to the "new" physical therapist. The tenor for logical and meaningful evaluation and treatment progressions is first established by the educator within both clinical and classroom environments.

This text is designed to facilitate that process. No effort or implication to replace or to rechannel the educational premises for teaching elements of clinical decision making is rendered within this book. Rather, the contributors firmly believe that an analysis of the thoughts and concepts embodied herein will assist educators in helping to appropriately mold the thought processes of their students within the context of existing teaching methodologies. Within this book, one will find analytic approaches to patients spanning five specialty areas, as well as the development of several philosophic issues that require necessary absorption and discussion among teachers, students, and clinicians if future directions of the profession are to follow the paths clearly laid by the membership of the American Physical Therapy Association.

By incorporating these treatment and philosophic components into classroom and clinical teaching, we believe that the educator's role in preparing "basic" physical therapy students to enter the profession will become greatly expanded. These students will have thus been exposed to issues that they will directly confront upon embarking on clinical practice. By providing basic entry-level students with specific content (e.g., decision trees, documentation, psychosocial aspects of treatment, and so forth), we feel that their abilities to more effectively communicate with their future colleagues, contribute to the profession, and support their rationale for treatment approaches will be substantially enhanced.

The text may be used in many different ways for basic physical therapy students. The sections dealing with decision making within specific specialties, by necessity, are best appreciated by experienced clinicians (or "advanced" physical therapy students). However, basic students will, at least, glean a preliminary insight into how some of the most respected therapists in our profession think and problem solve. The influence that that initial exposure to the words of these master clinicians will have upon the intellectual development of our basic students has yet to be determined. One cannot help but speculate that this influence can only be positive. The more broad-based contributions made by Watts, Hislop, Stockmeyer, Ramsden, and Johnson do not necessarily require advanced clinical training in order to facilitate student appreciation for the diversified components contributing to professional competence. Ultimately, each educator will find the most effective manner in which to incorporate parts of the text or its totality into his or her own unique teaching style.

Steven L. Wolf

A NOTE TO CLINICIANS

Our profession is expanding in scope and responsibility at an exponential rate. The necessity of graduating more physical therapists to meet the health demands throughout the remainder of this century has been articulated by many governmental and professional voices. Concomitantly, we are faced with escalating health care costs—a situation that has clear implications for financial reimbursement of physical therapy services within this country and abroad. Payment for services rendered is already under close scrutiny; clearly, future decisions on reimbursement for treatment provided by physical therapists hinge upon demonstrable efficacy and defined cost-benefit ratios.

Essential to promulgating our stance—and with it, our destiny—are the development of a sound rationale upon which evaluative and treatment decisions are made and the incorporation of contemporary elements (e.g., cost-analyses, documentation, applied research, interprofessional consultation, and so forth) into professional practice. This text attempts to address both of these issues by exposing the reader to the thought processes espoused by some of our master clinicians and by presenting information relevant to the expansion of our professional responsibilities in the future.

It is hoped that by digesting and utilizing the contents of this text, clinicians will be able to augment and diversify the bases for their clinical practices in a manner that promotes professional growth and better prepares us for our future responsibilities. Unlike texts of past, such as *NUSTEP,* this book does not attempt to explain clinical therapeutic applications by outlining or reiterating in step-like manner procedures for treatment within the five specialty areas addressed by the contributors. Certainly, sufficient numbers of texts and workshop offerings already provide such a service. Rather, the contributors view the basis for our clinical growth, and its resultant success, as an ability to more effectively integrate essential evaluation and treatment in an ongoing and continuous manner. Their thoughts on and methods of attaining such essential skills are presented in case presentation formats. We believe that by studying these approaches, all clinicians will be able to more adequately develop their own internal and external resources to better meet the demands and responsibilities facing us as we attempt to continue our professional growth in a manner compatible with the goals that we have set for our future autonomy. In this regard, this text is indeed unique from any of its predecessors.

We offer apologies to those clinicians whose special interests are not represented within this book. Time and physical, as well as fiscal, constraints prevented us from including other clinical specialty areas. Nonetheless, we believe that because this is a text about problem solving and the integration of evaluative and treatment methodologies, *any clinician* can enhance clinical competence through absorbing the process embodied within these pages.

Steven L. Wolf

ACKNOWLEDGMENTS

The success of the conference that formed the basis for this text could not have been achieved without the unique talents and unlimited energy of several physical therapists, each of whom deserves special accolades. The multitalented Bonnie Blossom undertook the planning and coordination of this effort. She was ably assisted by the following chairmen and their outstanding committees: Randy Walker (Finance Committee); Jody Tomberlin (Program Committee); Jim Church (Properties Committee); Stuart Binder-MacLeod (Publicity Committee); Nina Jo Byrd (Registration Follow-up Committee); Lynda Woodruff (Communications Committee); Glory Sanders (Resource Development Committee); and Lois B. Wolf (Social Committee). Considerable appreciation is expressed to the faculty of the conference and contributors to this text, who took one weekend of their time in October 1981 to fly to Atlanta to participate in the planning of the conference.

Financial support offered by the Physical Therapy Association of Georgia, Inc., several private practitioners, the Emory University Regional Rehabilitation Research and Training Center, the Shepherd Spinal Center, and numerous local vendors and rehabilitation equipment companies is greatly appreciated. The diligent typing efforts of my secretary, Gloria Bassett, are responsible for the final cohesive form of all contributions. Finally, the participants at our conference are acknowledged for their insightful analyses and active involvement throughout the four-day experience.

CONTRIBUTORS

RAYMOND L. BLESSEY, M.A., P.T.
Program Director, Cardiac Rehabilitation
Ross Loos Medical Center
Los Angeles, California

SUZANN K. CAMPBELL, Ph.D., L.P.T.
Associate Professor, Division of Physical Therapy
Department of Medical Allied Health Professions
School of Medicine
University of North Carolina at Chapel Hill
Chapel Hill, North Carolina

CAROL E. COOGLER, Sc.D., P.T.
Associate Professor, Department of Physical Therapy
School of Health Science
Georgia State University
Atlanta, Georgia

PHILLIP B. DONLEY, M.S., P.T., A.T., C.
Head Athletic Trainer
Professor, Physical Education
West Chester University
West Chester, Pennsylvania

HELEN J. HISLOP, Sc.D., F.A.P.T.A.
Professor and Chairman
Department of Physical Therapy
University of Southern California
Downey, California

MAUREEN K. HOLDEN, M.M.Sc., R.P.T.
Assistant Professor
MGH Institute of Health Professions
Clinical Specialist in Neurology
Department of Physical Therapy
Massachusetts General Hospital
Boston, Massachusetts

SCOT IRWIN, M.A., R.P.T.
Director, Physical Therapy
Clayton General Hospital
Riverdale, Georgia
Assistant Professor
Georgia State University
Atlanta, Georgia

GENEVA RICHARD JOHNSON, Ph.D., F.A.P.T.A.
Associate Professor
Department of Rehabilitation
Baylor College of Medicine
Houston, Texas

RICHARD NYBERG, P.T.
Clinician, Atlanta Back Clinic
Orthopedic Physical Therapy and Training Center
Faculty Member, Division of Physical Therapy
Emory University
Instructor, Institute of Graduate Health Sciences
Atlanta, Georgia

STANLEY V. PARIS, N.Z.S.P., M.C.S.P., P.T.
Professor, Manipulative Therapy
Institute of Graduate Health Sciences
Atlanta, Georgia
Visiting Lecturer
Massachusetts General Hospital
Institute of Health Professions
Boston, Massachusetts

WALTER PERSONIUS, M.A., P.T.
Department of Physical Therapy
School of Allied Professions
Medical College of Virginia
Virginia Commonwealth University
Richmond, Virginia

RONALD G. PEYTON, M.S., P.T., A.T., C.
Director, Sports Medicine Education Institute and Rehabilitation Services of Atlanta
Atlanta, Georgia

ELSA L. RAMSDEN, Ed.D., R.P.T.
Associate Professor and Planning Associate
Office of the Provost
University of Pennsylvania
Philadelphia, Pennsylvania

SHIRLEY SAHRMANN, Ph.D., P.T.
Associate Director for Research
Program in Physical Therapy
Washington University School of Medicine
St. Louis, Missouri

SHIRLEY A. STOCKMEYER, M.A., R.P.T.
Associate Professor
Department of Physical Therapy
Sargent College of Allied Health Professions
Boston University
Boston, Massachusetts

NANCY T. WATTS, Ph.D., R.P.T.
Professor and Director
Physical Therapy Graduate Program
MGH Institute of Health Professions
Massachusetts General Hospital
Boston, Massachusetts

STEVEN L. WOLF, Ph.D., R.P.T.
Associate Professor
Department of Rehabilitation Medicine
Assistant Professor
Departments of Anatomy and Surgery
Emory University School of Medicine
Atlanta, Georgia

JANET E. YOUNG, M.D., P.T.
Chief, Developmental Pediatrics
Department of Pediatrics
Fitzsimons Army Medical Center
Aurora, Colorado

CONTENTS

INTRODUCTION

STEVEN L. WOLF, Ph.D., R.P.T.

In the summer of 1966, a grant from the Vocational Rehabilitation Administration helped subsidize a 4-week conference known as the Northwestern University Special Therapeutic Exercise Project (NUSTEP). This project's major objectives were exploring and analyzing the "state of the art" of therapeutic exercise. Subsequently, the proceedings from the conference were published *(American Journal of Physical Medicine,* Volume 46, February, 1967, 1191 pp). Assembled for this Chicago meeting were clinical and research notables whose teachings and philosophies were often viewed with dogmatic enthusiasm. A considerable portion of the program was devoted to a review of the psychomotor skills underlying therapeutic exercise. This program included a limited amount of "basic information," primarily concerning motor control and muscle activity, that was provided by scientists and physicians with an identified allegiance to the rehabilitative process. In retrospect, conspicuously absent from the basic information section was any concerted attempt to relate scientific fact to clinical relevance. Furthermore, clinical-"technique"-oriented presentations appeared unrelated and fragmentary. Occasionally, when the umbrella of empiricism was let down, the few persons who provided relationships between application and basic, underlying neurophysiologic mechanisms had not subjected the latter to any form of external validation. Such was the "state of the art" in 1966. Clearly, physical therapy could justifiably have been labeled as a technology by other medical professions viewing our activities and actions.

Ironically, the June 1966 issue of *Physical Therapy* (Volume 46, listing 24 continuing-education courses, in contrast to 145 such courses listed in Volume 63, June 1983) contained an editorial by Helen Hislop, its editor at that time (and a contributor to this text), and entitled *Today and Beyond* (p. 584). In her typically profound and prognostic manner, Hislop wrote:

Specializing in the techniques of physical therapy will not be enough—we will have to specialize in the problems of our patients. . . . The future cannot be planned by tired, rigid minds. Those who challenge the present system will bear the wounds of the challenge. But wounds heal and the scars that remain may serve as useful reminders that achievement is made only by those who are dissatisfied. Achievement is made only by those who are willing to advocate changes in institutions to keep pace with progress and enlightened thinking.

We progress by difference. We regress by conformity. We advance by originality. We retreat by submission. We succeed by distinction. We fail by imitation. We achieve recognition through our maturity. We are bypassed through our inadequacies.

In the 17 years following NUSTEP, many of Hislop's thoughts have emerged as actions. Physical therapy has advanced primarily through the efforts of its past few generations. Individuals who had become dissatisfied with the knowledge base that dictated things as they were sought more sophisticated basic and clinical education, often outside the realm of physical therapy—only to return to enlighten and advance the knowledge base of more recent graduates.

Those physical therapists who sought change through advanced education have clearly contributed new clinical theories and techniques that are truly diversified. Yet, these people, several of whom are contributors to this book, shared some common elements. Each had learned to think critically, to decide rationally, and to seek additional information appropriately. Indeed, such components must stand as the cornerstone of professionalism.

Concurrently, policies were enacted and philosophies adopted that were, and continue to be, consonant with the maturation of physical therapy. Internal educational accreditation systems, post-baccalaureate educational entry levels, and specialization competency boards could be initiated only if definable and precise bodies of knowledge were becoming recognized both from within physical therapy and in the eyes of the medical community. Of equal significance was the fact that changes within state practice acts were underway. Such revisions enabled physical therapists to evaluate and/or treat patients autonomously. Implicit in these revisions were at least two assumptions: (1) Physical therapists have the depth of knowledge to be primary medical-care providers; and (2) elements of maturity, wisdom, and inquiry abound with enough significance to warrant the public's trust.

Of these emerging changes within physical therapy, unquestionably the last is the most awesome. In discussing professional standards, Philip Elliot, in his book *The Sociology of the Professions* (Herder and Herder, New York, 1972), wrote:

The scope for the development of independent professional standards is correspondingly lower. This would seem to be the one reason for the lack of interest such professions show in theoretical knowledge or academic learning, whatever academic definitions of a profession may have laid down as necessary for professional status. (p. 146)

To be deserving of voluntary participation within autonomous practice and for physical therapy to emerge as a profession, clinicians must engage in an ongoing pursuit of knowledge and reason. Inquiry and rational decision making within the context of comprehensive, not fragmented, treatment for all patients are mandatory. Toward this end, a survey of continuing-education courses will reveal that programs advocating instruction in specific motor skills or "techniques" regrettably persist, but their number and intensity have diminished since 1966. At the same time, the variety and frequency of courses designed to "integrate" approaches or to "analyze" the bases for treatment protocols have multiplied. In short, such changes in practice and education refortify the notion that physical therapy is evolving into a conglomerate of unique and esoteric skills complemented by documented and rational approaches. We are in transition from technology to profession.

Precisely these points of view were being articulated one pleasant night in the spring of 1980 when physical therapists within Georgia had gathered for a weekend meeting. From these casual discussions emerged profound introspection and the realization that who we are and what we can represent had not been intensely documented since the NUSTEP conference in 1966. Certainly, ongoing changes within physical therapy required a sharing of ideas through a collective wisdom greater than our own and an expression of comprehensive decision making by outstanding clinicians representing several of our emerging specializations. From these concerns was borne *Toward Excellence in Physical Therapy Practice: A Conference on Comprehensive Clinical Decision-Making,* which was held in Atlanta, Georgia, September 22 to 26, 1982.

Recognizing that clinical evaluation and treatment must be comprehensive, integrative, and ongoing, this conference sought, as its primary goal, a vehicle to assist physical therapy practitioners to develop and improve clinical decision-making skills. Specific objectives were as follows:

- to identify initial and ongoing evaluation processes and purposes
- to identify how and where to initiate treatment based on evaluation results
- to identify the need for and timing of re-evaluation and modification of the treatment program
- to assess personal limitations in the evaluation and treatment processes
- to improve the ability to interpret clinical signs
- to identify resources to improve the clinician's base of knowledge and skills.

The contributors to this text have attempted to provide both a series of multidimensional considerations underlying clinical decision making and insight into the thought processes undertaken during problem solving. Within the text, models for decision making are provided. Psychosocial, educational, and research issues are presented. The reader is given perspectives from clinical specialists with the hope that practice at assimilating their approaches will be congruent with professional clinical responsibilities, without sacrifice of one's unique interactions with patients.

The text begins with a comprehensive discussion of decision analysis presented by Nancy Watts. She refortifies the notion that such analyses are complex, broadly scientific, and valuable. At the same time, formulations of clinical decisions can be intuitive, uncertain, and expensive. A "decision tree" format is discussed, and the reader is reminded that although systematic derivation of decisions is important, such a process should not produce a loss of the uniqueness dictated by patient diagnosis and the individuality of each practitioner.

Helen Hislop provides a perspective on the role of education in clinical decision making. She makes an articulate argument for the clinician's need to integrate isolated pieces of data within the evaluative process. The importance of the patient is emphasized, for present and future clinicians cannot be taught or learn how to make meaningful decisions outside the clinical environs. In the second phase of her presentation, Hislop discusses risk. Within this concept, she implores the clinician to always question data and explanations. Higher education should not be feared by clinicians, but challenged in terms of relevance of information and applicability of knowledge. Last, her discussion of people and data demonstrates sample methods for data acquisition that are easily retrievable and clinically useful.

Geneva Johnson provides an insightful chapter on the collection and use of documentation within the treatment setting. She emphasizes that contemporary technology provides a rapid, easy, and efficient vehicle for data acquisition. Such accumulation need not require computers but must follow a systematic approach. The growth and maturation of physical therapy have already been addressed in this Introduction. Johnson discusses a frequently overlooked and underestimated phase of that growth—marketing. Our ongoing compliment of new people and novel clinical practice environments implies a responsibility in marketing our skills. This concern, argues Johnson, necessitates responsibility for the presentation of meaningful, accurate, and timely data acquisition and analyses. She reminds us of an ongoing need to be politically active at local, state, and national levels to attain the maximal and best representation for our skills and contributions to society.

A unique approach to decision analysis is offered by Shirley Stockmeyer, who emphasizes a need for clinicians to understand homeostatic mechanisms as a basis for clinical judgments and reactions to any aspect of treatment. She argues that the effects of a treatment intervention, designed to restore homeostasis, should be reassessed *between* treatments to differentiate prolonged responses from secondary physiologic or psychologic compensations. In this regard, clinical decisions must be, in part, based upon the timing, dosage, and nature of the intervention.

A meaningful discussion of the psychosocial aspects of patient-therapist interaction within the context of decision making is offered in the chapter by Elsa Ramsden. She provides a seven-phase (receive, infer, feel, feel-about-feeling, determine, decide, and act) process important to assessment *about* patients as a step preliminary to initiating clinical decisions. The reader is given a perspective on the clinician's role that emphasizes a comprehension of social and cultural components unique to each patient and that pleads for clinician determinations to identify and manage available resources *to effect the best* possible decisions. Ramsden concludes her chapter with a relevant discussion on therapists' responsibilities to themselves and the profession.

The second phase of this text exposes the reader to the thought processes used by superb clinicians in the areas of cardiopulmonary, neurologic, orthopaedic, pediatric, and sports physical therapy. Apologies are offered to readers with other clinical interests, such as geriatric or electrophysiologic physical therapy; however, limited financial resources prevented the inclusion of such essential areas of specialization within the conference and, ultimately, this text. The same explanation is rendered for why each specialty area is addressed by only two clinicians.

It should be noted that within each clinical presentation, the authors have attempted to reveal decision processes within the context of case studies. No attempt was made to impose a uniform style or format on clinicians, for to do so would detract from the unique presentation of each and limit the versatility and variance between specialties and specialists. Each author has chosen to draw upon information presented in the previous portion of the text in different ways.

Edited transcriptions from an extensive question-and-answer period within the conference are provided. This inclusion enables the reader to appreciate the concerns expressed by the faculty participants and the attending clinicians. Generally, the topics are approached within the context of the future of physical therapy. Concepts such as education, specialization, general practice, data acquisition, referral resources, and clinical training are presented in an intense and enlightening manner.

A summation is offered by Wolf, who attempts to differentiate between common and unique aspects of clinical decision making across specialties. Items identified for future exploration and development are highlighted. Unique considerations that emerged through presentations and discussions and that could potentially alter the approach to patient assessment and treatment are addressed.

Finally, Geneva Johnson shares her glimpses into the future of physical therapy practice. The basis of her concern centers about a necessity for a commitment to life-long inquiry and learning among clinicians within a climate that dictates a need for a greater variety of physical therapy services and renewed emphasis on prevention of illness and maintenance of health.

Chapter 1

DECISION ANALYSIS: A TOOL FOR IMPROVING PHYSICAL THERAPY PRACTICE AND EDUCATION

NANCY T. WATTS, Ph.D., R.P.T.

How can we improve clinical decision making in physical therapy? Let us begin by asking, "What is clinical decision making, and why do we feel it needs improvement?"

As I think about the decision process physical therapists use when they work with patients, six characteristics stand out.

CHARACTERISTICS OF CLINICAL DECISION MAKING

First, the process is *complex*. Treatment of even the most straightforward disorder requires a series of very different choices: choices about the problems to be addressed, goals and priorities, the timing and intensity of treatment, the methods to be used, the degree to which patients will be made responsible for their own treatment, and about where and by whom treatment should be given.

The process is also highly *evaluative*. In order to make these many choices wisely, we base them on a careful assessment of each patient's needs. We evaluate the patient's potential for response and the likelihood that the response will include unwanted side effects. Then, as treatment proceeds, we assess its effects, sometimes on a moment-to-moment basis. While much of the data base on which we build a therapeutic plan is collected before treatment begins, much that is important can be discovered only while treatment is in progress. This is especially evident during therapeutic exercise and functional training. We give a direction or start a movement and then see and feel the patient's response. Acting on this information, we adjust the pressure of our hands, the tone of our voice, or the speed of the movement in order to modify or maintain the patient's response, to shape it into the pattern we seek. At such moments, evaluation and intervention occur almost simultaneously in a rapidly reverberating circuit that links our performance to that of the patient. This is one of the skills I think of when we speak of the "art of clinical practice."

At the same time, our decision making is broadly *scientific.* We interpret the patient's signs and symptoms using a conceptual vocabulary drawn from years of study of the structure and function of the human body. We draw on studies of disease process, research on human development, and theories of human learning, perception, motivation, and pain. Our therapeutic choices are guided not by whim or custom, but by logical application of this rich, scientific lore.

Next, we must concede that our work is both *expensive and valuable.* Although charges for a single physical therapy treatment may seem modest compared with those for many other health services, our contacts with an individual patient often extend over many months. The sheer volume of our services creates an impressive national bill for physical therapy each year. This cost is balanced by the potential value of the goals we can help our patients achieve. What we do truly matters. The stakes are high: comfort, independence, dignity, even survival may depend heavily upon the correctness of the decisions made by the physical therapist.

Therefore, it is sobering to realize that our clinical decisions often are also highly *uncertain.* Each patient we treat is unique—different in important ways from all the others we see who share the same general disorder. The patient's needs, concerns, priorities, and potential for response are influenced by a network of interrelated factors. Some are known to us; others, however, may be entirely unsuspected. Even careful selection of treatment represents, at best, an educated guess. Although this uncertainty is difficult to tolerate, we know that if we were to attempt to eliminate it by identifying and evaluating every factor that might have a significant effect on results, neither we nor our patients would live long enough for treatment to begin.

Finally, as I examine this complex, evaluative, scientific, costly process we call clinical decision making, I am struck by how much of it is done *intuitively.* Delineation of the patient's problem, selection of goals, review of treatment options, interpretation of observed results, establishment of priorities, and all other major clinical decisions are made only in part through conscious, verbalized analysis. They also rely profoundly on what scientist-philosopher Michael Polanyi has called "tacit knowledge." If we examine human knowledge, suggests Polanyi, we find:

> . . .we can know more than we can tell. . . . Take an example. We know a person's face, and can recognize it among a thousand, indeed among a million, yet we usually cannot tell how we recognize the face we know. So most of this knowledge cannot be put into words.[1]

How well this describes the way a master clinician senses, recognizes, and responds to each patient's problem. The perception and integration of tactile and visual cues, and our sensing of the patient's mood and level of motivation, seem particularly reliant on intuitive skills borne of long clinical experience.

The clinical judgment of a physical therapist is clearly an elegant mixture of art and science. Complex, costly, and important decisions, based on careful evaluation and an array of scientific principles, also rely heavily on knowledge and judgments of which even the therapist is largely unaware.

We have good reason to feel proud of this decision-making process. However, the importance of these decisions for our patients, and the cost and scarcity of our services, oblige us to examine the process critically to search for possible flaws. Let me point out some problems I find particularly troubling.

HAZARDS IN CLINICAL DECISION MAKING

First, although even the simplest clinical problem presents the therapist with a number of potential choices for management, we are often tempted to ignore many of these decisions and to substitute a routinized approach to care. This is especially true for problems we see often. We develop "our way" of treating the hemiplegic patient with a painful shoulder, "our approach" to teaching transfers, our "pet tricks" for motivating the elderly arthritic patient. We cross some methods off our list of possible tests or treatments, dismissing them as being not really very effective, too time consuming, or "not the way we do it in our department." These general decisions sharply limit the range of options we consider for each patient. Carried to extremes, this leads to therapeutic programs based on habit and convenience rather than on rational, individualized selection of the best approach for each patient. This loss of openness is fostered by the fact that our standardized methods are often reasonably successful. When I ask clinicians what other methods they are planning to try besides the one they are using now, they often answer with surprise, "None. This is working fine." My next question, "How can you be sure something else wouldn't work even better?" is regarded as something only an aging teacher would ask.

Narrowness of vision is a challenge all decision makers face. Herbert Simon, in his analysis of the decision processes used by administrators, writes:

> All behavior involves conscious or unconscious selection of particular actions out of all those that are physically possible. . . . The term "selection" is used here without any implication of a conscious or deliberate process. It refers simply to the fact that, if the individual follows one course of action, there are other courses of action he foregoes.[2]

When choice is unconscious, the risk of narrowness is especially great. We are likely to simply accept the first promising possibility that occurs to us and reject all others by default. Yet, fully rational, conscious decision making is laborious. To be fully rational, Simon proposes, we must begin by identifying *all possible* courses of action. Then, these must each be evaluated in terms of the resources they will require and the results they promise. Only through careful comparison of such a detailed projection of costs and benefits can we expect to choose the *best* alternative. Simon recognizes that in reality this is usually impossible. Of all the possibilities actually open to us, only a few actually come to mind even when we make our most important decisions. Our knowledge of the consequences and costs of these alternatives is fragmentary and often inaccurate. We are limited in our efforts at rationality by our own knowledge, skill, values, and views of the purpose of the endeavor, and we are constrained by the practical limits of the system in which we work and by our own time and energies. Honest and accurate assessment of probable costs is particularly difficult for many therapists. Techniques for doing this have not been emphasized in our professional curricula, and concern with the business side of health care seems foreign, and even distasteful, to many dedicated clinicians. In reality, therefore, we compromise. We consider not all possibilities, but only those that seem most promising and feasible. We do not compare the possibilities in terms of all associated costs and benefits, but only in terms of those that seem most important and are most easily assessed. The risk, of course, is that we will compromise unnecessarily. If we and our profession are to thrive and grow, we must have tools to combat the many pressures that foster narrowness, tools that protect us from mindless routine and therapeutic tunnel vision by reminding us of the many choices we can make in patient care.

The evaluative component of our clinical decision making carries with it a different sort of risk. Here I believe the danger is not so much that we will be too narrow, but that we may be wastefully broad. We pride ourselves on the thoroughness of the subjective and objective data base we develop for each patient, and on the precision with which we can assess even subtle and complex problems. Many therapists have a battery of tests they feel should be completed on certain types of patients before any treatment is begun. This orderly thoroughness helps to ensure that potential problems will be picked up at an early stage and allows us to individualize each patient's treatment. However, I believe in many cases, a great deal of the evaluative data we collect are never actually used in designing treatment. In some cases, information we collect on all patients proves to be useful only for a few. In other cases, marked differences in findings are never translated into differences in the type, intensity, or timing of the treatment we select. In still other instances, we repeat evaluations already carried out by a colleague in order to get a more precise or complete picture of some aspect of the patient's problem even when this degree of thoroughness and accuracy is really not necessary in order for us to make a wise decision about care. The cost of these unused evaluations is difficult to justify. The minutes, hours, and days we spend in evaluating a patient are costly not only in terms of the charges they create, but in the demands they make on the patient's time, energy, and spirit. Most important of all, these wasted evaluations may have high "opportunity costs." These are the foregone benefits of the things we might have accomplished had we done something else with this time: the value of beginning treatment earlier, of treating the patient more often, of expanding our services to new patients. Of course, there are many times when thorough evaluation is essential, when choosing treatment without it is pointless and wasteful. The essential thing is that we use evaluation selectively. We cannot take pride in this part of our decision making unless we consistently ask ourselves:

"Will the results of this evaluation really make a difference in the treatments I choose?"

"Will knowing this help me improve my treatment decision enough to be worth what getting this information will cost?"

"Do I need to know this now? Could I wait until I'm more certain this information is relevant for this particular patient?"

> "What should I find out first? How should I begin my workup in order to decide what other information I need?"

This is not a defense of inadequate or sloppy evaluations. It is a plea for selectivity, frugality, and conscientious use of all the information we do collect. We have several tools that help us to do this: screening tests that help us decide in what area a patient needs more detailed assessment; evaluation strategies that follow a branching pattern, with findings at each stage determining what evaluations will be done next; problem-oriented records that highlight the relationship of data base to treatment plan. The problem is troublesome enough, however, to call for additional tools to guide our selection of evaluation methods.

The scientific theory that supports our professional practice can help us to achieve the openness and efficiency we seek. Our scientific knowledge can suggest new courses of action, help us predict response to treatment, and explain why unwanted side effects may appear. However, scientific theory alone does not automatically provide a clear guide to action for the clinician. Theory of a different sort is needed as well. Chris Argyris and Donald Schon,[3] in their analysis of professional action, describe three different types of theories. Some are *explanatory* and propose mechanisms that account for the phenomena we see. Others are *predictive* and describe the consequences associated with specific actions under specified conditions. It seems to me the scientific theory that makes up so much of our professional curriculum falls largely in one or the other of these two categories. The third type of theory Argyris and Schon label *theory of control or action.* Such theory states, "If you want to produce this result, under these circumstances, take this action." These action guidelines may be logically derived from theories of explanation and prediction, but the translation is not automatic. Particularly when we draw on scientific theory developed through laboratory studies on nonhuman subjects and use it to formulate theory to guide our actions with patients, the resulting theory of control must be carefully stated and rigorously tested. In physical therapy, we have done very little clinical theory building. Perhaps this is true in part because so much of the decision making of our finest clinicians is intuitive. Their judgments do appear to be guided by consistent theories of action, but these have not been fully spelled out so that they can be analyzed and tested. We do, of course, have many rules of thumb that we teach our students and follow ourselves in day-to-day patient care.

- Use diagonal, spiral patterns to facilitate motion.
- Wrap the stump so pressure is greatest distally.
- Work for proximal stability before distal mobility.
- Decrease the work load if the patient's heart rate exceeds the target level by more than four beats a minute.
- Bend your knees when you lift a heavy weight.

We have logical reasons for these clinical commandments, and much of our rationale is carefully derived from the findings of basic science. However, only a handful of these guidelines have ever been rigorously tested through clinical research. Even though our logic is impressive and experienced clinicians agree that such rules are true, we should mistrust them. Too many opportunities exist for us to fool ourselves through wishful thinking, self-fulfilling prophecies, and confusion of correlation with causation for us to be comfortable until our principles of action have been scientifically tested. Until then, our decision making will be guided not by a sound theory of action but by a body of professional folklore.

This sounds as though I believe that if we really set our minds to it, physical therapy could one day possess a series of tested rules that would tell a clinician exactly what to do with each patient. Not so! The sort of theory building I envision can help us to weed out many of the false rules of thumb we now follow. It cannot hope to eliminate all of the uncertainty that accompanies practice with varied and unique human patients. In an extraordinary recent book, *Medical Choices, Medical Chances,* Harold Bursztajn and his colleagues explore this uncertainty and its sources. They point out that:

> . . . a world that is made up of causes and effects is still an uncertain world. It is not simply that we cannot know all the causes; it is that causes themselves operate to some degree by chance . . . a particular effect may have many causes and a particular cause may have many effects . . . the same effects may not always have the same causes, and the effects of a given cause (and vice versa) cannot be isolated with certainty.[4]

Under such circumstances, a therapeutic plan represents a sort of "principled gamble" that the result we want will occur if we follow the most logically promising course of action. Yet, once our plans are implemented, we often fail to treat them as the uncertain ventures they are. We neglect to build into our treatments a carefully planned system for continuous monitoring of whether our gamble succeeds. To do this would require us to set objectively measurable targets that spell out how much we believe we should be able to accomplish within specific time periods. Instead, we are often content simply to say that our goals are to increase the patient's endurance, to relieve pain, to normalize tone, and to improve functional independence, without committing ourselves to how much achievement of each goal we hope for and by when. We also often neglect to specify the identifying characteristics of negative reactions or unwanted side effects we think may occur. This means we may be dangerously slow to recognize when our uncertain therapeutic gambles are not paying off. We tolerate failure to progress that should concern us and miss many signs of developing problems simply because we have not established a practical early warning system. Because we are uncertain in our expectations, we are reluctant to commit ourselves to definite standards for judging progress. However, it is this very uncertainty that makes such standards necessary.

As in other aspects of clinical judgment, the highly intuitive nature of practice impedes efforts to specify clear short- and long-term goals. One of the skills that distinguishes old-timer from newcomer is the ability to sense how rapidly each patient will progress. However, these predictions are often based on a complex integration of a variety of tacit clues. They are thus difficult to explain, and even the confident clinician may prefer not to write explicit time-based treatment goals.

The intuitive nature of clinical judgment creates other serious problems. It limits master clinicians in teaching their skills to the novice. It blocks us from challenging and comparing theories of action followed by our colleagues. It prevents us from coordinating our care with that of other disciplines. It discourages our patients from working with us to help design their own therapy. Our decision making, however splendid, is shrouded in inarticulate mystery. Argyris and Schon comment on this mystique, saying that the professional who practices in this way:

> Knows that he knows something, knows that students do not know it, knows that he cannot tell others what he knows, but knows they should come to know it. How then do they come to know it? In mysterious ways, perhaps by a kind of osmosis through proximity to a master, as in apprenticeship.[5]

Within this text, we have the privilege of sharing the ideas of a group of distinguished physical therapy scholars and clinicians who do not tolerate such mystique. They have tried to translate their intuitive skill into explicit theory that we can share. This is a rare privilege. If they succeed, we should be far better prepared to teach our own students and to collaborate in planning treatment with our colleagues and patients.

These are ambitious plans. How do we go about creating these improvements? What methods can we use to:

- remain consciously open to new options for treatment
- be selective and efficient in our evaluations
- develop tested theories of action to guide our practice
- monitor the success of our uncertain choices
- reduce the mystery in our decisions
- and do all this in a way that recognizes both the costs and the benefits of our actions?

Fortunately, these problems are not unique to physical therapy. They are common to all fields in which men and women make important and potentially costly decisions about action under conditions of uncertainty. The fields of business, public policy, and long-range planning have felt a particularly great need to develop decision-making techniques that deal with these challenges. Their literature can be of help to us.

DECISION ANALYSIS METHOD

The most useful approach I have found is one developed by Howard Raiffa[6] at the Harvard Business School, and recently adopted and applied to health care by Milton Weinstein and his colleagues[7] at the Center for the Analysis of Health Practices at the Harvard School of Public Health. The method is called decision analysis. It is a process by which the sequence of decisions and events involved in management of a problem is diagrammed over time using a branching format that takes into account the uncertainty of events at each step. Because I think this method has great promise as a tool for improving clinical decision making in physical therapy, let me describe it briefly.

As do other formal evaluative activities such as clinical audits and research, a decision analysis begins with careful delineation of the problem to be addressed. Analysis focuses on one aspect of management that is particularly critical, controversial, or uncertain. The starting point is usually a somewhat vague feeling of concern about this aspect of care. The process for reducing this concern to a problem for analysis is similar to the process by which a diagnostician converts a patient's chief complaint and presenting symptoms into a probable diagnosis. Arthur Elstein and his coworkers,[8] in their studies of the clinical reasoning process, point out that before problem solving can begin, the problem must be represented cognitively in the mind of the problem solver. For the diagnostician, this is accomplished by early generation of a limited number of provisional hypotheses about the nature of the problem. These serve to limit and guide the clinical workup. Although medical students are usually cautioned to ''keep an open mind until you have collected the facts,'' in the studies reported by Elstein and his associates, nearly all experienced physicians doing a diagnostic workup formulated specific, though tentative, diagnostic hypotheses long before most clinical data had been collected. These formulations then defined the ''problem space,'' or focus for later data gathering. The effect of this focusing on subsequent actions is profound.

Consider a simple, nonmedical example. Suppose that as you read this, you begin to notice smoke pouring from a wastebasket in the corner of the room. You feel interest and concern, which quickly are translated into one or more of a series of action questions:

- You might think, ''How can I get out of here if it gets worse?'' You will begin to look for doors and windows.
- Or you may ask, ''How can I put the fire out?'' You will begin to look for blankets, fire extinguishers, and water faucets.
- The more scientific thinker will wonder, ''What's burning?'' or ''Is it getting worse or about to go out?'' You will begin to crane your neck and edge over to look in the smoking basket.
- If your interest is in human behavior, you may ask, ''I wonder if anyone else noticed it?'' and begin to look around the room to see if other people are also concerned.

This only begins to exhaust the list of possible questions. While the example is trivial, it is clear that each action question represents a markedly different conceptualization of an initially vague problem situation. It is also clear that the problem formulation you choose will determine your subsequent actions. Both in attempts to carry out a formal decision analysis and in our day-to-day work with patients, we must begin by deciding what sort of problem concerns us. In physical therapy, this step is made difficult by the lack of a widely accepted, therapeutically relevant system for conceptualizing the disorders we treat. This is one aspect of the still incomplete body of clinical theory I mentioned earlier. Therapeutic thinking often begins with classification of the patient's problem in terms of one of the established medical specialties, such as orthopaedics or neurology. Or we may focus on a diagnostic label, such as asthma or emphysema. I suspect that our decision making might be strengthened if we began, instead, from a conceptual base that has more relevance to the types of therapeutic choices we need to make. For example, when I hear Shirley Stockmeyer describe a functional basis for viewing movement problems as disorders of mobility or stability, this seems to me a far more powerful starting point for therapeutic thinking than such conceptual labels as osteoarthritis or hemiplegia. I hope that after reading this text some new conceptual models for thinking about both the problems we treat and the therapeutic methods we use will emerge.

Whatever sort of problem model we use, the first step in a formal decision analysis should be to *narrow and delineate the problem focus.* Decision analysis is a detailed and time-consuming undertaking, and we will make more progress if we do not try to analyze all aspects of overall management of the patient's problem at once. For example, in the sample decision tree shown in Figure 1-1, the problem focus is summarized in the upper left hand corner. As you begin to look over this diagram, you may say to yourself, "I wonder what she thinks should be included in each level of treatment. I'd like to analyze that." Fine. That would certainly be a worthwhile focus for analysis. However, it is not the aspect of the problem addressed by this tree. This analysis is concerned simply with the question of how to determine readiness to progress from one level to another.

By the time the problem delineation is completed, it should specify the type of patients to whom it can be applied, the characteristics of their disorder that are of greatest interest for this particular analysis, and the specific action decision to be addressed. For example, the sample analysis in Figure 1-1 is concerned with otherwise healthy adults who have just had a total knee replacement, for whom the goal of treatment is to secure pain-free, functional range of motion and independence in function activities within a 2-week period. The analysis further assumes that all patients to whom it is applied will be receiving physical therapy, and that their program will consist of progression through a series of graded levels of exercise and functional training. It also assumes a context for physical therapy practice in which the orthopaedic surgeon referring the patients ordinarily will manipulate the knee if 90 degrees of pain-free motion has not been achieved within 2 weeks. The action problem addressed is, "How should the therapist decide when a patient is ready to progress from one level of treatment to another?" The time period for analysis begins with the second day after surgery and ends 2 weeks later, when a decision about manipulation will be made.

The next step is to *structure this decision process over time and diagram it* in a way that makes it easy to see what choices must be made, what options could be considered at each decision point, what intermediate consequences these decisions might have, how these consequences would influence subsequent decisions, and what outcomes might be expected at the end of the time period being analyzed. Definitions of key terms and explanations of commonly used conventions for making a graphic diagram, or decision tree, summarizing the analysis are provided in Figure 1-2.

My sample decision tree is modeled after a much more elegant analysis drawn up by an able and experienced Boston clinician, Bette Ann Harris.[9] Her original analysis included considerably more detail, particularly in the section concerned with evaluation and modification of treatment for patients who do not respond well during early treatment. I have pruned and reshaped her tree ruthlessly to make it easier to point out some of the features that are of general importance in diagramming decision analyses.

First, there are at least two branches at each choice point and chance point. In earlier drafts, many choice points included a much larger number

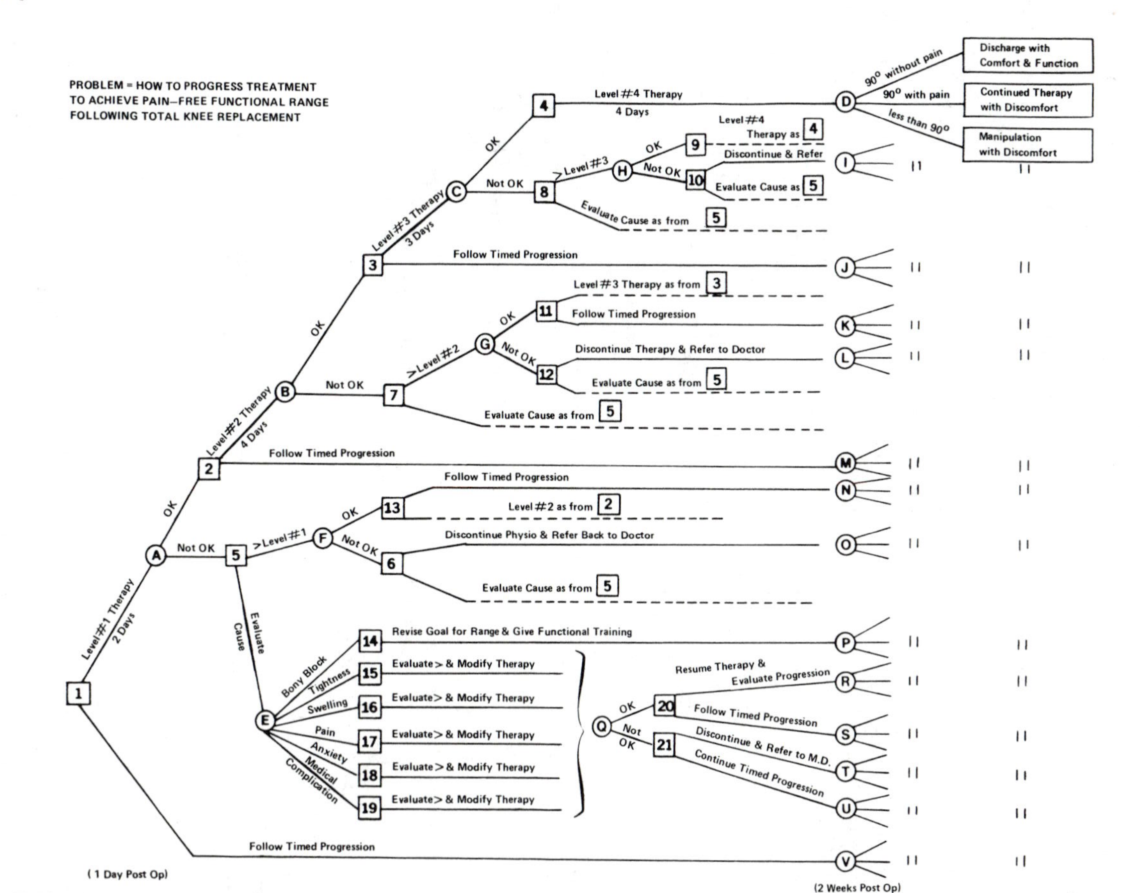

FIGURE 1-1. Early draft of a decision tree. *Problem* analyzed: When to progress postoperative treatment for total knee replacement patients. *Time period:* from 1st to 14th postoperative day.

Decision Tree — A diagram showing the relationship over time between the decisions made by the clinician and the unfolding of events such as the results of evaluation and the patient's response to treatment. Decisions and events associated with each approach to management of the problem are laid out in the sequence in which they occur, reading from left to right.

Choice Point — A point in the management process at which the clinician must decide which of several alternative actions to take. Actions considered may include:
- therapeutic interventions and/or
- evaluative information-gathering activities.

Choice points are indicated in the decision-tree diagram by the symbol □.

Chance Point — A point in the process at which events occur that are beyond the full control of the clinician, and thus are uncertain. These are points at which two types of "consequences" occur:
- the consequences of intervention become known
- the consequences of information gathering are revealed.

Chance points are indicated in the decision-tree diagram by the symbol ○.

Path — A particular sequence of actions and events leading from the point in the case at which analysis begins to an end result as the point where analysis is completed. Paths are shown by lines connecting the sequence of choice and chance points.

Outcomes — The possible end results of each path of action. Outcomes are described in terms of attributes of value to the patient, such as survival, changes in level of function, amount of discomfort, and are written at the far right of the decision tree. They are identified in the diagram by enclosing them in a box.

Survival

Strategy — Specification of the action to be taken at each choice point depending upon which events have been revealed at the preceding chance point. Strategy is described through a series of contingency statements which say, "If _____ is the situation, take _____ action; but if _____ is the situation, take _____ action instead."

Probabilities — Estimates of how likely it is different consequences or outcomes will occur. These are expressed as decimals or percentages. The probabilities for all possible consequences at a single chance point must total 1.0 if decimals are used, or 100% if percentages are used. The same is true for the total of outcome probabilities associated with each path of action.

FIGURE 1-2. Definitions and conventions used in making a decision tree.

of branches, reflecting the variety of options that, in fact, are open to us in most clinical decisions. This is a "pruned" tree in which all but the most promising choices have been deleted. You might feel the choices should be quite different. Analysis of these would be valuable. One purpose of such a tree is to provoke and structure discussion of different approaches to treatment.

The branches following each chance point reflect the uncertainty of our decisions. However confident we may feel about the probable results of our evaluations and interventions, we can never be entirely certain what will occur. In drafting a decision tree, I find it easiest to begin by outlining the actions I am most likely to take and the consequences I believe are most likely to occur. Then I go back and add the alternatives, the second thoughts, and the possible surprises and disappointments. Simply getting all this down on paper can help to stimulate thinking and provoke questions about things that have previously been done intuitively or as a matter of routine.

Next, notice that the diagram makes it easy to see the relationship between information-gathering activities and intervention decisions. We can inspect the tree to see if points exist at which it fails to branch appropriately. For example, if we were to find that intervention strategies do not branch although intermediate consequences or results of evaluation are different, we should question why treatment seems unresponsive to individual differences in the patient's condition. This may lead us to add new treatment options or help us to recognize that this consequence is unimportant for treatment planning. Evaluations that are not used to lead us into different paths of treatment are unnecessary and should be omitted.

The diagram also makes it easy to see when and under what conditions we will actually need different types of information. This can help us decide which evaluations to do first and can allow us to wait to collect other information until we are sure it will be needed. Our evaluations will then be more strategic than if we simply carry out every evaluation that might conceivably be needed at the very start. Clearly, such strategy calls for us to make many educated guesses. For example, in the sample analysis, if the problems listed after chance point E are, in fact, unlikely to occur in most patients, we would be sensible to gamble on this and begin treatment without checking each patient to make sure none of the problems are present. So long as our plan for managing these patients recognizes the uncertainty of this decision and includes a monitoring system to pick up problems quickly if they do occur, such selective initial evaluation can be safe as well as efficient.

By now you should be feeling irritated by the ambiguity of the terms used on the sample decision tree to describe consequences at many of the chance points. What on earth do "OK" and "Not OK" mean? Unfortunately, these are not unlike the very subjective judgments many clinicians make about their patients' progress; but in an analysis such as this, these terms clearly call for a much more precise definition. A decision tree is usually accompanied by a set of explanatory notes, covering such things as the exact nature of alternative therapeutic interventions and the objective basis for classifying chance point consequences. For example, at chance point A we might define "OK" by saying, "By the end of the second day of treatment, the patient should be able to: (1) move the affected knee through an arc of at least 35 degrees with minimal discomfort if the leg is supported; (2) do straight leg raises with the aid of a knee splint." Anything less than this would automatically be interpreted as "Not OK." In some analyses, we might want a greater number of categories for classifying results than the simple pass-fail system used in this example. However, we should be careful not to add categories unless these gradations in consequence really do make a difference in our subsequent decisions about treatment.

Regardless of the number of categories we use for classifying consequences at a chance point, we obviously need unambiguous operational definitions for each one. Thus, we will need to set measurable targets for what we hope to accomplish at each of a number of intermediate points in the time period covered by the analysis. This is an essential part of this tool for coping with uncertainty. These intermediate targets make it easy for us to tell whether treatment is succeeding, and they remind us at an early point to rethink our plans if the results we expect are not achieved.

Few people have argued the need for this sort of objective monitoring more forcefully than Alvan Feinstein[10] in his book, *Clinical Judgment*. In clinical medicine, he complains, a "pernicious, appalling, and widespread custom is the reporting of therapeutic accomplishment by means of judgmental or interpretive terms for which no criteria are given." Feinstein, who believes that the care of individual patients should be carried out using intellectual processes similar to those employed in valid research, argues:

> When a laboratory investigator makes decisions in conducting an experiment, we require that the ingredients of his reasoning be explicitly stated. We insist that he be able to specify his methods, his data, and his interpretations of the data, and that the specifications be precise and reproducible. When a clinician makes decisions in the experiments of therapy, we generally assume that the procedure is too complex for scientific documentation. The clinician is usually permitted to justify his work on the basis of "hunch," intuition, or a nebulously defined previous "clinical experience." His decisions are allowed a rationale that need not be overtly rational, and reasons that need not be particularly reasonable. If the clinician seems knowledgeable and authoritative, and if his reputation and results seem good, he can be condoned the most flagrant imprecisions, vagueness, and inconsistency in his conduct of therapy. The clinician does not even use a scientific name for his method of designing, executing, and appraising therapeutic experiments. He calls it *clinical judgment*.[11]

One purpose of decision analysis is to reduce this sort of fuzziness and make our clinical judgments more truly scientific.

Once the decision tree has been drafted and explanatory notes added to define choice point alternatives and chance point possibilities, two major steps remain in decision analysis: estimation of probabilities and valuation of strategies and outcomes. Both are complex processes, and I will describe them only briefly. However, such references as those by Weinstein and Bursztajn provide a wealth of theoretical background and practical guidelines on both steps.

The process of *probability estimation* is a curious blend of objective and subjective reasoning. At each chance point, we are asked to estimate the likelihood that each of the possible consequences we have listed will actually occur. If we do this for all individuals in the problem category, these estimates will draw principally upon whatever objective relative-frequency statistics are available from past clinical and scientific studies. However, in many cases, few objective data are available. In any event, the sources of variation in response among individual patients make the uncertainty of response too great to rely on statistics alone. When the analysis is applied to the individual patient, the clinician also must consider the many factors that make this case unique. Decision analysis, therefore, makes use of some unusual statistical methods developed by the English clergyman-mathematician Bayes—methods that let us combine our scientific logic and clinical hunches about the individual patient's unique potential for response with objective data about results observed in similar patients. The result is a subjective probability estimate—a sort of bet on the likelihood of different consequences occurring. For example, in the analysis shown in Figure 1-1, at chance point A, I might predict that among all patients in this group there is an 80 percent probability the response to treatment will be "OK" and only a 20 percent probability it will be "Not OK." However, for an individual patient who appears anxious and reports a great deal of discomfort the first day after surgery, I might be less confident of success and set my probability at 60-40 instead. Similar estimates must be made at the end of each path of action to express our belief that each possible outcome listed for that path will occur. This may appear to be a foolhardy and even unethical exercise. Since so much of our judgment is subjective, and the accuracy of our guesses is so uncertain, how can we put these guesses on paper as if they were real? Yet, in fact, clinicians do this same sort of thing intuitively each time they decide how to treat a patient. Drawing upon past experience with similar cases, and their clinical "sizing up" of the individual patient, they consider the "odds" that particular treatment methods will be both safe and effective. Without such thinking, clinicians would be unable to act. Or else, instead of attempting to make a rational choice, they would be forced to rely on flipping a coin or following a completely arbitrary and standardized program of care. Decision analysis does not impose an alien process on the clinician; it simply requires us to spell out the processes we already use and allows us to step back and look at them with a critical eye.

One benefit of such a critique is the direction it provides for setting clinical research priorities. The uncomfortable process of estimating probabilities makes painfully obvious the weak points in our basis for decision making. Research can then be concentrated on the points at which key choices about treatment are now being made on a dangerously uncertain basis, on areas where little objective data exist to guide or justify selection of a preferred approach. Without such analysis, we risk irrelevance and diffuseness in even the most carefully designed studies. Investigators will always be tempted to study those variables that are most conveniently quantified unless critical analysis of practice directs attention instead to the questions of greatest significance for improving patient care.

The final step in analysis is that of *valuation.* It, too, requires quantified yet uncertain estimates. Once the possible outcomes of treatment have been projected, we must try to judge their probable utility by estimating how much these results will matter or be worth to the patient and to society. Once alternative courses of action have been described, we must try to predict what types and amounts of resources each will require. While many of the techniques used to carry out these valuations come from the field of economics,[12] the focus need not be exclusively on costs and benefits that can be expressed in monetary terms. Cost analysis, for example, should take into account not only the charges made for equipment, services, and other components of care, but also the demands different approaches will make on the patient's emotional and physical resources. Cost estimates will provide a misleading analysis for treatment selection unless they consider the discomfort, inconvenience, frustration, boredom, and embarrassment treatment may impose on the patients and those close to them. Valuation of benefits will be similarly distorted if we overlook such outcomes as patients' real enjoyment of their relationship with the therapist or their increased ability to accept a disability that cannot be reversed.

The ultimate purpose of decision analysis is to make wise choices in selecting a path of treatment. Our goal is to choose not merely a good approach, but the best one available. Estimates of probabilities and values can help us see that the best approach is not always the one that promises greatest success in achieving therapeutic goals. Nor is it always the strategy that requires the fewest resources. Selection of the "best buy" usually involves complex and subjective tradeoffs, as we look for the strategy that will let us:

- achieve as much as possible of the outcomes that matter most to the individual we are treating, and
- minimize the risk of particularly dangerous or unpleasant consequences,
- while still limiting as much as possible our use of scarce resources.

Decision analysis begins with careful delineation of a problem. It ends with selection of a strategy for solving that problem. This strategy is not simply a predetermined list of steps to be followed during treatment. It is a flexible contingency plan that helps us anticipate and respond to the varied consequences we may encounter when our initial plan is implemented. Even if we decide not to use the decision analysis technique per se, such flexible planning must characterize our clinical judgment if we hope to achieve excellence in practice.

SUMMARY

My purpose in leading you on this whirlwind tour of decision-analysis methodology has not been simply to evangelize for this particular technique. Decision analysis is interesting primarily because it helps point out both the many admirable qualities of our clinical judgment and some of the ways in which it still needs to be improved. In our teaching, research, and clinical practice, other, quite different techniques can help us make the same improvements. The important thing is to recognize that our profession has a major task of theory building ahead. We now have decision processes that are:

- complex but often disorganized and narrow
- based on science but lacking in tested theory of action
- evaluative but often wasteful

- expensive but sometimes oblivious to cost
- uncertain but frequently unmonitored
- intuitive and thus difficult to critique or share.

Our job is to hold fast to the strengths in our present decision process while we seek ways to make it more open, frugal, accountable, strategic, and organized. I do not dream that success in making these improvements will bring with it standardized methods of treatment that have been proven to be the best. Even the soundest clinical theory cannot tell us exactly what to do for each patient. Far from it. We may reduce uncertainty and learn to cope with it, but we will never eliminate it altogether. So long as therapists continue to work with human beings in all their rich variety, the guidelines provided by theory will need to be interpreted, adapted, and redesigned for each case. In fact, the most important goal of our efforts to improve clinical decision making should be to make it more individualized, more rationally responsive to the varied needs, preferences, and characteristics of our patients. As we expand and employ the science of clinical practice, we must remember it is akin to the science of war as Stephen Vincent Benet described it in his poem, *John Brown's Body.*

> If you take a flat map
> And move wooden blocks upon it strategically,
> The thing looks well, the blocks behave as they should.
> The science of war is moving live men like blocks.
> And getting the blocks into place at a fixed moment.
> But it takes time to mold your men into blocks
> And flat maps turn into country where creeks and gullies
> Hamper your wooden squares. They stick in the brush,
> They are tired and rest, they straggle after ripe blackberries,
> And you cannot lift them up in your hand.[13]

We strive for excellence in physical-therapy practice knowing that each individual we treat is unique, yet believing that our judgment can be educated by experience and guided by principle.

REFERENCES

1. POLANYI, M: *The Tacit Dimension,* Anchor Books Edition. Doubleday & Co, Garden City, NY, 1967, p 1.
2. SIMON, HA: *Administrative Behavior,* ed 2. The Free Press, New York, 1957, p 3.
3. ARGYRIS, C AND SCHON, D: *Theory in Practice: Increasing Professional Effectiveness.* Jossey-Bass, San Francisco, 1975.
4. BURSZTAJN, H, ET AL: *Medical Choices, Medical Chances: How Patients, Families, and Physicians Cope with Uncertainty.* Delacort Press/Seymour Lawrence, New York, 1981, pp 32–33.
5. ARGYRIS AND SCHON, op cit, pp 183–184.
6. RAIFFA, H: *Decision Analysis: Introductory Lectures on Choices under Uncertainty.* Addison-Wesley, Reading, Mass, 1968.
7. WEINSTEIN, M, ET AL: *Clinical Decision Analysis.* WB Saunders, Philadelphia, 1980.
8. ELSTEIN, A, SHULMAN, L, AND SPRAFKA, S: *Medical Problem Solving: An Analysis of Clinical Reasoning.* Harvard University Press, Cambridge, 1978.

9. HARRIS, BA: Unpublished project for a graduate course in clinical decision analysis at the Graduate Program in Physical Therapy, MGH Institute of Health Professions, Boston, 1981.
10. FEINSTEIN, A: *Clinical Judgment*. Robert Krieger, Huntington, NY, 1967, p 250.
11. Ibid, p 16.
12. DRUMMOND, MF: *Principles of Economic Analysis in Health Care*. Oxford University Press, Oxford, 1980.
13. BENET, SV: *John Brown's Body*. Holt, Rinehart, & Winston, New York, 1927.

Chapter 2

CLINICAL DECISION MAKING: EDUCATIONAL, DATA, AND RISK FACTORS

HELEN J. HISLOP, Sc.D., F.A.P.T.A.

EDUCATION FOR CLINICAL DECISION MAKING

The subject of excellence in practice, education, and research has been around for a long time. The situation is not unlike the nephew who had not seen his elderly aunt for several years and dropped in to see her while on a business trip. She was delighted to see him and asked innumerable questions about his family and work. When given the opportunity, he asked what she had been doing. She was most voluble and said she was having an interesting and exciting time in her weekly Bible class. She had just returned from such a meeting at which the Book of Revelation had been discussed.

Being moderately versed in the Bible himself, the nephew was surprised and said, "But the Book of Revelation is one of the most difficult in the Holy Book. Had all the class studied it, and did they understand it?" Her reply was given without hesitation. "Oh, no! Oh, no! No one knew anything about it, or understood it, but they had such a wonderful time discussing it."

Perhaps this is true of our topic. We comprehend when excellence has occurred in practice and education and research—but very often as the outcome of a process and not via an understanding or appreciation of what the elements are that have created an excellent end product, be it patient performance, student or therapist performance, or assimilation of new knowledge into everyday use.

These are, indeed, troubled and trying times. Humanity has passed through many ages not unlike the present. With each time of trial, humankind has emerged, like the phoenix, better and greater. Physical therapy is one microcosm in the full scope of humankind. We stand today on the threshold of unbelievable achievement if we can only preserve it. Before us lie vistas so promising, so full of hope, and so full of great potential that even the intellectual giants in our midst question our ability to comprehend the future.

In this time of rocketing change in the pattern of society, a highly unified physical therapy profession can and may play a greater role in bringing health and well-being to our fellow human beings.

John Donne[1] said that "no man is an island." No man stands alone. In physical therapy, we must increase our awareness that we are not entire in or of ourselves. We live and exist to serve. When or if that service is no longer paramount, we place at risk our unity, the respect of others, and the purposes of our existence.

The times we face now are times of testing—times of stress from economic, cultural, and technologic unknowns. Challenges are flung by terrorists, troubled youths, the elderly, the disabled, and the disenfranchised. Physical therapy is vulnerable because it is a relatively new profession, one whose educational institutions are insecure and face threats to support and growth that sometimes border on extinction. Yet, this is occurring in an environment where there is the greatest relative demand for physical therapy services and personnel since the early 1950s.

I need not face you with a litany of the problems facing our educational programs:

- obsolete facilities
- outdated curricula
- laboratory impoverishment
- economic poverty
- inadequate teaching clinics
- weakened faculties.

Dire predictions are not the intent here; nor are they an expectation for the future. But the educational foundations of this profession must be bolstered from within and without if we are to face our time of testing with faith, good cheer, and high anticipation. Let us find in our problems our opportunities.

People must come to grips with their concept of masses of information, just as physical therapy must come to recognize that its transition to an adult science demands relevance of available information, imposes a need for new and improved information, and increases reliance on the meaning of this information.

Computer systems and on-line technology have caused a quasi-religious scientism whose tenet reads: If you can get at the facts, you can control everything. Unfortunately, this credo places an inordinate value on efficiency and an inconsequential value on thoughtful analysis.

Indeed, with the coming of modern microtechnology and in this climate of social upheaval, our ideas of time have undergone a major cultural crescendo into "instantism."

Beginning in World War II with the breakthroughs with sulfa drugs and penicillin, the first of the wonder drugs, there was instant curing of previously fearsome diseases.

Our instant society now provides us with:

- *instant foods:* at the expense of leisurely dining and human interaction, we have gained indigestion and antacid pills

- *instant communication:* wherein West Coast people shun voting in national elections because the results are predicted before the polls close
- *instant sex:* via birth control measures at the expense of maturing human relationships
- *instant credit:* where paying up debts and interest charges replaces the exhilaration of "saving up" for a wanted treasure
- *instant euphoria:* via hallucinogenic drugs whereby reality is lost to the "pastel twilight zones"
- *instant data analysis:* via computers rather than the more contemplative approach, which, although more fraught with errors, imparts more intimacy with the meanings of the data sources.

We claim to search for meaning and strive for excellence—and yet we choose to pollute these quests by expecting instant gratification, instant results, and instant interpretations.

I fear that unless tempered, our tampering with maturational intellectual processes may deprive us of a great deal of human wisdom—wisdom that comes from the understanding of history and human development, which is the one unique feature that separates humankind from all other species.

An expectation of instant education is the real pollution crisis of our age. The natural follow-up is demand for instant status and societal accolades. How does this instancy phenomenon affect our universities, and, more specifically, what is its influence on physical therapy programs? Education (instant or protracted) is very expensive. But if you think education is expensive, try ignorance. Physical therapy holds claim as a health science that includes a search for improved knowledge. If you think scientific research in physical therapy is expensive, try chronic disability.

Thus, it seems clear that education and science are the redemption of humankind in the age of the shoddy. Neither of them is a charity to be indulged; both are great forces to be liberated in physical therapy. But such removal of restraint will not be realized unless we assign greater priority of our collective energies to those ends.

Conviction, commitment, concern, and contract are the operative words that must drive the academic and clinical worlds together if excellence is to be a believable, achievable goal. It cannot come instantly.

Our educational goal is "Homo investigans," the scientifically astute clinician—not "Homo arachnoides," the dilettante who creeps into all areas of endeavor without a clear focus.

THE TOWN-GOWN CONCERN

In the view of most people, education takes place in the university; patient care takes place in the clinic. The values of the university differ from those of the health care system, and these differences need to be appreciated before any effective cooperative activity can occur. Close cooperation between the university and the clinical community seems a natural and desirable thing. I believe it is, but the value systems are not consonant—they are in conflict.

For longer than the current recession has been going on, academic centers have been looking over their shoulders in a state of dis-ease because of their great dependence on governmental funding. It has been reported that only a handful of colleges and universities operate in black ink. Declining governmental support, waning enrollment, inflation, and greener fields for faculty away from the university have caused apprehension, retrenching, and cutbacks in programs—including the demise of some in physical therapy.

For the university's faculty, there are the eternal one-upmanship and grantsmanship games that must be played; internal university politics do not differ significantly from the politics of other groups. But the faculty does coalesce in its common goals of the pursuit of knowledge and the education of the students. The majority of faculties have sought out this milieu because these goals have greater personal meaning than does personal wealth. Scholarship is a calling and a consecration, not a job.

In the clinical world, the ethic of the patients' needs above all others remains—but it is moderated considerably at the present time by the irrevocable necessity to bring in enough money for the institution (i.e., the hospital) to continue or for the clinician (i.e., private practitioner) to turn a profit. Thus, economic survival is higher than the patient's needs on the scale of values, and the length of the scale is measured by desired income over expenses for both institution and individual practitioner. But patient care is also a calling and not just a job.

The coin of academia is the published paper and completed students. The coin of the health care agency is the balanced ledger and the number of patient treatments. The feature common to both is the reason for our existence: people who need physical therapy. *This* must be the basis for easing the tensions and the problems that arise when common ventures are sought or expended collaboration is desired between university and clinic.

Faculty practices are springing up that are excellent for two reasons: they can increase the professional relevancy and credibility of the faculty, and they can provide a long-needed source of community consultation on patient management. Most universities have provisos for faculty engagement in external consultation and in patient care, and this is supported for full-time faculty to generate additional income while offering a valued service in the university's behalf.

It would benefit our academic programs if outpatient clinics and inpatient beds could be assigned to the physical therapy faculty within the teaching hospital or university clinic; a heretical concept when "beds" are totally controlled almost equally by physicians and fiscal policies. But it is an idea whose time must come, and soon, if physical therapy is to rise in stature as a provider of professional education. A guaranteed source of patients to participate in the teaching process, but not to be exploited by it, is an essential corollary to quality education, for without such there can be little student exposure to clinical decision making prior to the internship. It is no use saying "we are doing our best." We have got to succeed in doing what is necessary.

CURRICULUM CONTENT

The secret of care of the patient is caring for the patient. Both the science and the art of patient care are required in order to put to use the untold quanta of knowledge known to us. Indeed, the stockpile related to physical therapy alone threatens to engulf us, but we must not allow it to subvert our interest in the patients themselves. The patients know what they feel but do not know what their problems are; whereas physical therapists know what the problems are but do not know how the patients feel.

Keeping this in the forefront, we can avoid training a robot generation of merely adequate practitioners. In the classroom, the scope of science taught becomes wider and wider, while the interest of the investigator becomes narrower and narrower. The clinician's scope becomes broader and broader, so curricula are added to, and added to, and added to, until the force-feeding of facts becomes counterproductive.

Where does it stop? One way to stop it is to identify what *is* and what is *not* physical therapy. Input of knowledge just because it is available, when time is so precious, does not enhance our goal of excellence in physical therapy. Clinical decisions are based on knowledge readily understood, readily recalled, and commonly encountered. Procedures, instruments, drugs, and tests can be standardized. The patient cannot. Thus, those things about which we are expected to make decisions must have ascendancy in curriculum content. Need to know. Nice to know. Marginal to know. Irrelevant to know. Hardheadedness and adoption of a realistic working definition of physical therapy are essential to the development of sound, clinically based, patient-oriented curricula. It is bad enough to become obsolete in practice, but it is worse to be the recipient of an obsolete education.

TEACHING CLINICAL DECISION MAKING

Fact finding and decision making and analytical thinking—the kind of intellectual endeavor these demand is no different in physical therapy than in medicine or the law. The scientific method is the basic tool, for each new patient is an experiment, just as each law case is an experiment, in the search for truth.

As they struggle to use the scientific method, physical therapy students will, for a time, dismember their patients. They will, for example, isolate the patient's heart, parietal lobe, knee, or obturator nerve and observe its action under very specialized conditions. But in the end, students must put the parts back together in their evaluations and program plans if they are to be successful and stand up to the test of time.

For the evaluation by the physical therapist—just as the diagnosis by the physician—must display a total concept of the unique relationships between one patient as a person, the disorder or disease as a part of the patient, and the patient as a part of the community in which he or she must live. There is *evidence:* the limp, the arrhythmia, the pain, the spasticity. But evidence is not collected in a vacuum—it is examined and divided into variables that do not change under any given circumstance (e.g., hemorrhage) and those that can be manipulated or altered (e.g., intensity of pain with different positions). These are then examined in light of general rules (symptom analysis). The sources of information used to reach a *clinical* decision may vary widely. This is in striking contrast to the law, where hearsay evidence is ruled out as improper.

The physical therapist may gather information on a firsthand basis by evaluating the patient. If data are inconsistent, corroboration by other tests or another examiner may clarify the issue. This principle is similar to laboratory scientists collecting their own data in their own experiments. Their results, like those of clinicians, must be able to be replicated by others.

On the other hand, physical therapists will routinely honor information given to them by colleagues—from the physician, the nurse, another physical therapist—and often will accept such data without corroboration.

Another variable of clinical decision making is the failure to rule out bias. Excluding bias is the heart of the scientific method; and yet it is the *art* of the clinician. Bias allows physical therapists to intrude their mind-sets, attitudes, and values as part of the clinical decision-making process. These patient/therapist interactions play a significant role and not infrequently lead to conflict between the scientific and humanitarian approaches to disability.

In the laboratory, there are strict rules regarding the suitability of data. In the clinic, there often is an unstructured, ambiguous situation, the very uncertainty of which is an important variable.

Because of the uncertainty principle that intrudes into every human interaction between patient and therapist, it requires years for the clinician to develop intuitive decisions. This required clinical maturing cannot be telescoped into the period of time of the current basic curriculum (commonly 2 years). Only an experienced, knowledgeable practitioner can handle the subliminal knowledge that derives from years of experience and that leads to intuitive, and most frequently, correct, clinical judgment.

Thus, I hammer at the thesis that clinical decision making can neither be taught *nor* learned in the absence of the patient. Head, heart, and hand are the three Hs of clinical decision making; and the combination, when ripened, enables us to recognize solvable problems.

Caring about, caring for, talking with (not at), and *listening* are themes we must impress as part of an educational program. After the rudiments are taught, the rest of the learning comes from self-instruction motivated by the patient. No physical therapist, student, or clinician can ask more of destiny or should be content with less.

FROM WHOM WE LEARN

George Bernard Shaw said: "Those that can, *do;* those that can't, *teach.*"[2] Theodore Fox said it a bit differently: "Those who can't teach, like to talk about teaching, especially after dinner."

Teaching is not the focus of the university. Learning is. Learning is the compelling focus, and it takes place between teacher and student; student and student; and student and books. But in physical therapy, these are not the focal relationships.

> A teacher cannot be a teacher without a student.
> A woman cannot learn to be a mother without a child.
> A man cannot learn to be a husband without a wife.
> A student cannot learn to be a physical therapist without a patient.

It is only by listening and looking, trying and revising that we learn the nature of patients and their distress. Patients teach us reality tinged with humility. In spite of exponential increases in information and demands for knowledge, and the acquisition of new skills with new technology, we often are confronted with problems that make us realize how limited is our understanding, how imprecise are our interventions.

There is a dilemma all clinicians face: at one end, we know the limits of our knowledge and skills; at the other end, we must act promptly in the patient's behalf. We are not spectators with leisure to peruse human comedy and tragedy like the philosopher or the historian or the cellular physiologist. Clinicians must act, using the best knowledge and tools available and known to them. This is the dilemma that must be taught and learned. Our patients, young and old, black and white, harsh and gentle, rich and poor, are the ennobling teachers of us all.

In our time, more than any other in our brief history, there is a special and urgent need to ensure that the physical therapy student has those learning opportunities afforded only by direct interaction with patients.

I read a brief story that, when paraphrased, illustrates my point. A physical therapist had been on leave, and the first morning of her return, she was met outside the hospital by the Asian-born wife of one of her patients. "You come see my husband now," she was requested. Protestations about signing back in, looking at schedules, and updating patient progress and discharges were flatly turned aside by the wife. She was adamant. "Other PTs come look. Others come do *things.* You come look-*see.*" Those of us in this profession must not only look at our patients, we must have the vision and foresight to *see* (i.e., to understand) them as they are. Here lies the germ of clinical decision making—the voluntary association of two persons, one giving and one seeking relief. Such is the heart of physical therapy, and education without that component is hollow.

LISTEN

Listen to the patients stories. They are telling you their problems.

The importance of this dictum was brought forcefully home several years ago when one of our students was sitting for her third patient evaluation and treatment analysis. She was at the top of the class, with only a rare grade below an A, and her clinical practicum reports appeared faultless. Consequently, a difficult patient was assigned to her. We were amazed when she appeared in less than a half-hour, seemingly pleased and smiling proudly, with supreme confidence in the evaluation summary she had completed.

I asked her how she could be so confident, to which she replied that she had remembered the good advice of the faculty to "listen to the patient." She walked up to the patient and, in kindly and empathetic terms, softly asked him, "What troubles you?" His reply was a radial nerve injury at the elbow, complicated by bilateral carpal tunnel entrapment of ulnar and median nerves and an older history of repaired trigger fingers. She remembered. She listened. She quickly found her answer. She got an A.

Bonnie Blossom recognized the imperative need for student-patient interaction on a special plane when she conceived and implemented a student clinic at West Haverstraw Rehabilitation Center (now the Helen Hayes Hospital in New York) in which students experienced full responsibility for patients referred, using staff only for consultation. Obviously, this is an example of an idea before its time, for, despite its demonstrated value, it has not been widely emulated.

Curricula in physical therapy schools from coast to coast are striving to determine their destiny within their institution, trying to plan entry-level master's programs, and striving to move beyond the 1960s Worthingham[3] report to meet the needs of a society that demands instant gratification and resolution of health problems.

The students in the physical therapy programs seek relevance as they perceive it and frequently ask for learning rather than teaching. There is a wonderful excerpt from a book by Leo Buscaglia that is apt:

> There is a wonderful story in education that always amuses me. It's called "The Animal School." I always love to tell it because it's so wild, yet it's true. Educators have been laughing at it for years, but nobody does anything about it. The animals got together in the forest one day and decided to start a school. There was a rabbit, a bird, a squirrel, a fish, and an eel, and they formed a Board of Education. The rabbit insisted that running be in the curriculum. The bird insisted that flying be in the curriculum. The fish insisted that swimming be in the curriculum, and the squirrel insisted that perpendicular tree climbing be in the curriculum. They put all of these things together and wrote a Curriculum Guide. Then they insisted that all the animals take all of the subjects. Although the rabbit was getting an A in running, perpendicular tree climbing was a real problem for him; he kept falling over backwards. Pretty soon he got to be sort of brain-damaged, and he couldn't run any more. He found that instead of making an A in running, he was making a C and, of course, he always made an F in perpendicular climbing. The bird was really beautiful at flying, but when it came to burrowing in the ground, he couldn't do so well. He kept breaking his beak and wings. Pretty soon he was making a C in flying as well as an F in burrowing, and he had a hellava time with perpendicular tree climbing. The moral of the story is that the person who was valedictorian of the class was a mentally retarded eel who did everything in a half-way fashion. But the educators were all happy because everybody was taking all of the subjects, and it was called a broad-based education. We laugh at this, but that's what it is. It's what you did. We really are trying to make everybody the same as everybody else, and one soon learns that the ability to conform governs success in the educational scene.
>
> Conformity continues right on into the university. We in higher education are as guilty as everyone else. We don't say to people, "Fly! Think for yourselves." We give them our old knowledge, and we say to them, "Now this is what is essential. This is what is important." I know professors who teach nothing but one best "way," they don't say, "Here are a lot of tools, now go create your own. Go into abstract thinking. Go into dreaming. Dream a while, find something new." Could it not be that among their students there are greater dreamers than themselves? So, it all starts with you. You can only give what you have to give. Don't give up your tree. Hold onto your tree. You are the only you—the only magical combination of forces that will be and ever has been that can create such a tree. You are the best you. You will always be the second best anyone else.[4]

And so the curriculum must be in focus and the combinations known to achieve our goals:

CURRICULUM IMPERATIVES (OBJECTIVES)

1. The patient must be the major stimulus for learning.
2. A unified concept of physical therapy must be evident.
3. Basic clinical skills are essential as a preparation for significant clinical responsibility.
4. Scientific thinking must occur in a clinical setting.
5. Skills and habits of self-instruction must be instilled.

To achieve these objectives, I believe there are some curriculum modifications that are worthy of consideration; they focus on one entity, not the whole educational spectrum.

1. Use more clinical role models from the practicing community for physical therapy students. Accept students as unpaid volunteers in the clinic, and in return give them the benefit of a full-time clinician's viewpoint, service, empathy, and detachment as patients are cared for. This is what I call the "Adopt-A-Student" program.
2. Use community clinicians as tutorial directors of small groups of students in a patient-care environment. Tutorial clinicians will need some guidance and preparation by the core faculty to properly fulfill this roll.
3. Use clinicians as demonstrators in clinical skills laboratories on the campus.
4. Use clinicians to teach the process of patient evaluation, program planning, treatment, and record keeping. There is nothing like variety to add spice to life and to prevent students from thinking that the approaches to care are singular.
5. Sponsor Physical Therapy Grand Rounds on a monthly basis in the clinic, and invite students and faculty to attend and participate in discussing or presenting "textbook" cases.

Easy, you say? Try it, say I. The clinician has no time. Time away is money lost. Me teach? I'm only a clinician! Me on the clinical faculty? I have nothing to offer and more important things to do! What is the pay?

Easy, you say? Try it, say I. Academicians *know* what their students need to know—exactly what *they* themselves know. It is interruptive to have guest clinicians in the classroom. "Just give me a videotape of the clinician's talk and I'll put it in the library," will be a common faculty response.

Easy, you say? Whose challenge is it if it isn't the challenge of us all?

The plan, the concept, and the development of education for clinical problem solving and for the use of clinical judgment, their recognition, and their accomplishment, are possible. The stages need to be identified to achieve a higher level of excellence in practice than is currently the mode.

The responsibility for providing the ways and means and for mapping them is a joint one between the university and the clinical community. With a firm resolve, we can have confidence that our joint efforts will be successful.

PEOPLE AND DATA

Let me introduce myself as a citizen of the modern world. I am 128-47-8855 for Social Security and investment purposes; I am known as number 7238 by our payroll department; the post office recognizes me only as a resident of 90242. If you telephone me, I am known as 213-923-5591. My bank knows me as 20333-004489, as long as this number on my checks is sufficiently magnetized.

I came to Atlanta under various numbers on my airline ticket, but at least I used my own card to pay for this ticket. I am known to my airline friends as 312-087-888. In fact, they recognize me by this number the world over, except, perhaps, behind the Iron Curtain. Even while in the hospital, I may be known as Room 424-A instead of as a person with pains and ills.

As we move into the technologic world, individually we are in danger of becoming magnetized numbers on a card, magnetized impulses on a tape, or holes in a card that passes at incredible speed through transistorized devices that create electronic impressions.

Artificial intelligence is not the future. It is the now. Modern technology means Pac-Man and Apple computers; on-line systems and automation; Telstar satellites and space shuttles. But who will speak for people?

Thus this topic: People and Data.

Before addressing the people-data interface directly, let me briefly comment on why the topic has relevance by posing a few questions and giving them rhetorical answers—if, indeed, there are answers.

WHAT IS CLINICAL SCIENCE?

- Is it merely a derivative of pure or basic research?
- If that is so, the corollary is that *clinical* science is not important, and given time and interest, basic scientists will answer our questions.
- There is possibly some credence to this view, but let me direct your thoughts another way.

Clinical science is the parent of today's basic science—not the child, legitimate or illegitimate depending on your vantage point.

Duchenne's observations of applied electrical currents and intimations of bioelectric events were the *forerunners* of the science of neurophysiology and the technology of electroneuromyography.

The basic physiologic laws of the heart were not dreamed of prior to Harvey's clinical observation of the circulation of blood.

Just so, clinical physical therapy is the mother of the science of pathokinesiology.

Studies of physical disability or disordered motion cannot occur until the disorder is adequately described, the pain demarcated, or the motion pattern circumscribed.

Real knowledge of problems is derived only from recognition of the problem itself—the stuff of which clinical physical therapy is made.

There are many problems in the elucidation of human disease and disability that require early- and middle-state study to be diverted to animal experimentation. But the term with which we must come to grips is *clinical science* and, logically, the *clinical scientist.* For regardless of what must precede, work relating to human disease and disability must be done on people themselves.

No disability or disease is reduced or cured until humankind has been freed of it.

Who, then, are clinical scientists? They are first clinicians, but ones who at the same time are dissatisfied, pestering, curious, questioning—pains!

Do clinical scientists exist in physical therapy? A few.

Do we need clinical scientists? Do we wish to continue to exist?

What do clinical scientists do in physical therapy? They provide us with raw data about the patients who are cared for by physical therapists. They direct their accumulated experience (call that data!) toward ends that will improve physical therapy practice. They are perceptive and know the questions that need to be answered, but they are tentative and unsure about their ability to find the answers to their questions. Consequently, the only person of whom they ask their questions is apt to be themselves.

What advantages do clinical scientists have?

1. Access to the people, the patients, the problems.
2. A sum of information obtained as a by-product of the clinical care of sick and disabled people—huge amounts of empirical factual information about the causes, complications, courses, and outcomes of clinical problems.
3. Time to look and wonder.

But they have not, heretofore, had the opportunity to organize this information for sharing with others.

What handicaps the clinical scientist?

1. The natural variation of human beings—everything from genetics to blue jean preference makes one patient different from every other even if they have the same disorder.
2. Ethical constraints on human experimentation.
3. Lack of know-how in using available technology to organize day-by-day observations into what we call a data-base, but what you call clinical experience. Adding what *you* know and find to what others know and find.
4. Potential physical therapists–clinical scientists are awed by the rapid advances in technology and thus lack some of the self-confidence or cockiness needed to advance their efforts. They often have an over-exaggerated appreciation of what clinical research really is, and a diminished confidence in how much they actually can accomplish with just a little push.

Thus, my challenge is to give you a nudge and to try to illustrate that you have within your grasp and *well* within your capabilities the raw materials from which clinical science is drawn.

Evaluation, prognosis, goals, treatment planning, and actual therapy are the inextricably bound components of physical therapy practice.

These elements of care traditionally are briefly noted in the patient's chart and possibly expanded upon in special physical therapy records. The traditional progress note, regardless of its translation into computer storage in many institutions, remains the basic record of *what* the physical therapist does to and for the *single* patient and is the official record of the outcome of that service.

Beyond the stored patient progress note, computers are used widely for literature searches, hospital inventories, billing, laboratory tests, diagnostic radiology, and electrocardiogram interpretation, to name a few of the more common functions.

The very fact of the existence of this book leads to an observable fact: While evaluation, program planning, and treatment are better today than ever in the past, there is still widespread dissatisfaction with the general level of what physical therapy can or should be. It is appropriate, then, to address the people-data interaction with a view toward stimulating a greater striving toward excellence.

There are today no effective, multicenter computer interactive programs in physical therapy designed to serve either as data banks or as aids to clinical decision making.

Some would suggest that the lack lies with faults in basic physical therapy education. They would argue that there are unrecognized and untaught distinctions among the acquisition of information (memory), the synthesis or interpretation of information (knowledge), the use of information (competence), and the actual day-to-day management of patient care (performance).

These four factors, memory, knowledge, competence, and performance, can be used in concert to reach excellence.

But physical therapy education—largely, not entirely—stops at the first two steps: memory and knowledge. We do hear a lot of words about problem-solving curricula, but these usually are measured in terms of the competence of students to solve test problems on paper rather than in terms of actual performance. No one would argue that *actual* performance is the ultimate objective upon which excellence is based.

The goal is clear: to create the maximum likelihood of "correct" decisions about evaluation, program planning, and treatment methods. Such decisions depend upon the physical therapists' fund of information (memory), and their ability to synthesize the information they collect so as to apply it to planning and treatment, that is, problem solving.

The exponential expansion of biomedical knowledge makes it impossible for the curriculum model in vogue today to offer to the students all available facts and concepts and their interrelationships. Similarly, even the most expert clinicians, regardless of how dedicated and hardworking they may be, cannot assimilate the potential information available to them and use it to make good clinical decisions. It is a very sad thing nowadays that there is so little useless information.

Following this line of reasoning, we turn to the computer, with its massive information-handling capacity, as a logical expander of the clinician's capability. The models we look to are available to a limited extent in the field of medicine. In medicine, just as in physical therapy, development of computer assistance has been limited by lack of funds, lack of computer-wise physicians who will link with computer scientists for hardware and software development, and, not least, lack of acceptance and use of computer assistance by the clinician.

THE MEDICAL RECORD

The medical record serves a critical function in patient management. It is used by all professionals who come in contact with the patient, from the physician to the therapist, the social worker, and the clinical laboratory personnel. The record is the only defensible link between all factors and persons that affect the patient.

Weed[5] devised a computerized system called the Problem Oriented Medical Information System (PROMIS) that was designed to attack four major problem areas in the usual medical record:

1. inadequate coordination among the wide variety of persons (professional and supportive) responsible for the multiple aspects of patient care
2. excessive reliance placed on memory by these involved personnel
3. absence of a recorded rationale for actions taken or observations noted
4. inadequate feedback for improvement of care.

In Weed's PROMIS system, feedback is readily available with respect to a single identified problem that may be managed by four or five different professionals. For example, a locomotion problem may be treated by the surgeon by a tendon transfer, the physical therapist by mobility exercises and gait training, the occupational therapist via home modification provisions, and the vocational counselor by job retraining. Since the locomotor problem may be secondary to diabetes, a peripheral vascular insufficiency may be managed by the internist, nurse, physical therapist, and pharmacist. Interactions between the two problems and their resolution can be programmed into the computer so that at one time, any clinician can identify overlapping or interacting findings, thus adding clarity and relevance to each clinician's program for the patient. Retrieval can either be in chronologic outline, as a flow chart format, or be drawn out as a single- or multiple-problem analysis.

The strength of PROMIS lies in the obvious and undeniable availability of comprehensive information in a highly organized and reliable manner to all persons associated with a given patient. Where this, or another similar computerized program, is available, the performance attributes or shortcomings of health professionals are clearly identified and, therefore, earlier resolution of problems can be undertaken.

The library of displays available through PROMIS or similar systems encompasses most contemporary medical problems. Such massive programs are expensive to install and to train personnel to use. In concept, they should be cost-effective, but whether they really are may await a more computer-sensitized generation of professionals.

CATEGORICAL INFORMATION SYSTEMS

A variety of computer systems are available that serve specific diagnostic or medical management problems. Physicians faced with an electrolyte or acid-base disturbance can call upon a consultation system in which they interact in a question-answer mode to arrive at a successful diagnosis or treatment mode for a specific patient.[6] Diagnostic information computer programs are available on cardiovascular disease,[7] hypertension,[8] and renal disease.[9] Pople[10] and coworkers also have developed a computer-based diagnostic consultation that deals with a broad range of disorders seen by the specialist in internal medicine. Named "INTERNIST," the program relates likely clinical findings, frequency, and associated manifestations, and weights these to derive a hierarchy of likely diseases from which the practitioner can reduce the list to a correct choice.

PHYSICAL THERAPY DATA MANAGEMENT SYSTEMS

Although the technology and know-how are available, as are models-in-use such as those just mentioned, to date there is no such system either generated or adopted that will aid in physical therapy decision making.

I suggest that the following events are necessary before such a data-management system will become a reality.

1. Include in physical therapy curricula the teaching of both control system theory and methods of making clinical data computer-compatible.
2. Require elementary computer science as either a prerequisite or as part of the professional curriculum. I do not recommend making computer programmers or engineers out of physical therapists, but I do believe they need to know and understand that the computer is a logical extender of their practice, just as are exercise devices, electrotherapy instruments, and goniometers.
3. Purchase, as a beginning, one of the readily available microcomputers for the clinical department and one for student and faculty use in the academic department. Consult with the computer scientists in your institution to ensure that any purchased or leased hardware is compatible with the larger institutional computer systems.
4. Become acquainted with methods of data preparation so that organization can result in multiple uses of the data for such varied purposes as:

    - single case reports
    - analysis of groups of cases
    - epidemiologic studies
    - clinical research
    - institutional or departmental outcome assessment
    - reliability studies
    - personnel performance assessments.

One data collection/preparation system cannot satisfy all possible uses, but there is a general outline that can be adapted to a variety of clinical applications.

DATA PREPARATION

The clinician does not have time to design and maintain valid data collection forms and to use computer storage facilities unless the clinician has a reasonable idea of their immediate or eventual use. The more concisely the problem to be analyzed can be stated, the more clearly the questions can be phrased and the specific data to be collected identified.

How many patients' first episodes of low back pain are "cured" versus how much recidivism is there in the treated population? Are repeated episodes of low back pain associated with age? Occupation? Sex? Posture? Are there psychosocial factors that are common to the patients with chronic low back pain? Are certain treatment procedures more effective than others in reaching "successful" case closure? Are there any predictors in the routine physical therapy evaluation for length of treatment or success or failure?

Initial Activity

Once the purpose(s) of the data collection is defined, the sources of the data need to be spelled out: a personal history from the patient or patient's family; the comprehensive chart, including physician examination and test data; the physical therapy objective evaluation; and, finally, relevant information from published literature on the subject.

Are the data collected to be retrospective (chart review only) or prospective? If the former, then a preliminary and random chart review is essential so that provision will not be made for kinds of data that frequently are not charted. If the study is to be prospective, then data sheets and codes need to be designed and tested for validity, reliability, simplicity, and ease of recording.

The personnel who will collect the data (i.e., physical therapists) may be different from those who code and store it (i.e., department aide or clerk); therefore suitable training programs for both may be required.

Software (computer programs) to do the necessary retrieval or statistical manipulations should be available. Consultation with institutional computer staff is advisable from the onset.

Data Collection Document

After the project and its uses have been defined, and the computer hardware and software identified, a standard document (or form) to collect the necessary data can be devised. The form of data collection then will be compatible with the chosen computer.

The two most frequently used systems today are the punch card and the disk, and these may be interchangeable. The punch card often is used as the permanent record, especially when the disk is subject to inadvertent erasure.

The universal computer card with its 80 columns is known to all. "Do not fold, spindle, or mutilate" has become a dictum pervasive from womb to tomb. The punch card can accommodate only 80 coded items; if more are needed, as will be likely in most clinical studies, "trailer" cards are added. Each new trailer card, however, must use some of its columns to re-identify the case or the source of the data, an incredibly important fact when designing data collection sheets.

The data to be entered are either "nominal," that is, numbers which are themselves clinical data, or, alternately, codes to previously determined information.

In the most simple system, a clear format is devised on which the data collector enters numerical clinical data or circles or checks off the correct response to a specific question, each possible response having a designated code number.

The entered data and completed form are then funneled to the person who will fill out the computer entry portion of the document (i.e., the code portion), check for obvious errors, and identify inconsistencies or implausible answers.

The complete coded document may then be sent to a computer-center key punch operator or, if equipment is accessible, may be key-punched or disk-entered by department personnel. Key punch operators familiar with the project can most frequently detect translation or transcription errors.

Sample layout sheets, not complete because of time and cost, are presented as appendices at the end of this chapter.

Each collection document has a column that indicates both card number and the column(s) on the punch card where the code is to be entered. The document's second column is used to enter the raw data, and the third and largest column contains the actual questions and the responses entered by the data collector.

Data Coding

The system of coding information should be simple and unambiguous. This can be a headache when the data include subjective patient responses (e.g., what is your tolerance to pain?) as well as objective findings (e.g., range of knee extension). The range of responses must be sufficiently encompassing to ensure that important data are not obscured, remain identifiable, and represent discrete, discriminating responses.

If the data collector or coder cannot immediately identify the precise response, then the question should be subjected to further analysis and then re-coded.

In any study of low back pain, the last word, "pain," is the most painful to deal with—both as an item of clinical management and as an item of data identification. The pain occurs on "slight exertion" or only "during heavy labor"—or anywhere in between! The pain may be experienced during recumbency, or when sitting, or only when walking. Thus, the grading of pain in your document should subscribe to the convention in use in your institution, and collection of such data from patient to patient must be consistent.

Coding for missing, unknown, or otherwise unidentifiable data can take a variety of forms depending upon your computer program. It is important to code unidentified data, lest the computer treat a missing value as a zero and insert this into the statistical analysis, which could lead to false results.

Common conventions for missing data are (xxx) or (yyy), or the selection of a number code not apt to be used as a data collection value (9, 99, and 999 are used frequently). A negative number may be selected, such as (–9), or an asterisk (*) may be used if the program can properly identify that symbol. In the appendices, –9, –99, and –999 are used for coding missing data.

Clinical studies will, over time, usually require a revision of coding to remove ambiguous or consistently hard-to-record items, as well as to add new items as new insights are gained or new therapeutic tools become available.

Software and Form of Data Output

The programs to be used and the forms of data output vary; therefore, no concise discussion is possible here. Software to meet your needs may be available. If not, you may have to employ a programmer to write a program to meet your needs or to adapt incompatible software to your computer.

Outputs may be tabular, chronologic, graphic, or narrative. An experienced statistician or computer scientist should design or review your proposed analyses and test them against the stated purposes of your study.

A Caution

Blessed are statistical tables, for they delay the time of our thinking.

Run your eye and mind over the shelves and shelves of statistical data that are published yearly by the government, insurance companies, and the like. Lose yourself for a moment in the thickets of tables and numbers.

Is all this necessary?

Are clinical data so elusive? So subtle as to defy analysis? Is the problem so fatiguing and of such prolixity that it puts an end to genuine inquiry? Can we reduce the low back pain problem with a still greater explosion of data and papers?

This is a perplexing question for humankind and specifically for the physical therapist in search of more and better information to improve care. We are like, perhaps, a person caught in a philosophical confusion. A man is in a room who wants to get out but does not know how. He tries the window, but it is too high. He tries the chimney, but it is too narrow. If he would only turn around, he would see that the door has been open all the time.

Where is that door?

I suggest to you that the door is the adoption of logical modern information processing systems. And I further suggest that your institution study and implement the installation of computer systems for aiding clinical decisions. This is but one road to increased excellence in patient care.

RISK

Since its beginnings some 60-odd years ago, education for physical therapists has held center stage in our profession. The growth of the profession has been directly proportional to the maturity of the educational process. The fruits of physical therapy education are the profession's past, present, and future—and by these fruits shall we be known.

Very contemporary education issues are focused in several areas. To mention only the ones that are in everyone's mind at present:

- achievement of the APTA's established goal of a post-baccalaureate degree for all entry-level programs by 1990, a deadline that I do not believe we can achieve, but a goal that I do espouse

- development of curricula that will prepare the entry-level graduate for autonomous practice and all of the legal, moral, and professional responsibilities that encompasses
- accommodation to the escalation of newly developing programs in the face of ever-more-critical shortages of qualified faculty.

Clearly, our actions in these areas and others must be monitored by our pluralistic society, for we in physical therapy are in the public, and other disciplines do not possess the wherewithal to monitor our work as scientists and clinicians with the thoroughness, skepticism, and responsibility that we ourselves must. Clearly, posterity will not have that chance. Thus, it is important that you understand that we are in a position of enormous *trust* for the people of our country today and for generations to come.

In the deliberations that will continue as we pursue these goals, we must not run the risk of being blinded either by the threats or promises that will be raised. But *we* must constantly question the wisdom of our decisions in the light of our enormous obligation to posterity.

Education programs must offer a post-baccalaureate degree by December 31, 1990. A number of responses are possible: agree, disagree, indifferent, we can, we must not, we have the talent, we don't have the resources.

Practice should be entirely removed from the necessity for physician referral—or as an interim step, just put one foot in the water before plunging into shock.

Qualified faculty cannot be trained in adequate numbers to fill the need in existing schools, to say nothing of the dilution in quality caused by exponential openings of new programs.

What to believe? Whom to trust? How to decide? What sort of group persistently raises such questions? Are we in some ways emulating the deodorant commercial: "Don't be half safe!"—but is it desirable to be all safe?

In the midst of the richest, most productive time of our professional existence, protected by laws, respected by society, we are on our way to becoming frightened. Evidently, alarms are going off.

I submit to you that the arguments may be distilled to one word: RISK! What are the risks? Anger, fear, dissent, uncertainty, critical mass, knowledge factory, self-centeredness.

ANGER

The anger that our actions in education have generated is certainly almost totally external to physical therapy.

To think that we, a unified upstart group of approximately 45,000 physical therapists, had the temerity to make a decision about our education without the prior consent of a small number of deans, none of whom are physical therapists, and none of whom seem to have a reasonable notion of our function, place, or potential in health care. . . .

To think that we, as a group of mature adults, had the audacity to believe that we, more than any outside group, can best judge the quality and adequacy of our education programs via a superior accreditation process. . . .

To think that we had the unmitigated gall to decide that under given circumstances, physical therapists might be an entry point into the health care system and also practice autonomous of physician referral. . . .

What, you may ask, do the anger and reprisal generated by these clearly political issues have to do with clinical decision making? EVERYTHING. For anything and everything that retards the natural and planned development of our schools into acceptable, respected academic centers represents a reprehensible denial of our right to self-determination, and a denigration of the values that we have established for quality patient care over the last half-century.

The most inconceivable action comes from the total antagonism generated by the Southern Council of Deans of Allied Health, most of whom are physicians but certainly none of whom represents the disciplines that comprise that motley group called Allied Health.

In no other educational arena would groups such as ours tolerate being administered academically by persons with no background, understanding, or experience in the thing to be administered, with no commitment or obligation to the group being administered. Can you conceive of a medical school with a physical therapist as dean? Can you imagine a law school with an aeronautical engineer as dean? No, of course not. Yet, we have not raised our united voices in protest to university administrators who persist in this travesty of academic tradition and justice and who probably think that either we love and enjoy the situation or that *we* have no persons qualified to fill deanships. So we must pay the piper for our dereliction, and that price is the high risk to the continuity of our educational enterprise as we envision it should be.

The attitude of the contentious, angry deans is well expressed in one of Piet Heins' *Grooks:*

> I am the Universe's Center.
> No subtle sceptics can confound me;
> for how can other view points enter,
> when all the rest is around me?[11]

It would seem logical that deans could and should better direct their energies, support, and concern toward developing the professional disciplines under their aegis, rather than openly following a policy of repression and opposition.

The logical answer is to strive to place more physical therapists in deanships, in keeping with almost universal academic policy, and thus surmount not only benign neglect, but also unstable political pressures and overt underminings of progress and quality in physical therapy education. Education is, after all, not our present, but our future.

FEAR

And so we have anger from the outside. But fear from the inside is also a real risk. How extraordinary! Here we are. Growing. Financially sound. Resourceful. Protected. Possessing a considerable degree of sophistication. And on our way to becoming frightened of the future.

In times gone by, technology has generated fear. Would airliners crash into skyscrapers that would then topple over and kill thousands? Would nuclear energy plants explode or emit radiation that will maim millions? Will the carcinogen-of-the-month or a California earthquake carry us off? If entry level is raised, will students disappear and, finally, will support evaporate? Such fears as exist can be countered.

Know this: Each generation is richer in human ingenuity than its predecessor.

- The demand for physical therapy services will increase, not decrease.
- There will be increasing costs for physical therapy education, but the increased credible knowledge and skill to be applied in patient care will more than justify the financial factors.

Do we insist on removing the last possible risk before moving onward? The danger lies not here, but in undue caution that then is interpreted as the fear of all new things. That is the only fear that can spell failure. The world has not yet been inherited by the meek, but in physical therapy education it sure is being supported by the lot of us.

CLINICAL DECISIONS AND THE FACTOR OF DISSENT

Somewhere in the educational preparation for decision making there must be provision for the professional student to come to grips with what I would call productive dissent.

In each of us, the total of our life experiences confers a mantle of our individual selves—the concept of ourselves when we come up against, for the first time, ideas or feelings or communications that are different from those we have experienced. We experience and must deal with *dissent*. I use dissent here in the sense of an opinion that differs from our notion of behavior or is unpopular in our lifestyle or perhaps is just unseemly in light of our experience.

Our self-image, if I can call it that, gains consistency and integrity as we grow; but if we do not understand this carefully, it can lead to rigidity and resistance to dissent. It is easy to feel threatened when faced with patients who have widely different lifestyles, who have their own ideas of self-worth, who have other ideas of the *rights* of their worlds, and who have different *"true"* values. Unless physical therapists can feel secure, therefore, all dissent from their recommendations or ministrations is resisted, and they lose the ability to accommodate it.

For example, a few years ago, a member of the notorious Hell's Angels motorcycle club was a spinal-injured patient. The goal established for him by his physical therapist was wheelchair locomotion. His personal goal was motorcycle locomotion. The dissent between the two barred effective understanding. Each day was a new test of wills; convictions and feelings solidified on both sides until no accommodation was tolerable. Communication occurred as two opposing monologues, with dialogue absent. In the end, the patient left the hospital on a three-wheel motorcycle made and presented to him by his club—his life peers. His physical therapist felt only anger and frustration and failure because of the patient's risk-taking actions and because he could not bend to her will.

The ability to listen to opposing perceptions in a non-judgmental manner, to deal with different ideas with an open mind, can come only through exposure to wide varieties of patients as early as possible.

When physical therapists find themselves as the dissenters—with patients or colleagues or superiors—they must know not simply that they dissent, but how and *why* they dissent. For productive dissent is not simply an issue of intellectual freedom or brilliance, but the ability to suffer the intense pain of too much understanding and the willingness to give freely. Over the long course of history, dissenters are great people. It is a pity that we in physical therapy do not recognize this trait and encourage its positive development. To fail to do so is to increase the risk to our acceptance as a caring profession.

UNCERTAINTY AS RISK

Uncertainty about the timeliness of our decisions. Uncertainty about the value systems that provoked them. Uncertainty about the wisdom of increasing risk. Will these elements make it necessary to choose among risks?

Know this:

- The things that *do* occur in education and practice as a result of our actions will be so vastly exceeded by the virtually infinite things that *may* occur that our energies might as well be expended in the striving and the doing, rather than be dissipated in the worrying.
- In attempting to diminish possible losses, we may actually raise greater risks or displace them to other risks.

Consider:

- Nitrates are accused of being carcinogenic, but they are also excellent preservatives.
- Early and frequent sexual intercourse with a wide variety of partners appears to be related to cervical cancer, but the same phenomenon may be linked to lower rates of breast cancer.
- Entry-level graduate programs may cause an acute shortage of qualified faculty, but over time they will bring a greater measure of productivity in science and better patient care to society.

The tradeoffs are apparent!

A CRITICAL MASS FOR PHYSICAL THERAPY EDUCATION

The size of faculties in productive natural science departments in universities seems to be around 15 to 20 full-time faculty. This is the minimum size of the productive medical and biological science departments in top American universities. The best people may not wish to move to a smaller group because of lack of stimulation and services. I believe it to be true that one department consisting of 20 good people can gather more grant money, publish more research papers, garner more recognition, and train better students than can the same 20 people in groups of 5 people in four different schools. Even separation of a department into different, but adjacent, buildings lowers their power—to say nothing of dividing them between different campuses.

Is there a critical mass of similar size in physical therapy? This is hard to say because so few of our programs have a critical mass that reaches into double digits of full-time faculty. Thus, we are at risk with respect to minimal critical mass.

There are those who will argue that my thesis of the quality of the "big" is nefarious because the big programs are good not because of their bigness, but, rather, because they get a disproportionate budget, have lower teaching loads, have more clerical help, and pay bigger salaries. Partly true. But, again, these are the result of a critical mass as well as the cause. An intellectual chain reaction occurs. And as in any chain reaction, the faculty mass produces the conditions that produce the reaction that increases the reactivity.

Thus, we reach a point of *risk identification.* Perhaps our enterprise would accelerate if the small faculties would combine into fewer large ones. A few hot fires will burn more efficiently and with greater notice than many marginal ones.

It would be foolish to apply such an analogy blindly. But it is important to note the frequency with which a number of physical therapy educational programs with their little two- to four-person departments and with totally inadequate resources and equipment offer a few dozen or more courses to a few students. Amalgamation, if not merger, would better serve a geographic area, with improved faculty, better teaching conditions, better equipment, and with each person teaching his or her special subject yet having a lighter load with adequate time and resources for obligatory research and for patient care.

Foundations should be approached to consider giving incentive grants to facilitate either the merger of or agreement between institutions in order to hurdle the initial barriers and give them the necessary time to realize their greater potentialities. Risk reduction by innovation will yield rich dividends.

UNIVERSITY OR KNOWLEDGE FACTORY?

There is a tempting heresy loose in the land. Quite simply, it is the dangerous notion that in physical therapy and closely related disciplines:

a. There is no need for education beyond the baccalaureate level.
b. Indeed, education at the associate-degree level is probably satisfactory for what the physical therapist does.
c. The education of physical therapists is simply a production unit in the knowledge industry, a kind of specialized factory processing human beings for strictly utilitarian ends.

Why has this strange phenomenon developed? For it places our enterprise at grave risk. I believe there are some self-evident factors that contribute to, but do not thoroughly explain, the dangers. One such factor is the belief that our scholarly affairs are poorly managed and productively low, and that we are guilty of utilitarian and featherbedded usurpation of university functions. This is a harsh indictment, and it is pursued with varying degrees of fervor depending upon the kind of administrative unit within which the program resides and the philosophical bent of the administration.

The remedy is equally harsh. If self-regulation has failed, if the physical therapy programs cannot "match up," then we must consider the imposition of the classic remedy of external regulation or extinction. The power of decision on matters large and small in physical therapy curricula has moved upward from the department into the hands of deans and administrators, who have no feelings or concerns about where we have come from in 60 years and who have little or no understanding or could not care less about our *reasons* regarding where we want to go—reasons related solely to better patient care. We have only begun to grasp the consequences of this situation.

In shared innocence, we as a group, viable as the APTA, hassle ourselves about the issues and largely ignore the potential crippling influence of invasive, predatory external authority. The university's historical foundation of self-determinism frequently becomes for us a bitter irony. It is easy to focus blame on the physical therapy faculty when things go wrong. It is harder to fix responsibility on those whose actions result in the things that do *not* happen—for these are not measurable.

Everyone has a stake in the work of the university physical therapy program: parents, students, alumni, faculty, administrators, patients, clinical communities, and taxpayers. It will do us no good to rail at external meddlers. Instead, our challenge—and our opportunity—is to devise wider and deeper networks of support.

Universities are a very special kind of place. They are fragile as truth itself is fragile. They exist by public sufferance. And it is often a marvel that the public supports with its dollars an institution that is free-standing, openly critical to conventional wisdom, and enchanted with controversy. But in these last, the physical therapy component is weak; for we look to survive not by being friendly to disputation and hospitable to those who think otherwise than we do, but instead, we avoid the maelstrom of mainstream university turmoil and thus place our very existence at risk.

If I were forced to give an antidote for the risks I have mentioned, I would be forced to encapsulate my response into the watchword "Why?"

In the latter part of the 15th century, a child was born who was named Philippus Theophratus Bombastus von Hohenheim. A baby with such a name should certainly grow up to have a distinguished career; and this little child, given this big name in a remote part of Switzerland in 1493, did grow up to become a world-famous physician.

Early in life this boy, whom the world now knows as Paracelsus, decided that medicine was his vocation. An indefatigable student, he studied at one university after another; but he became outstanding as a learned man primarily through self-education. He was not convinced that the scientific medicine of his day was worthy of support. He learned more from people who were suffering than he did from all the text books and the professors. He was a man who constantly questioned. He remembered to ask "Why?"

Apparently, Paracelsus was not very diplomatic in his questioning, for he gained a reputation for being argumentative and for brawling in public. Bombastus, one of his names, is part of our language as the word "bombast"—inflated, pretentious language.

However, Philippus Theophratus Bombastus von Hohenheim had in him a major ingredient for scientific and clinical greatness: the ability to use the often forgotten word in physical therapy, "Why?" He was possessed with an insatiable desire to find the answers and to do something about them.

Our professions, our educational programs, do not stimulate or demand enough use of the word "Why?" The potentials are limitless in clinics and universities for physical therapists to ask "Why?" But they then must have the zeal and courage to search for the answers—in science, in education, in practice, and in the political process. And once they answer the why, they have the roadmap to the how and the when and the who and the where.

The spirit of physical therapy is a deep and far-reaching commitment to excellence. It is a stimulus, for it furnishes esprit de corps to our united efforts. Character is the sire of excellence. The high accomplishments of physical therapy to date and the greater ones to come are achieved by men and women of noble character. They give more than they take. They exemplify the good and the fine.

Clinical physical therapy is flourishing, and in that flourishing there is risk; but risk is the spice of life. If I may use this biblical quote, it puts risk into perspective:

> For unto whomsoever much is given
> of him shall be much required:
> And to whom men have committed much,
> of him they shall ask the more.
> (Luke 12:48)

If you have followed my meandering thoughts, you perhaps will agree with me that to take no risk is the highest risk of all.

REFERENCES

1. DONNE, J: *Devotions Upon Emergent Occasions.* 1624.
2. SHAW, GB: *Man and Superman: Maxims for Revolutionists.* 1903.
3. WORTHINGHAM, CA: *Study of basic physical therapy education.* Journal of the American Physical Therapy Association 48:7–20, 935–962, 1195–1215, 1353–1382, 1968, 50:1215–1332, 989–1031, 1970.
4. BUSCAGLIA, L: *Love.* Thorofare, NJ, Charles B. Slack, 1972.
5. WEED, LL: *Your Health Care and How to Manage It.* Essex, Essex Junction, Vt, 1976.
6. BLEICH, HL: *Computer based consultation: Electrolyte and acid-base disorders.* Am J Med 53:285, 1972.
7. BLEICH, HL: *The computer as a consultant.* N Engl J Med 284:141, 1971.
8. SCHWARTZ, WB, ET AL: *Decision analysis and clinical judgement.* Am J Med, 55:459, 1973.
9. GORRY, AG, ET AL: *Decision analysis as the basis for computer-aided management of acute renal failure.* Am J Med 55:473, 1973.
10. POPLE, HE: In *Proceedings 5th International Joint Conference on Artificial Intelligence.* Cambridge, Mass. 1977, pp 1030–1037.
11. HEIN, P: *Grooks 3.* Doubleday & Co, New York, 1970, p 6.

APPENDIX 1. Personal Data

Case Name ____________________
(not coded)

Card 1 Column	Code	Data Collection
1–2	_ _	Case No. ____________________
3–11	_ _ _ / _ _ / _ _ _ _	SS No. ____________________
12–16	_ _ _ _ _	Hosp No. ____________________
17–18	_ _	Eval No. ____________________
19–22	_ _ / _ _	Date mo/yr ____________________
23	_	Sex
		1. Male
		2. Female
24–26	_ _ _	Age at 1st eval _____ years
		−999 Unknown
27	_	Ethnic
		1. Caucasian
		2. Black
		3. Hispanic
		4. Asian
		5. Am. Indian
		6. Pacific Islander
		7. Other ____________________
		−9. Unknown
28	_	Marital
		1. Single
		2. Married
		3. Divorced
		4. Widowed
		5. Significant other
		−9. Unknown
29	_	Religion
		1. Protestant
		2. Catholic
		3. Jewish
		4. Hindu
		5. Buddist
		6. Muslim
		7. Other
		8. None
		−9. Unknown
30–32	_ _ _	Education
		Highest grade completed _____
		−99 Not educated (mentally retarded)
		−999 Unknown
33–34	_ _	Occupation
		1. Homemaker
		2. Unskilled worker
		3. Service (domestic, waitress)
		4. Skilled labor
		5. Craftsman
		6. Office (clerical, cashier)

APPENDIX 1—*continued*

Card 1 Column	Code	Data Collection
		7. Business (sales) 8. Professional 10. Student 11. Other ____________ −99 Unknown
35	_	Primary Language 1. English 2. Spanish 3. Italian 4. Japanese 5. Chinese 6. French 7. Korean 8. Vietnamese 10. Other ____________
36	_	Special Federal/State Program Participant 1. Veteran 2. Migratory worker 3. Public offender 4. Work incentive program 5. Severely disabled 6. None −9. Unknown
37	_	Job Incurred Disability 1. Yes 2. No −9. Unknown
38–43	_ _ / _ _ / _ _	Referral Date day/mo/yr ____________
44–45	_ _	Number of Dependents ____________ −99 Unknown
46	_	Living Status 1. Lives alone 2. Lives with "family" −9. Unknown
47	_	Work Status at Time of Referral 1. Civil service 2. Competitive labor market 3. Self-employed 4. Sheltered workshop 5. Unpaid volunteer 6. Not employed (student) 7. Not employed (other) ____________ 8. Homemaker −9. Unknown
48	_	Weekly Earnings at Referral (nearest dollar)

APPENDIX 1—*continued*

Card 1 Column	Code	Data Collection
		1. Less than 100
		2. 100–200
		3. 200–300
		4. 300–400
		5. 400–500
		6. >500
		−9. Unknown
49	—	Source of Income
		1. Self earning
		2. Public assistance (not disability)
		3. Retirement income
		4. Family support
		5. Disability (SS or Ins)
		6. Private relief agency
		7. Workmen's compensation
		8. Private insurance
		−9. Unknown
50	—	Major Disability Category
		1. Physical
		2. Mental
		3. Alcoholism or drug abuse
		4. Mental retardation
		5. Other ______________
51–52	— —	Secondary Disability Category
		1. Blind/visually impaired
		2. Deaf/hearing impaired
		3. Mental, psychoneurotic, personality disorder
		4. Learning disorder
		5. Cardiac/circulatory
		6. Metabolic, digestive
		7. Respiratory
		8. Cancer
		10. Orthopaedic
		11. Neurologic
		12. Genitourinary, renal
		13. Reproductive, gynecologic
		14. Endocrine
		15. Skin disorder
		−99. No specific information at referral
		Disabling Condition(s) at Referral
53–54	— —	Orthopaedic Deformity or Functional Impairment
		1. Poliomyelitis
		2. Arthritis/Rheumatism
		3. Muscle disease (dystrophy, etc.)
		4. Fracture(s); soft tissue injury

Card 1 Column	Code	Data Collection
		5. Amputation (UE) 6. Amputation (LE) 7. Collagen disease (SLE, polymyositis, etc.) 8. Cancer 10. Congenital malformation 11. Infection 12. Back pain (not specific) 13. Herniated intervertebral disk −99. No specific information
55–56	— —	Neurologic Deformity or Functional Impairment 1. Stroke 2. Multiple sclerosis 3. Epilepsy 4. Parkinsonism 5. Spinal cord injury 6. Head trauma 7. Cancer 8. Cerebral palsy 10. Myelodysplasia −99. No specific information −9. Unknown
57–58	— —	Other Disabling or Influencing Conditions 1. Allergic conditions 2. Diabetes mellitus 3. Cystic fibrosis 4. Asthma 5. Emphysema or other respiratory disorders 6. Old myocardial infarction 7. Recent MI or cardiac arrhythmias 8. Peripheral vascular disease 10. Hypertensive 11. Sickle cell anemia 12. Other anemias 13. Hernia 14. Ulcer (stomach, duodenum) 15. Nephritis or other renal disease 16. Colostomy 17. Aphasic or speech-impaired −9. Other ____________ −99. No specific information
59	—	Ambulatory Status at Referral 1. No equipment 2. Cane 3. Crutches 4. Walker

APPENDIX 1—*continued*

Card 1 Column	Code	Data Collection
		5. Wheelchair 6. Other ____________
60–61	— —	Previous Hospitalizations for Low Back Problems 0. None Number _____ −9. Unknown
62	—	Source of PT Referral 1. Orthopaedist 2. Family practitioner (M.D.) 3. Neurologist 4. Physical medicine 5. Physical therapist 6. Self-referred/friend-referred 7. Other
63–64	— —	Initial PT Evaluation conducted by 1. John Doe 2. Mary Smith 3. William Jones
		Case Outcome
78	—	Reason for Case Closure 1. Voluntarily left program 2. Unable to locate or moved 3. Transferred to other care/program 4. Failure to comply 5. Unfavorable prognosis 6. Death 7. No disabling condition (partial success) 8. Success/cure/restoration −9. Unknown
79	—	Work Status at Closure 1. Civil service 2. Competitive labor market 3. Self-employed 4. Sheltered workshop 5. Unpaid volunteer 6. Not employed (student) 7. Not employed (other) 8. Homemaker −9. Unknown

APPENDIX 2. Medical Evaluation

Card 2 Column	Code	Data Collection
1–2	__ __	Case No. ____________________
3–4	__ __	Eval No. ____________________
5–10	__ __ / __ __ / __ __	Date day/mo/yr ____________________
11–12	__ __	Physician ____________________
13	__	Confirmed Diagnosis
		1. Soft tissue impairment (sprain, strain)
		2. Discogenic
		3. Congenital malformation
		4. Ligamentous
		5. Postural
		6. Facet
		7. Neurogenic
		8. Other ____________________
		−9. No specific diagnosis
	1=yes 2=no	Problem Identification (write in yes or no)
14	__	Pain ________
15	__	Decreased motor function ________
16	__	Incontinence ________
17	__	Inability to work ________
18	__	Limp ________
		Radiologic Findings (write yes or no)
19	__	No positive abnormalities ________
20	__	Decreased intervertebral space ________
21	__	Confirmed disk abnormality ________
		(This information phase may be extensive or sparse, depending on purpose of study.) Columns 22–79 are available for additional data.

APPENDIX 3. General Psychosocial and Physical History

Card 3 Column	Code	Data Collection
1–2	__ __	Case No. ____________
3–4	__ __	Eval No. ____________
5–10	__ __ / __ __ / __ __	Date day/mo/yr ____________
	1=yes 2=no	Pain Exacerbated by the following (write yes or no)
11	__	Family problems (not marital) ______
12	__	Marital stress ______
13	__	Work stress ______
14	__	Economic stress ______
15	__	Changes in life pattern (e.g., retirement, relocation) ______
16	__	Other ____________ ______
		Life Satisfaction
17	__	Patient Reports Life to Be: 1. Very satisfying 2. Satisfying 3. Dissatisfying 4. Very dissatisfying 5. Will not evaluate
18	__	Patient Has History of Other Psychosocial Problems 1. Yes 2. No 3. None reported
		Prior Physical History of Complaint
19–24	__ __ / __ __ / __ __	When Was First Incident of Low Back Pain Date day/mo/yr ____________ (−9 Unknown)
25	__	Was There a Specific Event that Triggered Back Pain 1. Yes 2. No
26	__	Nature of Specific Initial Event 1. Work-related trauma 2. Home-related trauma 3. Pregnancy 4. Auto accident 5. Recreation-related trauma 6. No trauma; but sudden, spontaneous onset 7. Other ____________ −9. Unknown
27	__	When Do You Experience Pain 1. Always 2. Only when doing physical work 3. Only when walking

APPENDIX 3—*continued*

Card 3 Column	Code	Data Collection
		4. Only when sitting 5. Only when bending 6. Only when lying flat 7. Other ______
28	—	Prior Surgical History in Low Back? 1. Yes 2. No
29	—	Prior Physical Therapy 1. Yes 2. No
	1=yes 2=no	Nature of Prior PT Management (write yes or no)
30	—	Traction ______
31	—	Ultrasound ______
32	—	Diathermy ______
33	—	Passive exercise ______
34	—	Massage ______
35	—	Joint mobilization ______
36	—	Mat classes ______
37	—	Pool therapy ______
38	—	Biofeedback ______
39	—	Back care instruction and posture control ______
40	—	Back Supports or Braces 1. Corset 2. Back brace 3. Other orthotic device ______ 4. None
		(Columns 41–79 available for additional data.)

APPENDIX 4. Specific PT Evaluation

Card 4 Column	Code	Data Collection
1-2	__ __	Case No. ______________
3-4	__ __	Eval No. ______________
5-10	__ __ / __ __ / __ __	Date day/mo/yr ______________
		Muscle Test (Manual)
	right / left	Gluteus Medius (L-5) (circle correct grade)
11-12	__ / __	(right) 5. Normal 4. Good 3. Fair 2. Poor 1. Trace 0. Zero −9. Not tested (left) 5. Normal 4. Good 3. Fair 2. Poor 1. Trace 0. Zero −9. Not tested
13-14	__ / __	Gluteus Maximus (S-1) same as above
15-16	__ / __	Quadriceps (L-3) same as above
17-18	__ / __	Anterior Tibialis (L-4) same as above
19-20	__ / __	Extensor Digitorum Longus (L-5) same as above
21-22	__ / __	Soleus (S1-2) same as above
		Gait Analysis (−9, −99 not measured)
23	__	Limp 1. Present 2. Absent
24	__	Side of Limp 1. Left 2. Right
25	__	Type of Limp 1. Trendelenburg 2. Drop foot 3. Other ______________
26-27	__ __	Velocity (normal) ________ m/sec
28-29	__ __	Cadence ________ steps/min
30-32	__ . __ __	Stride Length ________ m

Card 4 Column	Code	Data Collection		
33–35	_ . _ _	Step Length (left) ________ m		
36-38	_ . _ _	Step Length (right) ________ m		
39–40	_ _	Single Stance Time (left) ________ sec		
41–42	_ _	Single Stance Time (right) ________ sec		
43	_	Foot-floor pattern 1. normal 2. abnormal −9. not tested		
		Energy Cost of Normal Walking (−99 not tested)		
44–46	_ . _ _	________ ml O_2/kg/min		
47–49	_ . _ _	________ ml O_2/kg/m		
50–51	_ _	________ % $\dot{V}O_2$ max		
52–54	_ _ _	Heart rate ________ beats/min		
55	_	Superficial Pain 1. Normal 2. Impaired −9. Not tested		
	1=yes 1=right 2=no 2=left 3=bilateral	Dermatomal Distribution Impaired (write yes or no)	(right side)	(left side)
56–57	_ / _	L-2	________	________
58–59	_ / _	L-3	________	________
60–61	_ / _	L-4	________	________
62–63	_ / _	L-5	________	________
64–65	_ / _	S-1	________	________
66–67	_ / _	S-2	________	________
		Peripheral Nerve Impairment (write yes or no)	(right side)	(left side)
68–69	_ / _	Obturator	________	________
70–71	_ / _	Femoral	________	________
72–73	_ / _	Superior gluteal	________	________
74–75	_ / _	Inferior gluteal	________	________
76–77	_ / _	Peroneal	________	________
78–79	_ / _	Posterior tibial	________	________

APPENDIX 5. EMG/NCV Analysis

Card 5 Column	Code	Data Collection
1–2	__ __	Case No. ______________
3–4	__ __	Eval No. ______________
5–10	__ __ / __ __ / __ __	Date day/mo/yr ______________
11–12	__ __	PT ______________
13	__	EMG Findings
		1. Normal
		2. Abnormal
		−9. Not examined
14	__	NCV Findings
		1. Normal
		2. Abnormal
		−9. Not examined
	1=yes 2=no	EMG Findings (write yes or no)
		L-5 Nerve root
15	__	Fibrillation potentials ________
16	__	Positive sharp waves ________
17	__	Myotonic potentials ________
		NCV Findings
18–19	__ __	Femoral n. ________ m/sec
20–21	__ __	Post. Tibial n. ________ m/sec
22–23	__ __	Peroneal n. ________ m/sec
24	__	Vertebral Mobility
		1. Normal
		2. Restricted
		−9. Not tested
	1=yes loc. 2=no no.	Location of Restriction (write yes or no)
25–26	__ / __	L2-3 ________
27–28	__ / __	L3-4 ________
29–30	__ / __	L4-5 ________
31–32	__ / __	L5-S1 ________
		Joint Proprioception
33	__	Hip
		1. Normal
		2. Impaired
		3. Absent
		−9. Not tested
34	__	Knee
		1. Normal
		2. Impaired
		3. Absent
		−9. Not tested
35	__	Ankle
		1. Normal
		2. Impaired
		3. Absent
		−9. Not tested

APPENDIX 5—*continued*

Card 5 Column	Code	Data Collection
	degrees	Range of Motion (right side) (−999 not tested)
36–38	_ _ _	Hip ABD active ________°
39–40	_ _	Hip ext. active ________°
41–43	_ _ _	Hip flex. active (straight leg) ________°
44–46	_ _ _	Hip flex. active (flexed knee) ________°
47–49	_ _ _	Trunk flexion ________°
50–52	_ _ _	Trunk extension ________°
53–55	_ _ _	Trunk lat. flex. (L) ________°
56–58	_ _ _	Trunk lat. flex. (R) ________°
59–61	_ _ _	Trunk rotation (L) ________°
62–64	_ _ _	Trunk rotation (R) ________°
65	_	Activity Profile 1. Mostly inactive, almost sedentary 2. Some physical activity (at least 4 hr/wk) 3. Regular physical activity (10–14 hr/wk) 4. Regular hard physical work for training, employment, recreation −9. Unknown
		Time Spent/Week (hr)
66–67	_ _	Sitting (TV, sewing, reading, desk work) ________ hr
68–69	_ _	Walking (daily routine) ________ hr
70–71	_ _	Bicycling ________ hr
72–73	_ _	Housework ________ hr
74	_	Light sports (e.g., bowling) ________ hr
75–76	_ _	Driving a car ________ hr
77–78	_ _	Other ____________________; ____.____ hr
79–80	_ _	Terminate record of case

Chapter 3

BASES FOR CLINICAL DECISION MAKING: ASSIMILATING DATA AND MARKETING SKILLS

GENEVA RICHARD JOHNSON, Ph.D., F.A.P.T.A.

COLLECTION, DOCUMENTATION, AND UTILIZATION OF DATA IN A TREATMENT ENVIRONMENT

My intentions are to: (1) present some purposes for collecting and documenting data; (2) identify sources that supply useful data; (3) state factors to consider in establishing a documentation system; (4) present a segment of a documentation system that makes use of the computer to store selected information; and (5) describe some of the ways that the information can be used for two kinds of research—clinical research and administrative research.

THE PROCESS OF PATIENT CARE

A philosophic principle that binds all physical therapists together is that the physical therapist provides an array of services that result in patient care. Patient care in physical therapy may be defined as a process that facilitates identification of the problems a patient presents and then provides mechanisms for assisting the patient to resolve those problems. The process, which is circular and continuous, is represented in Figure 3-1 and is based on the assumptions that the physical therapist is:

1. knowledgeable about

    - structures and functions of body systems
    - psychosocial behavior of an individual in health and illness
    - physical therapy services and the rationale for their use (science)

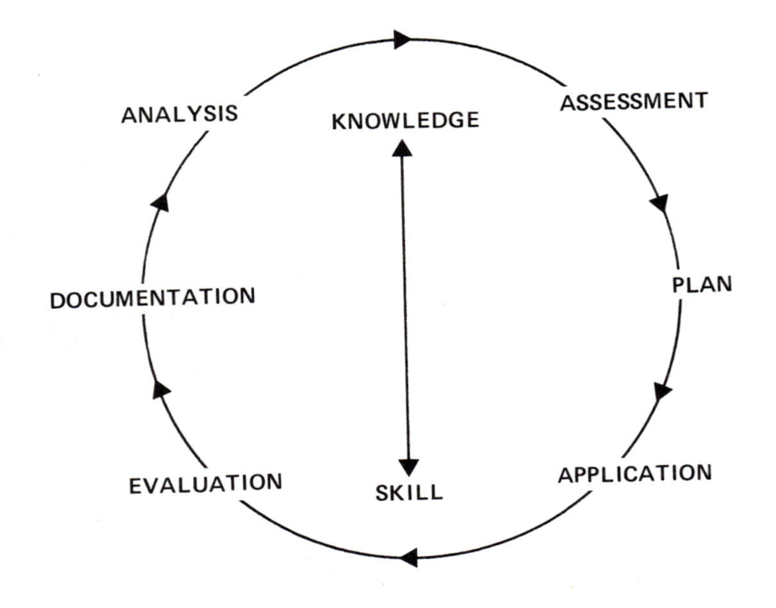

FIGURE 3-1. Process of patient care in physical therapy.

2. skillful and competent in the delivery of physical therapy services (art).

The process of patient care (see Fig. 3-1) is initiated by an *evaluation* of the patient's status. Information is gathered on the patient's physical, psychological, emotional, and social status, education, background, and employment history.

The next component of the process is *documentation* of the results of information gleaned from the completed physical therapy tests and measurements and from other sources. These documents are reviewed and interpreted in the *analysis* phase.

In the next phase, *assessment*, interpretation of the results of the various tests and measures, and information gathered from other sources are examined to determine the implications for the next phase, *planning*. Planning includes the setting of short- and long-term goals and a description of the actions to be taken to initiate the next phase, *application* of specific physical therapy procedures. As soon as application of treatment procedures is in progress, the process is repeated, beginning again with *evaluation*.

Obviously, each component of the process of patient care is important and all are interdependent to some extent. But the one component that is essential to every phase of the process is documentation. Documentation provides the reference information for each succeeding phase in the process, verifies services that have been provided, and reports the patient's response to those services.

PURPOSES OF COLLECTING AND DOCUMENTING DATA

The usual purposes for collecting information about a patient and that patient's response to intervention by the physical therapist may be grouped under four general headings:

- to establish the patient's status at any given time
- to plan care for the patient based on the information received from a variety of sources
- to monitor the quality of care being delivered to patients
- to determine the outcomes of patient care.

One clear implication of those purposes is that continuity of care will be a result. For example, if the physical therapist assigned to the patient is not present or leaves, another physical therapist can continue care based on the information in the patient's record.

Another implication is that we will use the information for research, that is, to study the outcomes of patient care. But that is not a usual purpose, so we most frequently excuse ourselves from the implication by saying such things as: "But I don't know anything about research methodology. Research is too complicated for me to do. I don't have time for that stuff. They won't let me do research. That is not in my job description. Research takes equipment and costs a lot of money. We do not have money for research."

I grew up in physical therapy thinking that clinical research was a natural, expected activity. Although I go back a long way, one of the earliest recollections I have upon entering a clinical setting was meeting a physical therapist on the staff who said, "I'm working on a research project." When I asked the nature of the project, she told me that she was collecting information on patients' responses to the use of progressive resistive exercise to strengthen musculature at the knee joint. As she treated patients, she used a simple procedure to record data systematically on three-by-five cards. I do not know the results because she never presented a report of that project. Even so, that example made an impact on me as a new physical therapist. I assumed that everyone was expected to do similar activities to determine the effectiveness of the procedures one chose to use. So I believed then, and continue to believe today, that a major purpose for collecting and recording information is for clinical research, that is, clinical research that is seen and accepted as a part of what we do every day in patient care.

SOURCES OF DATA

The first responsibility that a physical therapist has to a patient is to identify the problems that need the attention of personnel in physical therapy. The sources that can be used to collect information include:

1. *The Patient.* The patient can supply a history of the current illness or injury, if that information is not available in the patient's record. The patient or a family member can be asked to validate any information that is questionable and to give needed information that does not appear in the record. Records from other health care facilities, from

colleagues in the community, and from colleagues within your own facility often are valuable sources of data as well.

The most powerful source of data is the physical therapist's own evaluation of the patient's functional abilities, muscle strength and tone, perceptual abilities, endurance, coordination, and cognition. Of equal importance is what the patient tells you about the problems, how the patient defines and describes them, and what the patient tells you he or she wants to do about them.

2. *The Family and Friends.* For certain information, a valuable source may be family members or friends. Discretion must be used in accepting information from sources other than the patient. Although the information may be critical in making a decision about plans for patient care or the patient's discharge, if discrepancies are found, they must be reconciled without pitting the patient and family against each other.
3. *Health Care Professionals.* Colleagues in other health care professions (e.g., medicine, nursing, occupational therapy, social work) can provide information that will supplement and complement what has been gathered from other sources. Participation in patient care rounds with other health care professionals is an important method for getting information from them.

COLLECTION OF DATA

With so many potential sources of data, you can drown in facts, figures, and conjecture. You will need a carefully organized documentation system that can provide the means by which to determine: (1) the nature or kind of intervention used, (2) when the intervention occurred, (3) where the intervention occurred (setting), (4) the results of the intervention, and (5) the effectiveness of the outcome of intervention.

The design of a documentation system includes the content (what is to be collected), methods (how you will collect information), and materials (forms, format, instructions for use). Before you design your system, you should know why you need the information and how you plan to use any information you collect. Some criteria to use as guidelines in making these determinations are that information must be: (1) meaningful, (2) accurate, (3) timely, and (4) systematic. A brief discussion of each criterion will show the value of screening during data collection.

Meaningful. To be meaningful, information must be important in relation to its intended use, not just nice to have. If you cannot justify a need to know, you probably do not need to know. Identify specifically what you need to know about an area.

Accurate. Any information recorded must be accurate, both in content and in method of collection and documentation. Data collected must be reliable for the patient's record, for research, for governmental agencies, and for other financial sponsors.

Timely. Information that is not recorded promptly is not available for the benefit of the patient or for colleagues who may need to know what you have learned about the patient. For all practical purposes, unrecorded information does not exist. Delay in recording information can be costly in several ways, since financial sponsors do not reimburse us for undocumented services. We may lose revenue, and the patient may be burdened with bills for services that could have been reimbursed if a record of services delivered had been available.

Systematic. Collecting and recording accurate data in a timely fashion must have regularity. If data are to be used for making judgments, decisions, and comparisons, these data must be collected under specified conditions, for example, at the initiation of a care plan, every third day thereafter, and on the day prior to discharge.

The criteria cited above form an acronym that is familiar to all physical therapists and easy to remember: MATS. I say about records that MATS is a MUST.

An important aspect of data collection is the forms used to record permanent information for the patient's record. All documents should conform to minimal standards that require them to be:

1. *Identified.* The origin of the form should be readily apparent; for example, the name of the facility and the name of the department should be prominently displayed.
2. *Current.* Outdated forms may not allow for collection of comparable or adequate information.
3. *Easy to Use.* Forms that are crowded, unattractive, or have complicated instructions for completion may be either completed incorrectly or not completed at all.
4. *Dated.* The form itself should carry the date of any revisions. The user of the form should be required to sign the form and to record the date on which information is entered.

The minimal standards for a document give us another acronym that is easy for physical therapists to remember: ICED.

A COMPUTER DOCUMENTATION SYSTEM

Over the past year, we have designed, adopted, and initiated the first segment of a new documentation system that allows direct entry into the computer from a terminal in the department.* Although the present segment is designed essentially to generate charges, we can extract detailed information about patient services delivered. Analysis of those data over time can lead to the development of outcome standards for several classifications of patients with severe disabilities.

As a foundation for describing ways to use documented information for research, a brief description of the collection method we use in our department will be helpful. Then I will present several examples of how the data can be used for studies related to patient care and to management.

A sample of a record of charges for the Department of Physical Therapy at The Institute for Rehabilitation and Research (TIRR) is shown in Figure 3-2. The codes used to record the services delivered are shown in Figure

*Gayla B. Alexander, L.P.T., Associate Director for Administration, Department of Physical Therapy, The Institute for Rehabilitation and Research (TIRR); and Jaime Cuzzi, Director of Management Services, TIRR, deserve credit for development of the system.

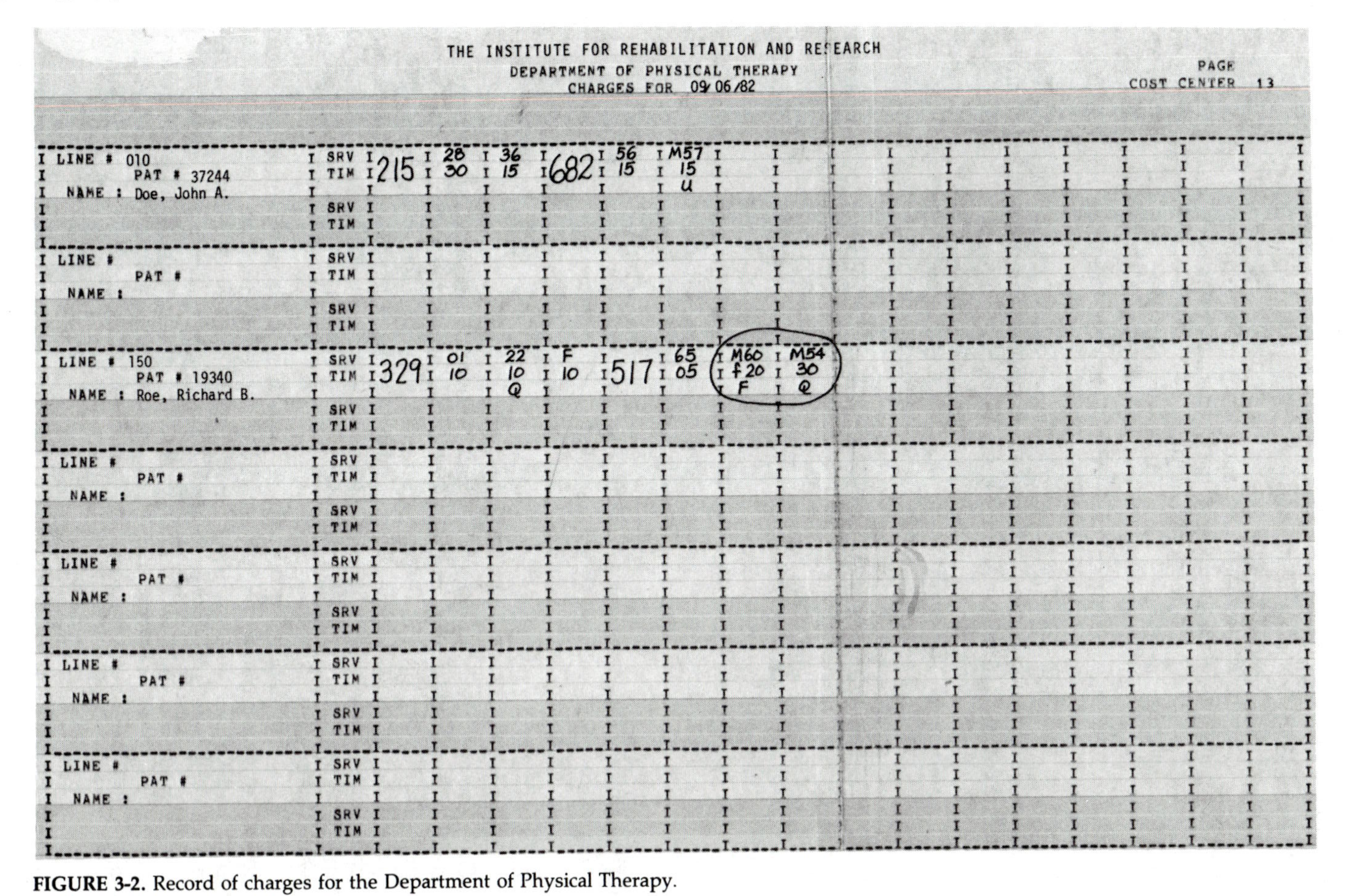

THE INSTITUTE FOR REHABILITATION AND RESEARCH
DEPARTMENT OF PHYSICAL THERAPY
CHARGES FOR 09/06/82

PAGE
COST CENTER 13

LINE # 010	SRV	215	28	36	682	56	M57		
PAT # 37244	TIM		30	15		15	15		
NAME : Doe, John A.							u		
	SRV								
	TIM								
LINE #	SRV								
PAT #	TIM								
NAME :									
	SRV								
	TIM								
LINE # 150	SRV	329	01	22	F	517	65	M60	M54
PAT # 19340	TIM		10	10	10		05	f20	30
NAME : Roe, Richard B.				Q				F	Q
	SRV								
	TIM								
LINE #	SRV								
PAT #	TIM								
NAME :									
	SRV								
	TIM								
LINE #	SRV								
PAT #	TIM								
NAME :									
	SRV								
	TIM								
LINE #	SRV								
PAT #	TIM								
NAME :									
	SRV								
	TIM								
LINE #	SRV								
PAT #	TIM								
NAME :									
	SRV								
	TIM								

FIGURE 3-2. Record of charges for the Department of Physical Therapy.

02-DEC-82
15:22

THE INSTITUTE FOR REHABILITATION AND RESEARCH
PHYSICAL THERAPY SERVICE CODES

Consultation

1 OUTSIDE CONSULTATION
2 PT CARE CONFERENCE
3 PT CARE ROUNDS

Evaluation

20 ARTICULAR
21 CARDIAC-PULMONARY
22 ELECTRICAL STIMULAT.
23 EQUIPMENT
24 FUNCTION
25 GAIT
26 HOME ASSESSMENT/PROG
27 MOTOR CONTROL
28 MUSCLE STRENGTH
29 ORTHOTIC
30 PAIN
31 PHYSICAL ASSESSMENT 1
32 PHYSICAL ASSESSMENT 2
33 PHYSICAL ASSESSMENT 3
34 PROSTHETIC
35 ROM
36 SENSORY
37 TONE
38 SKIN

Treatment

50 BRONCHIAL DRAINAGE
51 CLASS *
52 COLD *
53 DEBRIDEMENT
54 ELEC. STIMULATION *
55 EQUIPMENT MODIFICATION
56 EXERCISE, ACTIVE *
57 EXERCISE, RESISTIVE *
58 FUNCTIONAL TRAINING
59 GAIT TRAINING *
60 HEAT *
61 HOME PROGRAM
62 MASSAGE
63 MOBILIZATION
64 NEURO DEVELOPMENT
65 POOL ASSIST
66 ROM
67 STANDING *

Other

Equipment

A BIOFEEDBACK
B COLD PACKS
C CYBEX
D EMG
E FES
F HOT PACKS
G HUBBARD TANK
H JOBST
I KINETRON
J PARAFFIN
K PARALLEL BARS
L POOL
M PULLEYS
N STALL BARS
O STANDING TABLE
P TECA
Q TENS
R TRAINING ORTHOSES
S TREADMILL
T ULTRASOUND
U WEIGHTS
V WHIRLPOOL

Absence

A ILLNESS
B SURGERY
C PATIENT REFUSES
D SCHED CONFLICT
E NOT READY
F BOWEL/BLAD ACCIDENT
G DISCHARGED
H IVP
I NO SHOW (OP)
J OOTB
K LATE MEALS
L LOA
M STAFF SHORTAGE
N TRANSFER TO MIC/MAIN
O TRANSPORTATION (OP)
P WEATHER (OP)
Q CANCEL (OP)
Z OTHER (WRITE IN)

Therapist Codes

000M	001M	002M	106A	107M	109M	113A	114A	216A	220M
325M	327M	332C	334C	336M	338A	344M	349M	560A	562M
671M	672M	674M	675M	680M	689A	792M	794M		

FIGURE 3-3. Code numbers.

A.

SRV		28	36
TIM	215	30	15

B.

SRV		56	M57
TIM	682	15	15
			U

C.

SRV		01	22	F
TIM	329	10	10	10
			Q	

D.

SRV		65	M60	M54
TIM	517	05	f20	30
			F	Q

FIGURE 3-4. Sample documentation of patient services.

3-3. The system for entering information on the charge sheet is simple, requires minimal effort on the part of the individual providing services, and can yield an enormous amount of accurate data if used properly.

Each day, the department receives from the Department of Management Services a printout listing the patients who are scheduled to receive services that day. The patients' names and hospital numbers appear in alphabetical order, and each name is assigned a line number for the day. Assigning a line number facilitates any search for information about services given to a patient on any specific day.

Space is available to make 32 entries for each patient. If more space should be required, the patient's name and number can be listed again by hand on the daily roster. Throughout the day, the names of new patients are added to the daily roster by hand.

Each staff member is assigned a code number to be used when recording services provided. The number reflects the category of the individual (e.g., coordinator, clinical specialist, staff physical therapist, physical therapist assistant, technical aide). That classification is important if comparisons are to be made between individuals or between groups, or if a description is to be drawn of one group.

The following information is available about the services given to patient John A. Doe on 9/6/82. A clinical specialist (number 215) performed an evaluation of muscle strength (28) for 30 minutes, and a sensory evaluation (36) for 15 minutes (Fig. 3-4A). A technical aide (number 682) provided active exercise (56) for 15 minutes, and resistive exercise (57) for 15 minutes using weights (U) (Fig. 3-4B). The M preceding the type of treatment given (57) indicates the use of minimal supervision.

The second patient, Richard B. Roe, also received services from a staff physical therapist (number 329) who gave consultative service (01) for 10 minutes, and electrical stimulation (22) for 10 minutes with TENS (Q) (Fig. 3-4C). The remainder of the treatment time, 10 minutes, was cancelled because of a bowel/bladder accident (F). A physical therapist assistant (number 517) gave heat (60) for 20 minutes with hot packs (F), and electrical stimulation (54) for 30 minutes with TENS (Q) (Fig. 3-4D). Except for preparation (65) for 5 minutes, the time was charged at the rate for minimal supervision (the M preceding the service numbers indicates minimal supervision). The fact that the patient received heat (60) with hot packs (F) is recorded, but no charge is made for that service since the heat and electrical stimulation (54) were provided simultaneously. That is indicated by encircling the two treatments. The lowercase f preceding the recorded time for heat (60) indicates that no charge is made for heat as a separate treatment.

EXAMPLES OF UTILIZATION OF DATA COLLECTED

1. *Clinical Studies.* From the data collected daily in the department and from admission information, we have in the computer a substantial data base on each patient:

- patient's name, age, sex, diagnosis, date of onset of illness or injury, date of admission, date of referral for physical therapy services, date of discharge, and the discharge environment (e.g., home with family, independent living arrangements, nursing home, another hospital)
- kind and amount (time in hours) of physical therapy services delivered
- kind and amount of physical therapy services not delivered, and reasons for the failure to deliver those services
- personnel who delivered the services.

With these data, we can complete descriptive studies of any designated population (e.g., men, ages 18 to 24, with complete spinal cord injuries at the level of C-7).

A descriptive study would include: (1) all services received by each patient; (2) the total amount of time devoted to each procedure; (3) the changes in the patient's status over time; (4) the outcomes that can be assigned to physical therapy, for example, strength, flexibility, mobility; and (5) the total time required for the patient to reach established goals. The total time can be reflected in two figures: actual hours, and the number of days, weeks, or months from the initiation of services to discharge.

Descriptive studies on any patient population are important because they lay the foundation for the development of questions about the value of our interventions. Descriptive studies also allow us to compare the approachs to and outcomes of care delivered by two or more physical therapists.

2. *Management Studies.* Much of the same data collected for clinical studies are useful for a wide variety of management studies related to utilization of: (1) an evaluation or treatment procedure, (2) time by an individual or a group, or (3) equipment. Patient absences or cancellations can be tracked and related to an individual care giver, a patient care group, or a patient care unit. The results will determine if absences or cancellations are due to a

failure in the delivery system (staff shortage in the facility, illness of staff, over-scheduling), to patient illness, or to refusal of services by the patient for any reason.

I have cited the most obvious examples of the studies that are possible in our department. The cost for analysis of data can be justified because the results of studies can lead to precision in selecting and applying physical therapy procedures.

SUMMARY

The collection and documentation of information about our patients and the physical therapy services delivered to those patients are essential elements of excellence in patient care. Technology can make the collection, documentation, and utilization of data rapid and easy, once a system is established.

You do not need a computer to create a reliable system of data collection and documentation. But you must have the determination to initiate and maintain a system.

MARKETING

Most of us have more patients than we can manage comfortably, so the development of marketing strategies to attract patients is not high on our priority list at this time. Nevertheless, I would like to discuss some practical ways to market ourselves and the services we have to offer. Because I believe that we know more about motor behavior and motion enhancers than anyone else, I think that we need to let our colleagues in other professions, especially in medicine, and the general public know who we are and what we are about.

DEFINITION OF MARKETING

My stripped down, simplistic view of marketing in health care states that marketing involves determining community needs and comparing the requirements for filling those needs with the resources of the provider of services (e.g., a private practitioner, a hospital, an agency, or a school). Marketing also includes public relations (i.e., giving information about services to those who need to know it) and is initiated after a decision is reached that a fit exists between a community need and the ability of the provider to meet that need. Publicity and selling are other aspects of marketing.

PURPOSES

Marketing may seem to be a function of the facility, rather than the concern or responsibility of a single professional discipline or individual. But physical therapists can use the elements of marketing strategy (i.e., research, public relations, publicity, and selling) to good advantage both internally and externally.

A marketing program for physical therapy would have the following purposes: (1) to inform physicians and others in the facility and the community of the services available in physical therapy; (2) to increase the number of referrals within a facility; (3) to increase the number of referrals from physicians in the community; (4) to attract referrals from a specific medical or surgical service; (5) to inform physicians and other professionals about physical therapists, their academic and clinical preparation, and their skills in evaluation, treatment, and consultation; (6) to attract funds for special projects; (7) to recruit staff; (8) to expand or add to physical therapy services; (9) to add new positions; and (10) to inform the public about physical therapy services and the knowledge and skills of physical therapists.

ESTABLISHING A PROGRAM

A marketing program focuses on: *internal constituencies* (the board of trustees, physicians, nurses, and other health care professionals, other personnel in the facility, and volunteers) and *external constituencies* (physical therapists in other facilities, other professional colleagues in the community, agencies, schools, other potential users of services, and the general public).

ACTIVITIES DESIGNED FOR AN INTERNAL CONSTITUENCY

To achieve marketing purposes internally, we can use a variety of activities that may be classified as research, public relations, publicity, or selling. None of these categories is discrete; nor does that matter. The important point is to have a marketing plan that gives attention to the several segments. In that way, you will be prepared to focus on a particular segment as the need arises.

Research

- Collect and analyze data on the services provided, the recipients of those services, outcomes of services provided, cost of providing services, and income generated from the variety of services provided.
- Other data to be collected and analyzed would include items such as recruitment of personnel, staffing patterns, and termination of personnel.

Systematic documentation of meaningful, accurate data in a timely fashion will serve as a foundation for reports on the effectiveness of services delivered and for requests for expansion or addition of services.

To offer a different service or an additional service in the department, the approval of an administrator usually is necessary if operating costs will change. Justification of the need for the service will include descriptions of: (1) the service; (2) the kinds of patients who will benefit from that service; (3) the expected outcome for those patients; and (4) the financial implications, including cost of operation (e.g., personnel, space, equipment, supplies required), and an estimate of income to be generated by offering the service.

Public Relations: Examples to Use with Physicians

- In addition to convincing the administrator of the merits of your plan for expansion or addition of a service, you may need the support of physicians who refer patients to you as well as those who do not customarily refer patients to you. In either case, you will need to supply them with documentation similar to that which you prepared and presented to the administrator. The physician will be less interested in the financial aspects and more interested in the outcome of service, a comparison of those who received the service with those who did not, and the satisfaction of patients with the service.

- Learn and speak the language the physician understands when you are asking or answering questions.
- Make daily rounds to see your patients early in the morning. Visit those who may be referred, as well. Many physicians make early morning rounds, so you increase the possibility of seeing and talking with the patients' physicians.
- Prepare informative but concise status notes for the patient's record. Do not use abbreviations unless they are commonly known and accepted by everyone who records information for the patient's record.
- Invite the physician to be present during a patient's treatment time. Select a specific activity you want the physician to see. Raise questions and demonstrate the patient's functional status.
- Prepare and distribute attractive, eye-appealing brochures that describe your services.

Public Relations: Suggestions for Use in Facilities and Private Practice

- Announce all new appointments via a memorandum.
- Describe the new employee's educational preparation (give degrees earned, universities or schools attended), experience, and state information about licensure. Give the employee's title.
- Publish the same information in the facility's newspaper.
- Announce all promotions via a memorandum.
- Announce all staff achievements, especially papers published, presentations given at meetings, any degrees awarded, and participation in professional and community activities.
- Participate on committees or task forces (e.g., safety, infection control, special events, records, and so forth). Volunteer to serve on committees. Recommend other staff who have special interests or talents.
- Send notes of appreciation, congratulations, or condolences to staff.
- Send copies of letters of appreciation or commendation to appropriate persons, for example, employee's supervisor.
- Invite staff in other departments and physicians to join in a potluck lunch in your treatment area.
- Invite personnel in other departments to speak at your staff meetings.
- Volunteer to speak about physical therapy and physical therapists to others in the facility.
- Learn the names of people you see frequently, and address those persons by name.
- Smile—look happy.
- Dress so you look like you are there for business.

- Offer one hour a week to plan a fitness program for interested staff, if you can make the time for that.
- Hold an open house periodically. Plan activities that involve all visitors so that each one can try out selected equipment or be tested for strength or flexibility or feel an electrical current.
- Have exhibits in the treatment area showing patients receiving care or special projects in progress. These exhibits could be placed on public view later in the lobby or on the walls in the hallways.
- Distribute handouts to patients and visitors that tell the story of your treatment unit.
- Volunteer to help on the patient care unit if your assistance is needed while you are there (e.g., help transfer a patient).
- Organize special events programs that give staff the opportunity to present short papers, report research results, or present an interesting patient problem with the results achieved.
- Be prepared to tell members of your board of trustees and any other important persons about the department, the role of the physical therapist, the educational preparation required for practice, and your own contributions in physical therapy.

Often in the past, we have exhibited what I call the "basement mentality." Many physical therapists today are too young to remember when the department of physical therapy was usually located in the basement. No windows let in light. Many physical therapists sat in their private "mole holes" waiting to be discovered by physicians and patients. They were indignant when they were not consulted about matters related to physical therapy.

Some of that behavior is still exhibited in a different form by those physical therapists who refuse the challenge of today and the promise of tomorrow. These are the ones who do not participate in the activities of the American Physical Therapy Association at any level. They do not attend continuing education programs because they do not have time; nor do they seem to feel a need to add to their knowledge and skill in patient care. These same physical therapists can be heard saying things like, "Only a physician should evaluate a patient. I am not qualified to practice medicine." The danger they represent to the advancement of physical therapy is frightening. The negative image they create for the profession will be extremely difficult to erase.

ACTIVITIES DESIGNED FOR AN EXTERNAL CONSTITUENCY

Public Relations: Professional Public

Public relations activities designed for the professional public require careful planning and may require considerable time and effort on your part. Some approaches that can give you desired results are as follows:

- Prepare and submit articles designed to share your patient care results with others.
- Prepare presentations for local, chapter, and national scientific sessions.

- Present information about physical therapy to health care organizations in your community.
- Prepare and distribute brochures describing the services you can provide. Include the mechanism for referral: to whom, where, when; fees or arrangements for payment; parking situation; directions for reaching your facility; operating hours.
- Send letters to segments of the professional public announcing services—those in place or those to be offered. Include community agencies, rehabilitation nurses, selected physicians, and colleagues in physical therapy in your mailing.
- Hold an open house for professional colleagues in the community.
- Present Physical Therapy Grand Rounds for colleagues in your own and other facilities.
- Offer continuing education courses. Make some of these interdisciplinary in nature.
- Prepare tapes, slides, or films on subjects of special interest to your colleagues. Offer these for loan or purchase.
- Offer short-term, intensive clinical experiences for physical therapists who need a refresher or want to learn how you manage care for a specific patient population. Charge a fee to cover the cost of instruction.

Publicity: General Public

The general public can be informed through the media about physical therapy services in your facility. Although you are familiar with most of the approaches, I want to emphasize the following:

- Prepare and offer high-quality spot announcements of 30-seconds duration to your local television and radio stations. These spots, if accepted, will be aired as public service announcements without a charge for air time. Since you may need to consult a marketing specialist as you prepare these spots, the cost of preparation is a factor to consider when you choose that approach.
- Give human interest stories to your local newspapers. If possible, establish a working relationship with a reporter whose work you admire. Encourage the use of pictures as well as text for the story.
- Participate in the special fund-raising activities in your community.
- Volunteer to appear on radio or television talk shows to tell about your department and your role in health care.
- Hold an open house for selected groups once or twice a year.
- Invite school children to tour your department. Tell them about your activities.
- Establish a scoliosis screening day, or volunteer to participate in one that is already established.
- Encourage patients and their families to speak on behalf of physical therapy at community functions. Encourage testimonials about the quality of your services.

The activities suggested for public relations and publicity do not exhaust the possibilities but may serve as the impetus for you to generate your own list.

SELLING PHYSICAL THERAPY AND THE PHYSICAL THERAPIST

Value of Services and the Physical Therapist

A legitimate part of marketing is the selling of ourselves and our services. The commodities we offer are knowledge, skill, experience, and hope. No one else knows what the physical therapist knows or how to use that knowledge for the benefit of a patient.

To sell ourselves and our services, we must value what we know and what we do. We must believe in ourselves and in the hope we extend to those who use our services. The value we place on ourselves is reflected in the way we behave and in the language we use to describe ourselves. I think that physical therapy is a glamorous, vital, giving, caring profession and that the physical therapist as a teacher and toucher is unique among health care professionals. If you think about it, you, too, will realize that we are the health care professionals who do the most touching. Touching is a form of communication that signifies caring. As physical therapists, we have the opportunity to express our care and concern through touching because we have access to a patient's body in a most intimate way. That is a privilege most people do not give lightly. And yet, we are allowed that privilege each time we deliver any kind of service to a patient. We hold a patient, give support, move body parts, lift, and cradle. In short, we nurture the patient at a time when such caring behavior from us may be essential to the patient's recovery. One of the best ways to sell ourselves may be through the concern and care that can be expressed so clearly through touching.

Value of Reimbursement

In the past, we have allowed others to place a value on our services, to set our salaries, and to profit financially from our knowledge, skill, and dedication. Because what we have to offer has unique value, we have a right to expect fair and just financial compensation for our services. That in itself is a justifiable reason for a marketing program planned and executed by physical therapists for physical therapists.

All of us must guard against exploitation of the physical therapist. Exploitation demeans the person and the profession. You can be assured that if we are unwilling to be assertive in our own behalf, the exploitation will continue. As a group, and individually, we must expect to provide high-quality service and to be justly compensated, in salary and benefits or in direct income, for delivering those services.

Value of Descriptive Language

The language we use to describe ourselves is an important aspect of marketing. I hear physical therapists speak of "jobs and wages" and of being "hired." These terms make me think of an assembly line in a factory. As a professional employed in a health care environment, the physical therapist who uses the words "jobs, wages, and hired" to define a relationship with an employer may create an image that matches those words.

Another term that does little to promote the status of physical therapy is "chief" to designate the director of a service unit. The term "director,"

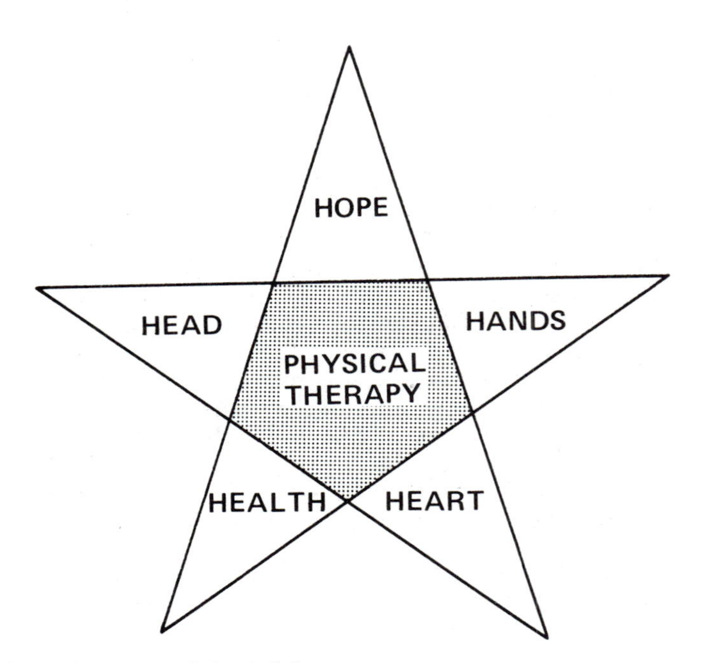

FIGURE 3-5. Vital aspects of physical therapy.

which appears in our early literature, is descriptive of the responsibilities usually assigned to an administrator or manager—planning, leading, organizing, and controlling.

Many other terms that may be used to describe us or our service units are less than complimentary. For example, in most facilities, physical therapy is classified as an *ancillary service. Ancillary* is derived from the Latin for "handmaiden." To whom are we handmaidens?

SUMMARY

Ours is a profession of service. We offer our services to the very young, to the very old, and to all of those in between. I see us as a bright star in the firmament of health care (Fig. 3-5). Each of the points of our star represents a vital aspect of physical therapy. We have a great deal to give. I think that we use our *heads* to make decisions about what to give, and we try to give high-quality care. Our *hands* are very important in what we do, and so are our *hearts.* We strive to help people to maintain or regain *health.* In the process, we offer *hope* that health will be the end result of the services we provide.

We have a responsibility to let others know about us as professional practitioners and about what physical therapy has to offer in the development, maintenance, and restoration of physical function. The task of informing colleagues in other professions and the general public is ours. That means that we must be highly visible in our places of employment and in our communities.

Creating change in the profession and expanding our services, as well as extending those we now offer into new and different environments, are our responsibilities, also. As we become a profession with a preponderance of independent practitioners, competition for clients will increase. I see that as a healthy part of our growth. Most of us will accept the competition as a challenge to maintain our services at a high level of quality.

To arm yourself for your responsibilities in marketing, I cannot overemphasize the importance of collecting and analyzing meaningful, accurate, and timely data in a systematic fashion. Data on the who, what, how, when, and where of the services you are providing will serve as the basis on which to make patient care and administrative decisions. Be alert to changes occurring in your practice. These may be the result of changes in state and federal legislation, population shifts due to openings or closings of industrial operations, or changes in referrers and the reasons for referral. With adequate information at the appropriate time, you will be prepared to make adjustments in your services to absorb either an increase or decrease in demand.

Knowledge about marketing and skill in the process of marketing will be essential to the establishment and maintenance of a productive practice in any environment in the near future. Without delay, physical therapists must acquire knowledge of marketing practices and develop skill in their use. The selected bibliography at the end of this chapter will merely introduce you to the extensive literature available on marketing in health care.

Each one of us has power to make change. Together, you and I are powerful enough to achieve whatever goals we set. We must learn about and use the political processes in our employment environments, in our local communities, and at the national level for our advantage and for the people we serve.

A fitting end to this chapter is a brief quotation from an unidentified source:

> To achieve all that is possible, we must attempt the impossible. To be as much as we can be, we must dream of being more.

The only limits we have are those we impose.

BIBLIOGRAPHY

CLARKE, RN AND SHYAVITZ, L: *Marketing information and market research—valuable tools for managers.* HCM Review/Winter, 1981, pp 73–77.

COOPER, P (ED): *Health Care Marketing: Issues & Trends.* Aspen Systems, Rockville, Md, 1979.

FALIC, J: *Humanistic design sells your hospital.* Hospitals, February 16, 1981, pp 68–74.

Taking health care to hospitals. Hospitals, June 1, 1977, pp 51–72.

KOTLER, P: *Marketing Management,* ed 4. Prentice-Hall, Englewood Cliffs, NJ, 1980.

LEE, JM: *Marketing ensures success of maternity care program.* Hospitals, December 16, 1980, pp 91–94.

WALTER, CM: *Academic medical center features image analysis in marketing audit.* Hospitals, August 16, 1981, pp 91–100.

Chapter 4

CLINICAL DECISION MAKING BASED ON HOMEOSTATIC CONCEPTS

SHIRLEY A. STOCKMEYER, M.A., R.P.T.

Many of the procedural aspects of physical therapy treatment can be described in terms of the application of stimuli. Procedures that use electrical, mechanical, or thermal modalities obviously involve stimulus applications. Therapeutic exercises, whether they entail handling by the therapist or the use of apparatus, can include such stimuli as touch, pressure, stretch, resistance, joint compression, joint traction, or head movement. Active responses by the patient further generate input from such sources as changes in blood gases and blood pressure, muscle tension, muscle shortening and lengthening, intrafusal muscle tension, and active head movement. Distance receptors and receptors in internal organs are frequently affected by the stimulus complex used in therapeutic regimens.

Those physical and physiologic inputs that are an integral part of treatment do not act upon a passive organism. At the time of treatment stimulation, the individual will demonstrate baseline values for the given function the treatment is designed to change. The effects of therapeutic stimuli interact with the individual's pre-stimulus level of a function and are further determined by how well the individual is organized to respond to the environment and then return to the baseline. The individual's pre-stimulus level of function is, to a great extent, dependent on the person's general state. Only an evaluation that takes into account these individual variables can form a reliable basis for decision making about the effectiveness and course of treatment.

GENERAL STATE OF THE ORGANISM: ITS INFLUENCE ON BASELINE FUNCTIONING IN AUTONOMIC AND SOMATIC SYSTEMS

In his holistic theory of the organism, Goldstein[1] emphasized that the effects of stimuli were determined by both the stimulus and the total state of the organism. The general state, in turn, affects the baseline values of many functions.[2,3] The relationships among state regulation, autonomic regulation, and somatic regulation have been described in a developmental theory proposed by Als.[4] If an infant has not achieved stability in the regulation of state and is not making smooth transitions from one state to another, the processing of external stimuli can be so difficult that autonomic and motor functions deteriorate. If somatic motor regulation is deficient, it can affect the general state of the infant and tax autonomic functioning.[4] For example, the premature infant who is barely maintaining a flexed posture can lose that posture completely, exhibit changes in autonomic functions, and become generally stressed in response to a tactile stimulus or to handling.[5]

Some of the neural bases for the interactions of state with autonomic and somatic control are founded in concepts about the reticular activating system. Dell[6] explains that "the reticular activating system has been described as the site of convergence of heterogeneous somatic and autonomic afferent activity and to it has been attributed the part of integrator of the different spheres of activity of the organism." The power of a given sensory message to activate the reticular system depends on the functional state of the reticulo-cortico-reticular loop at the particular moment the input is received. Reticular activity is monitored and controlled in part by the cerebral cortex, and cortical activity will be different for different states. The reticular system makes the adjustments necessary in autonomic functions (respiratory, circulatory, and humoral) for somatic activities to be effective.[6]

Dell[6] uses the term "critical reactivity" to define the results of a process in which homeostatic controls, through an adjustment in reticular activity, selectively place motor neurons of the "final common pathway" at the disposal of the systems that activate them. Keeping the somatic system and the autonomic system each in homeostatic balance involves setting the level of excitability of neurons so that there is adequate reactivity, while at the same time ensuring constancy in baseline tone, moderation in the range of responses, and a balance between antagonistic mechanisms. In the autonomic nervous system, there is a balance between sympathetic and parasympathetic mechanisms that needs to be maintained along with reactive capacity in each half of the system. In the somatic motor system the balance that is required for reactive yet stable responses could be between tonic and phasic mechanisms. It is also possible that the balance that is of most importance for the maintenance of control occurs between muscle groups of antagonistic patterns. Fine and ongoing adjustment in the baseline levels of various functions to the critical level of reactivity enables the organism to react with a high degree of efficiency and differentiation.

INFLUENCE OF PRE-STIMULUS LEVEL ON RESPONSE

The initial value (IV) of a function is the same as the baseline, the prestimulus level, or the pretreatment level. The IV of a given function changes as the general state of the individual changes. The closer to a sleep state, the lower will be the baseline level of such functions as somatic muscle tone, heart rate, blood pressure, and respiratory rate. As an individual changes to a state of alertness or stress, the baselines of such functions will be higher.

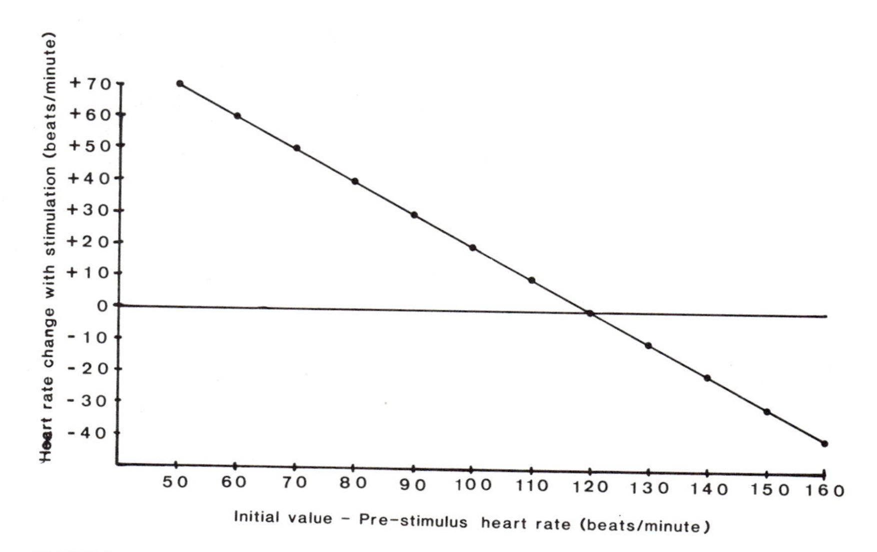

FIGURE 4-1. Correlation of initial value of heart rate with change in heart rate from stimulation. A hypothetical single case.

The principles concerning the influence of pre-stimulus level on response are embodied in the Law of Initial Value (LIV) as proposed by Wilder.[2,7] The Law of Initial Value states that: The *higher* the IV of a function the *less* change will occur in response to a function-*increasing* stimulus, and the *lower* the IV of a function the *less* change will occur in response to a function-*decreasing* stimulus. These rules hold true for IVs that are in midranges of the function. When the IV of a function is well beyond the midrange, there is an increasing tendency for no response or a reversal of response.

Figure 4-1 represents a hypothetical plot of the relationship between heart rate response to a function-increasing stimulus and the IV at which that stimulus was given. If a person's heart rate is low and a function-increasing stimulus is given, there will be a large increase in response. The same quantity of function-increasing stimulus given when the IV is high will yield little or no change; and at even higher IVs, the heart rate might be *lowered* in response to a function-*increasing* stimulus. If a person's heart rate is high and a function-decreasing stimulus is given, there will be a large decrease in function. The same quantity of function-decreasing stimulus given when the function is already low will yield little or no change. At very low IVs, a function-*decreasing* stimulus can actually *increase* heart rate. Further discussion of the reversal of response, or so-called "paradoxical reactions," will be presented in subsequent sections of this chapter.

The Law of Initial Value is comprised of regulatory rules for the size and direction of responses to stimuli, taking into account non-zero values of pre-stimulus baseline functioning. Any consideration of the LIV must take into account the fact that the response to a stimulus depends not only on the IV but on the dosage of the stimulus. A great many responses in a wide variety of systems follow the LIV. Wilder[2] has assembled and organized those findings and provided a critique of many studies in which the LIV was operating but went unrecognized. Several investigators,[3,8,9,10] studying autonomic functions in infants, have found response patterns consistent with the LIV. Some phenomena that were not understood at the time of their discovery can be explained by the LIV. Sherrington[11] discovered that the effect of electrically stimulating a muscle depends on the pre-stimulus state of contraction. In response to stimulation, a muscle that is contracting will relax and one that is relaxing will contract.

EFFICIENCY OF RESPONSE TO STIMULI

The LIV, in addition to being a set of regulatory rules for the size and direction of responses, also describes a mechanism that attempts to bring about an optimal level of response. If the IVs reflecting a wide range of states are correlated with the amount of changes induced by a stimulus applied at that IV, a regression coefficient can be calculated for that individual and that stimulus. For a detailed explanation of the statistics related to the LIV, see the work of Lacey and Lacey.[12,13] The responses shown in Figure 4-1 represent a relationship with no variation from the mean, a hypothetical but highly unlikely situation. Individuals show scatter about the regression line and differences in the slope of the line and the point of reversal.[3]

An individual with good homeostatic stability responds with a quantity of change that takes him or her toward the regression line, that is, responds by seeking an average level of response that is optimal. If the IV is already at that optimal level, no change takes place. If the IV is below optimal response level, homeostatic mechanisms will raise the function. If the IV is above optimal response level, the function will be lowered in response to a function-increasing stimulus. The extent to which an individual can achieve an optimal response level regardless of the IV (or state) may be a measure of homeostatic stability and the efficiency of the LIV.[3] Absolute values of change and absolute values of IV alone may not provide enough information. The variables of spread (deviation from optimal level), slope, and point of reversal may be needed to obtain an accurate picture of a patient's homeostatic status.

COMPENSATORY MECHANISMS: THE CONCEPT OF BIDIRECTIONAL SYSTEMS

There is a constant struggle in both somatic and autonomic systems between those forces that are working to keep the organism reactive, ready to change, and mobile, and those forces that are working to maintain stability and provide constancy. The range of changes that can take place in a system is constrained by biologic limits beyond which forces become destructive. Well within biologic limits, there are homeostatic limits that define the range of effective controlled responses. Demands placed on an individual may require wide ranges of function, but a return to a stable mid-value is essential as a reference point for subsequent responses. These concepts can be illustrated and elaborated upon by using as an example the function of somatic muscle tone. In the daily cycle of activity of a normal person, which includes periods of sleep, quiet wakefulness, alertness, fatigue, and stress, somatic muscle tone could vary considerably. In a healthy individual, tone returns to a mid-value after the factor initiating the change ceases or when compensatory mechanisms prevail. Normal tone has a baseline that is not a zero value. Some healthy individuals tend to have a baseline on one side or the other of average tone; that is, some healthy people are "high tone" or "low tone" without the state being pathologic. Depending on general state, an individual may return to a baseline that is above or below the mid-value, but not extremely so. That baseline can shift according to state but will remain in a homeostatic range where the system is stable.

In pathologic conditions, the baseline tone from which the person functions could be either extremely high or extremely low. Although an individual patient can have very high tone and little mobility, this does not mean the person is stable in a homeostatic sense. Rigidity is not extreme stability. Some abnormal states might represent a failure to stabilize around mid-value, with the result being very labile responses or fluctuating baselines of tone. Goldstein,[1] in his holistic theory, thought diseased states represented a lack of constancy of function around "middle values." Wilder[2] expanded on that idea and proposed that it was the constancy toward the LIV with which an individual complied that determined health.

When the mid-value of a function is considered to be the baseline, and responses occur in either direction away from that point, we are then dealing with a bidirectional system. The component halves of a bidirectional system do not act independently of each other, and what happens in one half influences the other. The halves of the bidirectional autonomic nervous system are the parasympathetic and sympathetic divisions. The component halves of the somatic motor system are less clearly defined. Several possibilities are worth consideration: tonic and phasic mechanisms, approach and avoidance controls, and flexor and extensor systems.

Selbach[14] has explained the relationship between the component halves of a bidirectional system in terms of a "rule of induction." A stimulus designed to activate one half of the system activates the controlling centers of both halves of the system. The initial response of the first-half center occurs against some resistance from the second-half center. The second-half center begins its influence with low intensity and may not be clinically observable. Its action continues and is manifest toward the end of the initial response. The role of activity in the second-half center is to counterbalance the action of the initial-half center. The more that the first-half center causes a deviation, the greater will be the counterbalance or compensation. Functions are maintained as the feedback from deviation in one half of the system automatically brings about a correction by the other half. Each half of the system induces a response in the other so that they "tune each other mutually inductively to a homeostatic level."[14]

Compensation that occurs as a secondary effect to a primary response is usually "silent" in that there is simply a return to pre-stimulus state or slightly beyond. The direction of the function is reversed to bring it back to the pre-stimulus IV (Fig. 4-2). This change is not a passive return to baseline, but rather one that is brought about by active homeostatic regulation. In somatic motor functions, the braking mechanisms are an example of counterbalance. As a contraction proceeds, there is induced in the antagonist a progressively increasing state of facilitation (Sherrington's[15] successive induction principle).

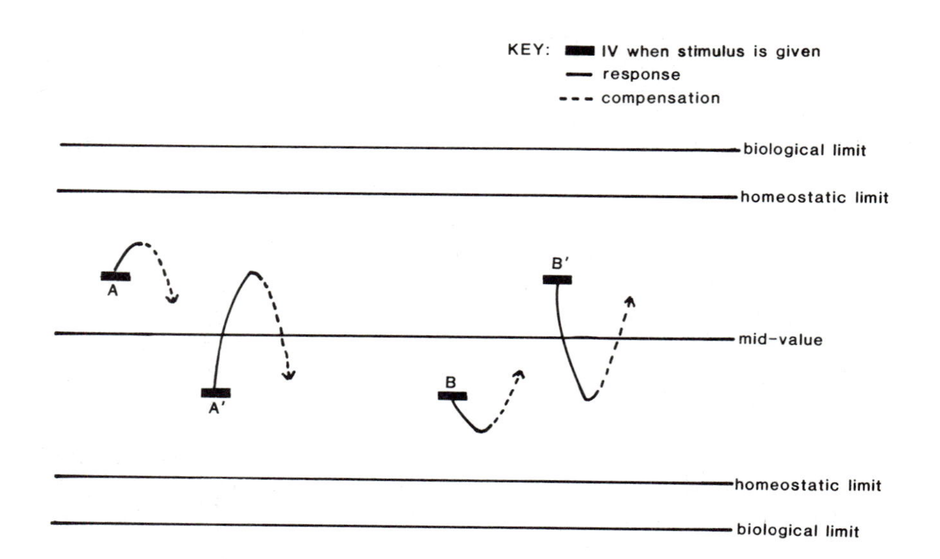

FIGURE 4-2. Compensation for deviations from the initial value occur back toward mid-values in a stable system. (A) IV high, function-raising stimulus yields small response. (A′) IV low, function-raising stimulus yields large response. (B) IV low, function-decreasing stimulus yields small response. (B′) IV high, function-decreasing stimulus yields large response.

When there is a very high IV and there is great stress on the organism as a whole such that it is pushed beyond homeostatic limits, there may be no observable initial reaction, and the secondary effect may be so exaggerated that it seems to be the main effect. When the secondary effect, an overcompensation, is seen, it is considered a paradoxical reaction. It is clinically very important to distinguish between a reversal that is a result of the system being pushed beyond homeostatic limits and a reversal that represents a normal system seeking an optimal level.

THERAPEUTIC IMPLICATIONS

Many variables that affect responses to therapeutic stimuli operate in every individual. Some of those variables that have been considered in this chapter are as follows: the pre-stimulus level of a function, a factor that can be constantly changing because stimuli of all types, in addition to therapeutically designed stimuli, are impinging on the organism; the state of the organism, a factor that can be affected by a wide range of sources from emotional and cognitive influences to organic disorders; and the general efficiency of an individual's homeostatic mechanisms in regulating reactivity and restoring levels of functioning through stabilizing compensations.

It may seem to be a difficult task to predict the responses of an individual or to generalize from combined data. In fact, the study of baseline measurement per se as part of physical therapy evaluation has not been dealt with in a comprehensive manner. The full usefulness and impact of therapeutic procedures will be, in part, dependent on the expansion of research efforts on homeostatic function and the accumulation of a body of knowledge that allows for more exacting use of therapeutic stimuli. Meanwhile, therapists will be alerted to the role homeostatic mechanisms play in response and can examine responses in light of those mechanisms. Some questions that could be useful as a part of evaluation and re-evaluation are considered in the following paragraphs.

Are compensations effective? Do they bring the function back to mid-ranges? The measurement of the effects of treatment usually extends only to the period immediately after completion of the treatment. For some patients and some treatments, it is quite important to measure responses over an extended period. Procedures involving thermal modalities often have secondary effects that are first manifest several hours after treatment. A very strong positive response to treatment may have a strong compensation that takes the patient back beyond the pre-stimulus level. That compensation does not necessarily occur immediately. For example, hot packs applied for a painful restricted shoulder might provide the patient with relief, and yet, several hours later when "the treatment wears off," the patient experiences a great deal of pain and loses the range of motion gained during treatment. It is possible that the treatment caused vasodilation and reduced muscle tone initially, but the "compensatory" secondary effects were too great and eventually brought about vasoconstriction and heightened tone or a return of spasm. Reducing the dose (decreasing the temperature of the packs) may not achieve as great an initial response, however, without secondary effects that are so great the patient may retain a greater proportion of each treatment's initial effects.

Patients who have a great deal of difficulty reversing out of a posture they achieved actively may have lost the ability to automatically activate the second-half center of a bidirectional system. The patients stay at the extreme achieved in the initial response and do not have the mechanism for quickly changing the balance between flexors and extensors in the direction of the antagonist.

Overshooting a target, a problem seen in ataxic patients, could represent a loss of the inducing capacity of a bidirectional system. The normal compensatory braking mechanism activated before the end of the movement is not functioning to decelerate the limb.

Is the response to treatment expected, absent, or paradoxical? The absence of a response to a treatment should not automatically be taken as a signal to increase the dose. The patient may be at that moderately extreme IV where no change takes place.

The use of some stimuli results in initial and compensatory effects where the second effect is the therapeutic one. For example, ice massage used to increase circulation will cause vasoconstriction and then vasodilation, which is the therapeutic goal. Activating the stronger muscle of an antagonistic pair first in order to facilitate the weaker one makes use of the activation of the second-half center and the compensatory response as the primary therapeutic effect.

If the response to treatment represents the reverse of what was expected, it is possible that the IV of the function was toward the high end of the scale for that patient. It would be worthwhile to attempt treatment with the patient in a less stressed situation.

One problem in interpreting paradoxical effects (reversals from the expected direction of response) is that without knowledge about the responses this individual makes at a variety of IVs, the examiner cannot tell if a response is a primary reversal to an optimal level or a secondary compensation that is exaggerated.

Is there homeostatic instability with wide fluctuations in response and difficulty returning to mid-value? An individual lacking homeostatic stability is unable to maintain functions within limits that are efficient and enable controlled reactivity. Selbach[14] has proposed that beyond the range of homeostatic regulation there is a "zone of lability." When patients are pushed by internal and external environments into that zone, paradoxical reactions occur that are extreme overcompensations. When patients are in that labile state and react with extreme reversal, they will be in a homeostatic "crisis." The dysreflexia or autonomic crisis that can occur in spinal cord injured persons is an example of an extreme reversal. The high IV and extreme reversal can also explain the course of vasomotor crises such as the migraine headache. Vasoconstriction of cerebral blood vessels gradually increases to a point beyond the normal homeostatic range. The control of tone becomes labile and a reversal to atonia of smooth muscle occurs in those cerebral blood vessels involved. The lack of tone allows the walls of vessels to be stretched by blood coursing through, and that stretch, which is greater than normal, stimulates pain receptors.

Because of the interaction of autonomic and somatic functions, knowledge of the status of both systems can provide the therapist with more information about each system than would be obtained by monitoring just one. For example, when using a procedure that is intended to affect somatic muscle tone, it is important to be alert to changes in skin color, perspiration, respiratory rate, and heart rate. Premature infants, elderly persons, and persons with some diseases can be very stressed by procedures that seem innocuous. Just the stress of being handled or the anxiety about illness and treatment can cause the loss of control that is tenuous. Bowel and bladder accidents could be an expression of the momentary loss of homeostatic balance between sympathetic and parasympathetic functions.

It is well known that a high-tone child cannot be forcibly and constantly held in a posture that puts overactive muscles in a full stretch without resulting in extreme disorganization of autonomic and somatic functions. In effect, the stretch represents a function-increasing stimulus for muscle tone that is already high. Initially, the child will resist and, more importantly, will show autonomic signs of stress such as increased perspiration, changes in skin color, and rapid, shallow breathing. Eventually, the child might exhibit extremely decreased tone. Although low tone in this case is a goal of treatment, the use of a crisis and the loss of homeostatic stability to obtain it is a very unsound practice. Extreme stress and its secondary effects may be life threatening to a patient with very inadequate homeostatic mechanisms. Inhibitory procedures that include a more dynamic movement component and do not evoke greater extremes in a function, which are already very high, provide a sound basis for treatment of the high-tone child by restoring the balance between inhibition and facilitation.

Is there poor reactive capacity? In contrast to the person who has too great lability and lacks homeostatic controls to bring the function back to mid-value, some patients have lost the normal range of responses and the ease of reaction necessary for adaptability. Usually, the loss of reactive capacity is seen in patients with very low or very high tone. The tendency would be to increase the amount and frequency of stimuli in order to "get them going." However, their low reactivity must not be taken as a sign that they have good homeostatic stability. Without thoughtful use of stimuli, these patients could be pushed into an overcompensation that is as maladaptive as their original condition. Inactive, low-tone infants who have been subjected to indiscriminate and excessive amounts of stimulation frequently become agitated and demonstrate problems with feeding and sleeping. They go from being underreactive to being overreactive and unstable. Moderation in the use of facilitating or inhibiting procedures could progress the patient further with control while avoiding the disorganizing effects of wide swings in reaction.

The concepts of homeostasis in somatic and autonomic functions help in the lawful interpretation of individual variation and lead to treatment decisions that are more effective for the individual patient. Treatment goals could take the following forms: development of homeostatic stability, establishment of compensatory responses that are appropriate in timing and amount, reduction of lability of responses, and establishment of normal reactivity. Clinical research efforts will be needed to develop means of obtaining data on the individual patient to profile homeostatic status and provide the tools for predicting the reactions of the individual to various therapeutic procedures.

SUMMARY

Decisions about treatment procedures and their dosages cannot be made effectively if they are based solely on general knowledge of the effects of a procedure and on the response frequently seen in patients with a given disability. Individual variations exist in pretreatment levels of function, in reactivity to treatment stimuli, and in the organization of the controls that return systems to a state of equilibrium after a response change. These individual variations in homeostatic mechanisms appear to be critical factors in determining the outcome of treatment. The limited state of our knowledge about how to measure these homeostatic variables sometimes prevents us from examining them prior to initial treatment. For example, it may be necessary to study a series of responses to treatment in order to understand how well the individual compensates for response changes and returns to a mid-value for a given function. Nevertheless, understanding homeostatic mechanisms can assist in making decisions as treatment progresses and in evaluating unsuccessful treatments.

The effects of therapeutic stimuli interact with the individual's pretreatment levels of those functions the treatment seeks to change. The patient with an initial value (IV) of a function that is very low may not respond the same as one whose IV is very high, even though both may receive the same dose. Treatment decisions leading to an adjustment in dosage to achieve a more desirable effect should be based on a consideration of the influence of the IV on treatment outcome. Paradoxical responses to treatment may indicate that the person has good compensating mechanisms or may indicate abnormal lability in a system. In the first case, it may be unnecessary to alter treatment, but instead it may be appropriate to consider if the patient's state may have pushed the IV up to the level where the stimulus evoked the paradoxical response. In the second case, it would be imperative to alter treatment in order that the patient not be thrown into a homeostatic crisis. The decision to alter treatment would depend on recognizing when a specific response to treatment was exaggerated and when more general changes in state and autonomic functions signaled a disorganizing and detrimental effect of treatment.

The general state of the individual patient can be affected by a wide range of factors, and state, in turn, can affect the pretreatment levels of many functions and, therefore, affect treatment outcome. Early treatment decisions might have to involve changing initial state before beginning procedures targeted toward a specific deficit. For example, treatment will have to be changed in time, or state changing procedures instituted, in an infant who is very agitated. In children and adults, anxiety about their illnesses and treatment experiences is a significant factor affecting treatment outcome. Therefore, the most important early decisions might well involve procedures to relax and reassure the patient.

Treatment is designed to bring about change in some system. This response change can last for varying periods depending on the treatment stimulus, its dosage, the systems affected, and the status of the individual. In addition, the timing of the secondary effects, or compensations to response change, appears to vary according to a number of factors. In light of these timing variables, there are decisions to be made about treatment groupings, frequency, and duration. If the patient is already into the compensating stage of a response to one treatment, it is important to consider if the application of the next modality is most effective at that time or cancels the effect of the first treatment. Repeating a single treatment very frequently, for example, every few hours, may be more effective than doing a single treatment once each day. Decisions regarding timing of treatment require ongoing monitoring of the patient's status, including evaluation between procedures and for longer periods after the completion of treatment.

Physical therapeutic procedures have the potential for being more powerful in their effects when their application takes into account the homeostatic factors of the individual's reactive capacity and equilibrating processes. As evaluation of the homeostatic status of the patient improves, decisions about the dosage, the timing, and the nature of treatment will become more tailored to meet the needs of the individual patient.

REFERENCES

1. Goldstein, K: *The Organism.* American Book, New York, 1939.
2. Wilder, J: *Stimulus and Response: The Law of Initial Value.* John Wright and Sons, Bristol, England, 1967.
3. Bridger, WH and Reiser, MF: *Psychophysiologic studies of the neonate: An approach toward the methodological and theoretical problems involved.* Psychosom Med 21:265, 1959.
4. Als, H: *Social interaction: Dynamic matrix for developing behavioral organization.* New Directions for Child Development 4:21, 1979.
5. Als, H: *Infant cues: The clinician/caretaker's guide to interaction.* A Workshop at Boston University, Boston, May 17, 1982.
6. Dell, P: *Reticular homeostasis and critical reactivity.* In Moruzzi, G, Fessard, A, and Jasper,

HH (EDS): *Progress in Brain Research, Vol 1, Brain Mechanisms.* Elsevier, New York, 1963, p 82.
7. WILDER, J: *Basimetric approach (law of initial value) to biological rhythms.* Ann NY Acad Sci 98:1211, 1962.
8. WOLFF, PH: *Observations on newborn infants.* Psychosom Med 21:110, 1959.
9. LIPTON, EL, STEINSCHNEIDER, A, AND RICHMOND, JB: *Autonomic function in the neonate.* Psychosom Med 22:57, 1960.
10. RICHMOND, JB AND LIPTON, EL: *Some aspects of the neurophysiology of the newborn and their implications for child development.* In JESSNER, KL AND PAVENSTEDT, E (EDS): *Dynamic Psychopathology in Childhood.* Grune and Stratton, New York, 1959.
11. SHERRINGTON, CS: *Man on His Nature.* Doubleday & Co, New York, 1953.
12. LACEY, JI: *The evaluation of autonomic responses: Toward a general solution.* Ann NY Acad Sci 67:123, 1956.
13. LACEY, JI AND LACEY, BC: *The law of initial value in the longitudinal study of autonomic constitution: Reproducibility of autonomic responses and response patterns over a four year interval.* Ann NY Acad Sci 98:1257, 1961.
14. SELBACH, H: *The principle of relaxation oscillation as a special instance of the law of initial value in cybernetic functions.* Ann NY Acad Sci 98:1221, 1962.
15. SHERRINGTON, CS: *The Intergrative Action of the Nervous System.* Yale University Press, New Haven, 1947.

Chapter 5

BASES FOR CLINICAL DECISION MAKING: PERCEPTION OF THE PATIENT, THE CLINICIAN'S ROLE, AND RESPONSIBILITY

ELSA L. RAMSDEN, Ed.D., R.P.T.

PERCEPTION OF THE PATIENT

> What I want to explain in the Introduction is this. We have been nearly three years in writing this . . . We began it when we were very young . . . and now we are six. So, of course, bits of it seem rather babyish to us, almost as if they had slipped out of some other book by mistake . . . So we want you to know that the name of this [chapter] doesn't mean that this is us being six all the time, but that it is about as far as we've got at present. . . .
>
> A.A. Milne

With those words as background, let me try to outline more formally the purpose of this chapter. The scope of our professional practice as physical therapists has increased in Gulliverian leaps as technology keeps bringing more information for application to our sphere of practice. A cursory review of professional curricula over the past 50 years is more than enough to convince anyone that the scope of physical therapy practice is multisystem, involving all aspects of human behavior. Nevertheless, the historic core of physical therapy practice is still present: working with patients to improve motor function. The physical therapist observes the movement of another individual. Aberrations in function are noted, priorities are established, and a problem-solving strategy of some sort is launched. That sounds simple enough! Indeed, it is terribly complex, as any physical therapy student in the final year of academic preparation would adamantly assure you. What it means is that before, during, and after any physical activity by the therapist, there is mental activity that has come to be called clinical decision making. The heart of that procedure is a process called *inference*. Inference is the pivotal point upon which all else depends. Increasing our awareness of this essential but complex concept can lead to greater facility in treating patients, supervising other staff, relating to nurses and physicians, or making any other decisions that affect our work or our lives.

My purpose in this section is to carefully examine the means by which we process incoming data to arrive at inference. I will briefly discuss some key current concepts related to brain-behavior relationships operating in the reception and storage of information. Based on this, I will outline how inference occurs and the steps leading to some form of action. In the process, I will illustrate these concepts with applications to clinical practice.

CONSCIOUSNESS AND OUR WORLD OF PERCEPTION

A patient is in the treatment area and you are the therapist seeing this person for the first time. What do you bring to this encounter? Professional experience? Specific professional skills? A sophisticated technical education? Yes, all of these. In addition, you bring your own experience of the world and your personhood, including your mind-sets and expectations for behavior. Of course, you would agree, the patient brings his or her own experience of the world and personhood, with expectations for behavior. Before either of you utters a sound, much has happened between the two of you and within each of you.

We could even say that you have seen more than you are aware of seeing. Because seeing so often starts the process, I will focus on the visual sensory system for now, although, of course, all the other senses get into the act. The eyes are a very active component of the human sensory apparatus. They are constantly moving to scan and inspect myriad details in the environment. As the eyes move, they pick up details via the fovea, the small central area of the retina that has the greatest concentration of photoreceptors. This movement allows access to the greatest amount of detail to be scrutinized. In normal viewing of a still object, the eyes alternate between rapid movement and fixation.

Vision begins with light striking the retina. In simple terms, this physical energy is changed into neural messages that move toward the brain via the optic nerve, optic chiasm, optic tract, thalamus, and the lateral geniculate body. The latter send axons to the occipital lobe. An image is constructed in the nerve cells of the visual cortex, in the form of neural activity, that is very different from the retinal image.

One way the cortical activity is different is that it begins to produce what we usually call meaning or labeling. When we see a patient for the first time, the patient's size, shape, position, arrangement and configuration of parts, and movement are not a totally new experience for us. We are able to recognize familiar patterns in our vision of the person new to us. To understand how this happens, we need to take a short excursion through the results of recent studies on memory, for they lead back to and illuminate how we process sensory data.

The capacity to remember things has been discussed in relation to cognitive processes by Miller,[1] Broadbent,[2] and Kesner,[3] among others. They hold that both memory and cognitive processes start with sensory input. The individual probably selects which data to focus on through a combination of an attending mechanism and existing interest at the moment of sensory input. Craik[4] suggests that there is a very brief "sensory memory" stage, milliseconds in duration, during which input experience is converted to coherent images that then move on to sensory regions of the brain.

Short-term memory (STM) is the second phase of information processing and is distinguished from long-term memory (LTM) by storage time and function. There is wide acceptance of the theory that STM acts as the conscious processing unit of the brain.[5,6] Cognitive processes require both STM and the data that is stored in LTM. It seems that STM is closely related to coding, rehearsal, thinking, retrieval mechanisms, and decision making.[5] It seems to be a temporary working memory used by these control processes. Further, STM encodes the data to be transferred to LTM storage. According to Craik,[4] the encoding involves tagging the data with cues to enable access for retrieval later. He found that the same cuing was used for both encoding and retrieval, as did Norman.[7]

There is wide speculation about the location of STM and LTM, with agreement on only one issue: the consolidation process, which enables data in STM to be transferred to LTM, takes place within the hippocampus. The well-known patient H.M.[8] had bilateral hippocampal lesions surgically produced in an effort to relieve intractable epileptic seizures. The patient could not consolidate material from STM for transfer to LTM storage following surgery, nor on subsequent follow-up over a period of 15 years.

This very brief excursion through neuropsychology is sufficient to provide background for the model below. Only one additional premise is needed, namely, all behavior is communication. We derive meaning from body movement, muscle tonus, and eye movement. Even in spoken language, the nonverbal aspects convey as much as 85 percent of the message received. The nonverbal components include both nonvocal gestures and such vocal cues as rate, rhythm, pitch, tone, and tempo, as well as the Ums, Hurumphs, Ers, Ahs, and Uh Huhs peppered throughout communication.

HUMAN INFORMATION PROCESSING AND INFERENCE IN DECISION MAKING

Having prepared the ground, we can now dig into a conceptual scheme to analyze the processing of information and identify some of the factors that contribute to distortion. This model builds on the neuroanatomical view of the human brain decoding information or messages that come from the environment, and encoding messages that are sent out to the environment. This model proposes seven stages in the decoding-encoding process. I will briefly identify and discuss each, illustrate its function and relationship to other stages, and suggest ways in which characteristic distortions may develop. Remember that the STM into LTM process means that at least the first four stages will occur—and may even be recycled—before any perception reaches our awareness.

Stage One: Receive

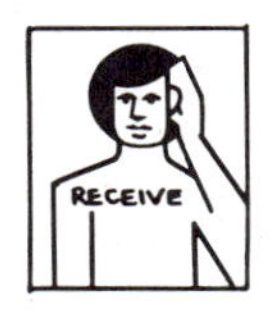

The first stage is the arrival of data through sensory organs and the transmission of that information to the brain. The neuroanatomy and neuropsychology of these processes were discussed briefly above using the visual system as an example. Let us continue with the visual system and reintroduce our patient, whom you are seeing for the first time.

The physical aspects of the setting affect the capacity of the eye to receive data. Dim lighting may obscure certain movements or facial expressions; bright glare may cast shadows. Both result in a distortion of the incoming data. The integrity of the sensory equipment itself can introduce distortion at several levels. Vision declines with age, but near vision particularly becomes impaired after age 40, when presbyopia is marked. Clouding and thickening of the lens decrease one's ability to adapt to changes in brightness or to discriminate in dim light. Impairment in function for physical or neuropathologic reasons anywhere along the visual system pathways from retina to sensory cortex will result in inaccuracies in data transmission.

Stage Two: Infer

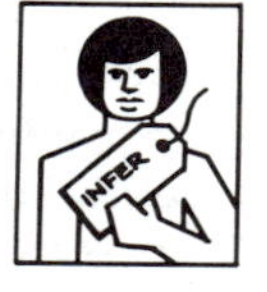

William James noted decades ago that on its own, sensory input represents a ''blooming, buzzing confusion.'' Input must be processed to determine meaning. When the appropriate region of the brain has received the encoded message from the hippocampus, some ''sense'' of it must be made. Input data are compared with stored data via the coding cues mentioned earlier. Information organized into complex patterns and stored in memory is referred to as cognitive maps.

One of the functions of the inference step is to determine which aspects of the input data will be the focus of attention, the ''figure,'' and which shall remain as ''ground.'' The attending behavior and the needs and interests of the receiver will influence this focus and override other factors. For example, the disheveled appearance of the patient and the strong odor that assails your olfaction may cause you to infer that this person is a derelict. The social context or background within which the encounter takes place certainly contributes to the meaning derived. If encountered outside of the treatment context, this same person could more readily be ignored and placed at a greater distance by moving yourself away.

The cognitive map analog of the inference process implies that the brain, like the computer, can be programmed with categories of information. We will look at four categories, or patterns, of cued encoded information: neural structure, individual experience, vicarious experience, and cultural and subgroup experience. Little is known about the breadth of the influence of predispositions on perceiving certain stimuli in particular ways, or even how it works. Neuropsychologists and psycholinguists attribute great potential significance to this concept, however. For example, Noam Chomsky[9] argues that the brain is constructed in such a way that the processing of language corresponds with the brain characteristics of grammar.

When you look at a patient whom you have never met before, and who reminds you of someone with whom you have had prior experience, you are prepared, probably at an unconscious level, to make inferences about the patient's behavior based on your own experience. Because of your ''mind-set," you may misconstrue portions of the incoming data to fit the cognitive map that developed from that earlier experience.

Vicarious experience, as well as direct experience, contributes to the neural activity associated with memory and learning. Therefore, items about which we have heard or read or of which we have seen pictures are also part of the memory bank, with categories and cuing mechanisms of their own. I may never have seen a patient with neurofibromatosis, but having seen films and read newspaper accounts, I would probably recognize the condition should a patient present the clinical signs, as did the Elephant Man.

The process by which each child learns from family and subculture what it means to be a person also supplies innumerable patterns against which to check the meaning of incoming data. Normally, when people unknown to me ask for directions, I feel at ease in responding to their requests for assistance. However, if these persons come from a culture in which strangers stand closer than in mine, they may move to a position within the space that I have learned is reserved for intimate friends. Then I would likely perceive them not as asking directions, but as violating my space or even "personally attacking."

When incoming data are somewhat vague, unclear, or unfamiliar, we frequently overattend to one aspect and correspondingly underattend to other aspects, thereby distorting the input to "fit" the meanings we have stored in memory. Similarly, when the exactly right cognitive map is not stored, we may alter the data to make them fit a map we have and thus be able to attribute meaning to it. In the process, we sometimes import data from a cognitive map and attribute them to the incoming information. As nature abhors a vacuum, so it seems that our psyche fills in empty places with information previously stored so that we may more easily relate to strangers or more comfortably deal with new situations. For these reasons, distortions are common in situations that bring together persons from different cultures or subcultures; the same behavior may mean different things to different persons.

Stage Three: Feel

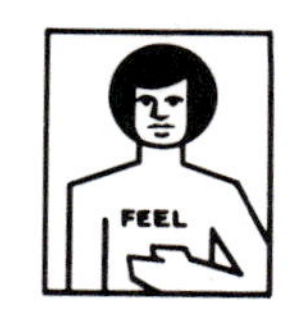

In the third step in this model, feelings are aroused by the meaning inferred. The range of feelings extends from positive through neutral to negative and may vary in strength from extremely strong to very weak. Inferring that a red octagonal sign that is seen while driving is an instruction to stop may produce feelings of annoyance when one is late for a meeting, or rather neutral feelings when that pressure is removed. Since the meaning associated with incoming data was transferred to LTM accompanied by some kind of affect, it seems reasonable to think that the visual image retrieved brings an affect component along with it.

The feelings identified at this stage are of two types: (1) primary or basic affect states, usually labeled with words like pleasure, sorrow, affection, or anger; or (2) somatosensory descriptions such as warm, cold, tense, tight, or loose. These feelings may influence the inference itself at least as much as the action taken in response. Since attention tends to focus more sharply on that aspect of our perception that arouses the strongest feeling, the impact of that feeling is magnified, perhaps affecting the accuracy of our perceptions. For instance, studies have consistently found that high anxiety reduces one's accuracy in perception, while a moderate level of anxiety enhances awareness of relevant information. At times, the feelings associated with aspects of the "ground" may be so strong as to cause a shift in focus to make them the "figure," thus producing a different inference entirely; one more in keeping with the feelings, even though it might interpret less accurately the actual information received.

Stage Four: Feel-about-Feeling

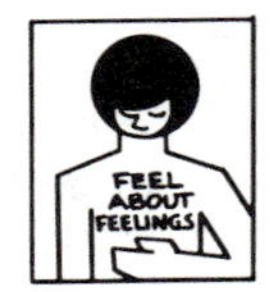

Up to this point, we have followed a piece of information as it was received via the sensory apparatus, matched for meaning with material cataloged and stored in LTM, until it produced an effect in the observer. Now we find the psyche comparing the inference and its associated feeling with the values and self-concept held by the individual. It is as if I ask myself, "How do I feel about myself feeling this way?" Or, in the terms made popular by transactional analysis, "Am I OK or not?" For instance, our patient with disheveled attire and strong body odor may elicit the inference that this person is a vagrant who is unconcerned about being offensive to others. This inference elicits feelings of anger and disgust. However, there is a countervailing strong value for health professionals to provide care irrespective of social class, age, or sex. This value, along with the self-concept that is related to it, collides with the feeling of disgust and causes us to feel badly about feeling disgust toward this patient. The usual resolution under these circumstances is to modify the data behind it—the inference—and, if necessary, to make it fit the value system and self-concept. Festinger[10] has identified and labeled this phenomenon "cognitive dissonance."

Stage Five: Determine

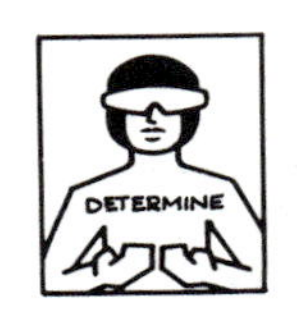

In this stage, one determines what is being perceived and felt, and this determination provides the basis for a response. It is the net result of the preceding stages finally entering awareness. However, even it often proceeds outside of awareness. In fact, the whole process from reception of data to the action or response made to the data may be played out in us without our ever becoming conscious of it. Problems with an interaction are a useful warning signal that distortion may have crept into the process. Acceptance of the conscious or unconscious determination may increase the risk that distortions will go undetected and may quickly lead to increased difficulties.

Stage Six: Decide

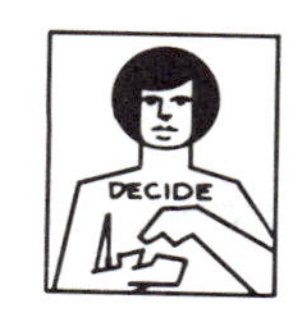

Having made a determination, the next step is to prepare to take action consistent with that determination. The question, whether consciously or unconsciously dealt with, is, "What effect do you want to produce on the other person, or on the environment?" in light of your inference, feelings, and feelings about feelings. If some part of the previous stages is consciously available to you, you have some options. For instance, if you are aware of feeling disgust or feeling not quite OK, you may decide to recheck your internal data to be sure that the determination is accurate, going back to check inference, feelings, and so on. If you see the situation as one in which it is critical for you to be correct in your inference and response, you would want to recheck at this stage. Similarly, if confusing aspects exist in the situation, such as differences in culture or subculture, rechecking is important.

The next order of options deals with responding. The response may be either to go ahead to some form of direct action, or to pause to test the perception with the other person. Careful observation of the patient's nonverbal and verbal behavior in response to your action will provide additional data that will contribute to validating or invalidating the inference you have made. A variety of communication skills can be used to facilitate such collecting of new data.

Stage Seven: Act

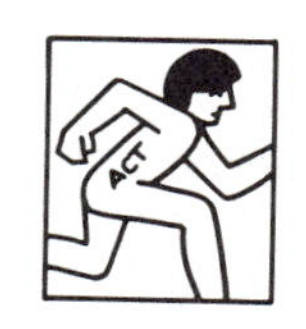

The final action may be automatic and spontaneous if the entire process has been outside of awareness. Whether conscious or not, the action will be strategic, that is, planned to achieve the impact you want it to have. In building a conscious strategy, you may choose to seek more information. Careful interviewing will elicit more data, and the process for you will begin again.

Whatever action you select will conclude the cycle of processing communication for the moment. Any response by the other person, whether verbal or nonverbal, will provide a new message for you to process, moving through the cycle from receiving to inferring, to feeling, to feeling about feeling, to determining, to deciding, to acting, and potentially to beginning yet again. This old rhyme comes to mind:

> A wise old owl sat on an oak,
> The more he saw the less he spoke;
> The less he spoke the more he heard,
> Why aren't we like that wise old bird?
>
> Edward Henry Richards

SUMMARY

A brief discussion of visual reception of data and processing that data through short-term memory and long-term memory provided a background for a developing model of inference, processing, and distorting. The conceptual scheme analyzed data processing within an individual and identified sources of distortion.

This model built on the theory that persons process data, decoding information that comes to them via sensory apparatus and encoding messages they send. Seven stages in this process were identified: (1) receive, (2) infer, (3) feel, (4) feel-about-feeling, (5) determine, (6) decide, and (7) act. Each stage was discussed, the visual system serving as the focal sensory apparatus, with a patient in a treatment setting as illustration. Relationships between and among stages were identified; the manner in which distortions occur and relationships to awareness were also specified.

THE CLINICIAN'S ROLE

> To assail the changes that have unmoored us from the past is futile and in a deep sense, I think it is wicked. We need to recognize the change and learn what resources we have.
>
> Robert Oppenheimer

> Change is inevitable. In a progressive country change is constant.
>
> Benjamin Disraeli

In very real ways, everything around us is changing. When we bring our attention from the world scene and international scope to the immediate present and interpersonal perspective we have only altered the magnitude of the change. In another sense, the world we live in is a different kind of world from that of our parents and grandparents. The prevalence of "newness" in our lives is greater; the changes have brought about alterations in the quality of things we thought we could count on as being stable, or fixed, such as morals, religion, family, and love. In a span of 20 years, the information about our planet has matched and surpassed all the knowledge of the natural world before. How can we hope to keep pace or cope with such monumental shifts in our data base? Or perhaps, more realistically, how can we pace ourselves to cope with the impact that this information explosion has in terms of human behavior—in terms of our practice as physical therapists?

Recognizing what we do in our practice, physical therapists deserve to be called change agents. Of course, all individuals are agents of change. Insofar as we have interaction with another human being, change is taking place, no matter how small the scale. The issue is not whether change happens, but whether it happens to us or happens spontaneously or happens because of our planning. Although all our lives are touched by change, my purpose here is to focus on the ways in which you as a physical therapist and health professional are an agent of change. I will try to suggest some observations that can help you to be a more effective change agent. However, I will need some special cooperation from you. I want you to experiment with adopting a "state of not knowing."

Although you are each an expert in your professional practice in providing care to patients, I'm sure you would agree that there is much about patient behavior, about human behavior, about which you know very little. We often find ourselves in a situation in which a question is put to us with the implicit expectation that we have the answer—that we *should* have the answer. Temporarily, try to accept a state of "not knowing." It is really OK not to have the answers to everything.

Indeed, you can use "not knowing" positively. Open your eyes to see more, tune your ears to hear more, and become more aware of the sensations on your body as well as those within it.

This sensory preparation of yourself is essential to a "state of not knowing" and to observing behavior well. It is a common tendency to move quickly from observing behavior to finding a rationale, or a "why;" but if we forestall "finding an answer," we may learn more. We may find that the observed behavior has a sequence, a cause-effect relationship with some other behavior that consistently leads to similar results or has a specific impact on another person or on the individual. In these ways, our openness discloses much richer data than our ready answers would have permitted. "Your ability to perceive is something that is learned and you can learn to do it better."[11]

STRATEGIES OF CHANGE

The literature on change is both old and young, both deep and broad, depending on the discipline through which you approach it. Psychology, sociology, and the applied fields of management and personnel relations will provide you with different perspectives. We can extract a set of four fundamental principles, or stages, that appear in each approach. I label them as identifying the need for change, establishing goals for change, selecting and using the means to bring about change, and evaluating the results of the change (Fig. 5-1). You may already have noted their similarity to the classic medical sequence of diagnosis, prescription, treatment, and evaluation. Let us use them to look at a treatment case and thus better understand how the physical therapist can function as a change agent. First, we must have a *need for change.*

> Maria T., a 55-year-old woman of Italian nationality, weight 190 pounds, height 5 feet 2 inches, has polyneuritis. She is married, has six children, all living, and resides in South Philadelphia. She has been transferred from acute care to rehabilitation for physical therapy.
>
> Evaluation findings identify generalized weakness, with all muscle grades in poor to trace range. She understands and speaks English but is fluent only in Italian. Some members of her family visit every day, usually bringing one or more home-cooked foods to her "because she looks too thin."

This brief amount of information includes several different problems (Fig. 5-2). Taken in order: (1) She is 40 to 60 pounds overweight. (2) She has serious neuromuscular problems that lead to severe disability. (3) She has a

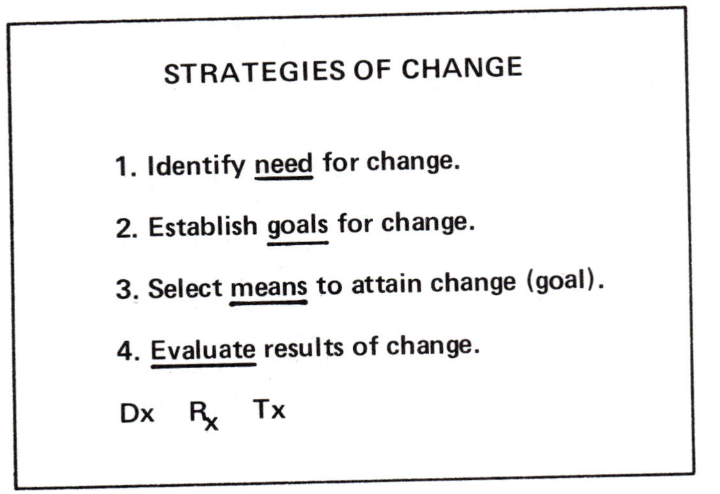

FIGURE 5-1. The four fundamental strategies of change.

mild to moderate problem in verbal communication with English-speaking patients and staff. (4) She has a solicitous and attentive family who are concerned that she is losing weight and are anxious to help her in any way they can. Each of these problems sounds very much like a diagnostic entity that we might identify in a problem-oriented medical record. Each can be restated in terms of a need for change. The first problem is easy to "translate." "She is 40 to 60 pounds overweight" becomes (1) "She needs to lose approximately 40 pounds." In none of the other three problems is establishing the need statement so simple, and accomplishing the goal may be exceedingly difficult. The respective need-for-change statements might be: (2) "She needs to be able to achieve functional levels in all aspects of activities of daily living." (3) "She needs to converse easily in Italian as well as English with selected patients and staff." (4) "She needs to understand and accept her diet and exercise program and her increasing independence and have family support and cooperation in this program." Having identified the needs, then priorities can be set. There is no guarantee that identifying a need and bringing it to awareness will lead automatically to a desire to make that change on the part of the patient.

The second stage in the change process is to *establish a relationship* between the patient and therapist to work toward some of the change goals *that they both share.* This process is similar to the chemist putting the right elements together to arrive at a stable compound or prescription. The patient may have learned to agree with the authority figures in hospital settings, but may not really agree at all that she needs to lose weight. Her husband's status and her role in the family are entirely consistent with her well-rounded figure. Putting Maria on a special diet is an appropriate course to take. Keeping her on it is another matter, especially when the family value system is different from that of the health professionals. It is doubtful that both therapist and patient share this goal.

Recovery from polyneuritis is a slow, tedious process involving a lot of hard work and perseverance. Maria and her family certainly want her to be

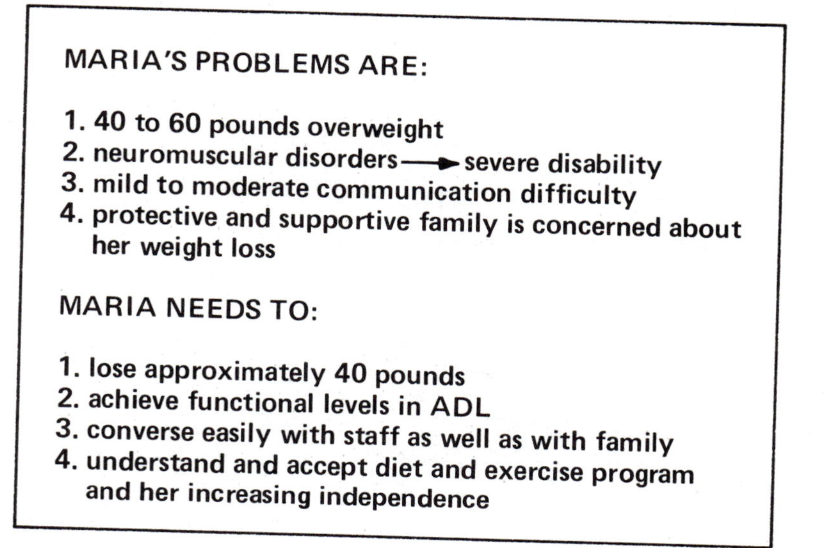

FIGURE 5-2. List of Maria's problems and needs.

able to move about her home independently. They would probably agree that some amount of hard work is necessary on Maria's part to achieve that end. But here again the value system of the family may conflict with the therapist's, since it holds that the grandparents are to be cared for, even catered to—it is their right! "And so much hard work isn't good for Mama." Perhaps the priority issue is now apparent. How *do* we get the family involved in the treatment program to the degree necessary to challenge their value system and even to change certain parts of it? We will come back to this question.

The third stage is the process of *selecting the appropriate course* and working toward the desired change or goal. An analog is the development of a tailor-made treatment program. There are more ways than one to achieve a specific goal, but which is the best? What are the pros and cons of each, and what is the best way to introduce physical therapy activity for this patient? We can agree that patient and therapist work together to achieve treatment goals. This relationship must be able to support negotiation if two people are to work together toward commonly held goals. Maria is going through a period of uncertainty, anxiety, and stress, experiencing constantly changing circumstances and new demands by new people. As information is collected and analyzed, the problem becomes more complex, not less. Vested interests begin to emerge from within the patient-family system as well as from the treatment system. For example, within the patient-family system we might find: (1) rivalry between two adult siblings for decision-making authority related to Maria's care; (2) her husband striving to have control but encountering resistance from the oldest daughter; and (3) Maria clearly relying on her family to make decisions she now cannot make. The treatment system brings its own concerns: (1) the number of staff and the treatment time available limit contact time to 30 minutes twice a day, but because of her size and emotional lability, little can be accomplished in this time frame; (2) no one on

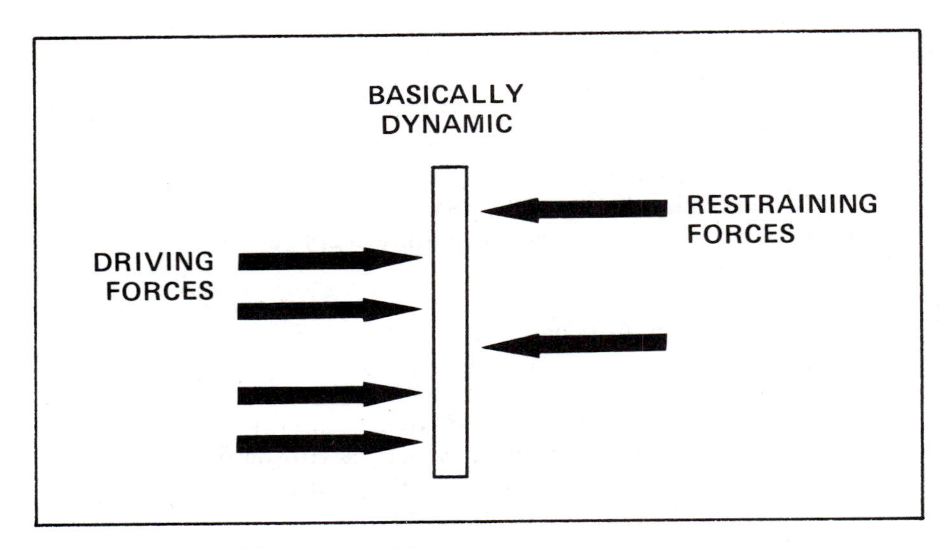

FIGURE 5-3. Force field analysis model.

the staff speaks Italian, so the time required for instruction in activities is doubled; (3) therapists, perceiving the patient to have a low level of motivation, prefer to redirect their energies toward other patients.

Given such an impasse, the patient may well begin to think that her problems are too great to solve, and she then may decide to give up. The resulting increased dependence and passivity would further reinforce the health professional's perception of poor motivation. A different patient might instead become hostile and resist the staff's efforts to develop treatment. Here is a case where treatment is going sour, but there is nothing wrong with the physical treatment. It is the interaction dynamics that are critical here.

If this patient is to show progress, the therapist must work for resolution of the interpersonal situation. Achieving resolution depends on some creativity and experimentation by the therapist, who might find help by working out a force field analysis (Fig. 5-3). Developed originally by Kurt Lewin,[12] this model suggests that all situations are basically dynamic, not static. Any condition is the present balance of the various forces acting on it. Using the model to plan change involves identifying two sets of forces. One set, "the driving forces," consists of those forces that push toward one's goal. The other set, "restraining forces," consists of those forces that push away from the goal. To create an imbalance, we can alter magnitude, change direction, or add a new force.

In Figure 5-4, the four driving forces on the left are balanced by the four restraining forces on the right. More factors could be added to this scheme; but these already show that to bring about a lasting change in Maria's condition, the therapist must find a way to intervene in the system and create an imbalance between the restraining and driving forces. This imbalance may occur by altering the magnitude of any single force, through a change in the direction of one of the forces, or by adding a new force. The trick is to pick one or two that you can influence and that will make a positive difference.

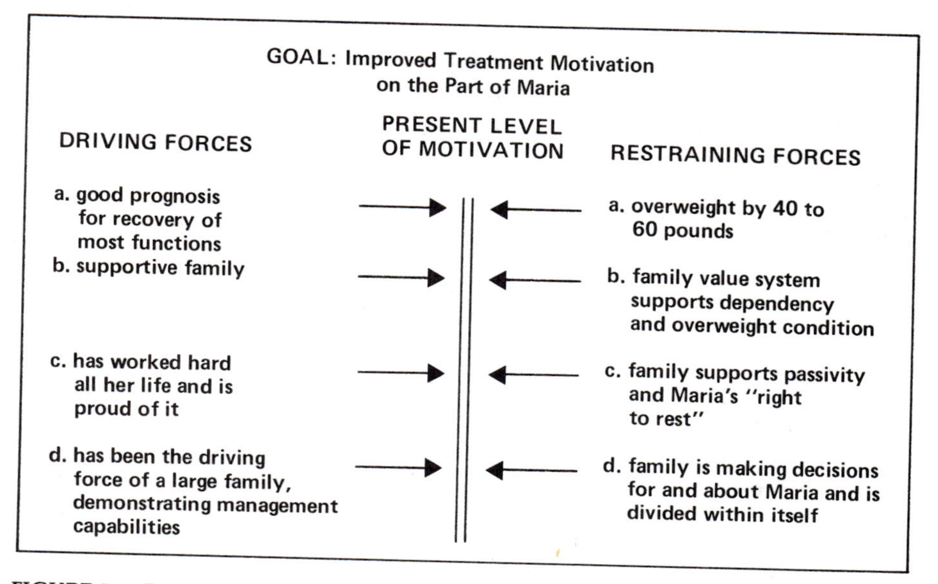

FIGURE 5-4. Force field analysis for Maria.

Innovation opportunities are usually numerous and provide openings for creative experimentation. If such chances are seized, the results will be exciting. For instance, in the case of Maria, the therapist adopted the overt behavior style of an Italian relative. This included fast-talking, emotion-laden speech, scolding, and excitability. The patient was more responsive to this style than to the earlier traditional professional one and even began to consider the therapist as an ally. I think the effective dynamic was that the patient gained the additional personal strength she needed to begin making her own decisions, invest more energy in her exercise program, stay on her diet, and tell her family how to behave. She walked out with a quad cane on discharge, which far exceeded the expectations of everyone in the department.

Unfortunately, the story does not end there, and the sequel drives home the point I want to make here. The therapist's intervention achieved change without dealing constructively with Maria's family. Consequently, when Maria went home, her family literally "loved her to death." The belief system that strongly valued Maria's "right to rest" after so many years of hard work soon resulted in decreased function, confinement to a chair, and then to bed. Maria died from too much care.

The final stage in any model of planned change has to include some form of *feedback, evaluation,* and *planning* for the next time. The primary test of the therapist's intervention is the stability and lasting effects of the patient's behavior when the therapist is no longer actively working with the patient. It was this point that showed the error of the strategy the therapist used in working with Maria. Tests that anticipate the postdischarge outcome can be built into the treatment program itself. Such feedback and evaluation prior to termination will show possible shortcomings in time to allow development of a new planning strategy that can have initial implementation before discharge. All too often, we lose track of patients following discharge.

For instance, in the case of Maria, several strategies could have been followed that might have revealed the family's "counterproductive" and "dangerous" demonstrations of love. A weekend visit home by the patient prior to discharge might have brought the issues into better focus. A home visit by the therapist, social worker, or visiting nurse similarly might have identified potential problems. Follow-up outpatient visits at 2 weeks, 1 month, and 2 months would surely have shown decreasing functional capacity, making further investigation imperative.

Compare Maria with patients with whom you have worked. I am sure you will come to the same therapeutic imperative: we *must* identify and manage information resources at every step in the process. At the first stage of *need for change,* the therapist chose the obvious physical needs of the patient while ignoring what was known about the family system. Consultation with the family, the social worker, or the parish priest might have highlighted the need to attend carefully to the family system. The results in this case clearly indicate an inadequate diagnostic process. At the second stage of *establishing a relationship of collaboration,* the therapist might have included key members of the family in that collaboration. They could have served as resources rather than adversaries in subsequent treatment. At the third stage of *selecting an appropriate course,* the therapist should have included some members of the family along with Maria. The resource management needed here is really people management. As the therapist works with these family members in treatment sessions with Maria or in consultations afterward, the key to the message is inclusion of family in the process. It then becomes the "trained" family members' responsibility to teach, indoctrinate, or win over in any way possible the rest of the family. Finally, at the *evaluation* stage, we must recognize that Maria might have lived. The analysis of more complete data would have yielded different results. Resources at this stage might include a range of hospital personnel: records administrator, quality assurance officer, social worker, physician, nurse, and others. Many can contribute to the design of a method to analyze the outcome of physical therapy intervention in patient and patient-family systems. We want to know if what we do makes a difference in the long run, as well as on a short-term basis. The five steps in the problem-solving process are shown in Figure 5-5.

I hope this discussion makes the point of treatment clear. I am sure you can see how it applies with equal force to working in a department, to relating to the wide range of health professionals and support personnel who work with you, to securing cooperation in your institution, and even to improving your "marketing."

SUMMARY

The physical therapist as an agent of planned change was discussed within the framework of clinical practice. Strategies for change included four steps: identify need, establish goals, select means, and evaluate results. Application to a patient situation was provided. In this instance, inadequate interpersonal dynamics posed a threat to success. Kurt Lewin's force field analysis was described as a useful tool in analyzing the forces in the interpersonal system and the potential direction of change for resolution. Finally, the

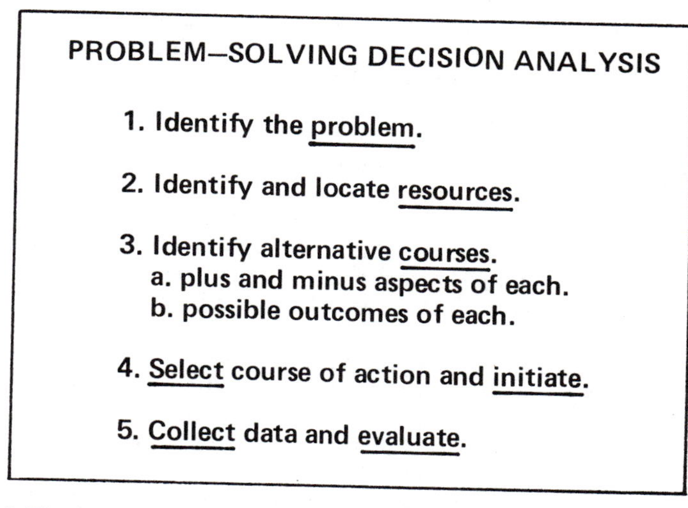

FIGURE 5-5. The five steps in the problem-solving process.

change process was placed within a problem-solving context of five steps. Emphasis was placed upon selecting the key problem to work with and identifying and managing resources. Application to the clinical case was made.

RESPONSIBILITY

As we draw to a close our discussion of clinical decision making, it is quite apparent that our task is well along in many ways and just begun in other respects.

> "Christopher Christopher, *where* are you going, . . ."
> "Just up to the top of the hill,
> Upping and upping until
> I am right on top of the hill."
> "Christopher, Christopher, *why* are you going . . .
> There's nothing to see, so when
> You've got to the top, what then?"
> "Just down to the bottom again."
> Said Christopher Robin.
>
> A.A. Milne

I think I can best help you face both ups and downs by focusing on the inevitable concomitant of decision making: *responsibility.* The implications of that reality are profound for the patient, the therapist, and the profession. Therefore, let us look at all three as interacting components of a larger system. Systems models have provided freedom and breadth of understanding for physical and biological scientists as well as social scientists. They have been used for relationships in small or large configurations. A systems approach assumes interrelationships among parts, organization, interdependency, and a structure and stability at a given period in time. It may be helpful to envision a circle within which are the patient, the therapist, and the profession. On the outside is the environment, with all it brings to bear on our system. We will look at the patient and therapist first, and then examine the impact of this combination upon the profession.

The patient provides the therapist with data in the form of body movement, in part or as a whole. From this, the observer formulates an impression. All behavior is communication in that it stimulates a meaning. That meaning is assigned through *inference,* as was discussed earlier in this chapter. In addition, all behavior has a reason, is purposeful or directed toward some goal, but is not necessarily conscious. In other words, there is a *why* for which we may search. For example, when we observe an ambulating individual who on weight bearing has marked adduction of the weight-bearing limb, we would ask why and might suspect gluteus medius weakness as one possibility. The same process pertains to analysis of interpersonal communication. As we gather more data, the internal formulations alter to accommodate the newer information. Of course, the same process is occurring for the patient with regard to the therapist.

A model we may use to show the interplay of communication and relationship is the Johari window, named after its developers, Joe Ingrim and Harry Luft.[13] As shown in Figure 5-6, the "window" is a grid comparing two sets of information—information known to the person and information known to others—which constitute the two axes. The *arena* is the place of public interaction. The patient's self-knowledge is available to the therapist. The *blind spot* is an aspect of the patient of which the therapist has some awareness, but the patient does not. As feedback is provided to the patient, the potential exists for personal growth, for the patient to learn more about self. The therapist may also learn as refinements are made in the manner of giving feedback in increasingly acceptable forms. The *facade* constitutes an aspect of the patient about which the patient knows but the observer does not. This facade decreases as interpersonal interaction permits the patient to disclose more and more. Finally, the *unknown* is that part of the individual that is not known by either the patient or the therapist. Even this part can shrink as positive relationships permit interaction of feedback and disclosure to bring new insights.

Our understanding of personal growth is enriched by understanding the epigenetic principle derived from the growth of an organism in utero. In general terms, this principle states that organisms grow according to a plan that guides the development of parts, time of appearance, and function, until the organism is whole, as can be clearly seen in the development of the human fetus. When an infant exchanges the biochemical world of the uterus for the social system of the culture, we can observe that the organism we see will follow several predetermined plans throughout the life span: neuromuscular, biochemical, psychosocial, and so forth. Erikson[14] suggests that the healthy individual who is provided with a reasonable amount of guidance from family and cultural group will follow the "inner laws of development" that result in a series of new potential growth areas, both motor and social.

Erikson's grid is well known for its representation of the human life cycle. Imagine a grid eight squares high by eight squares across. On the left, from bottom to top are arranged an elaboration of Freud's five "sexual"

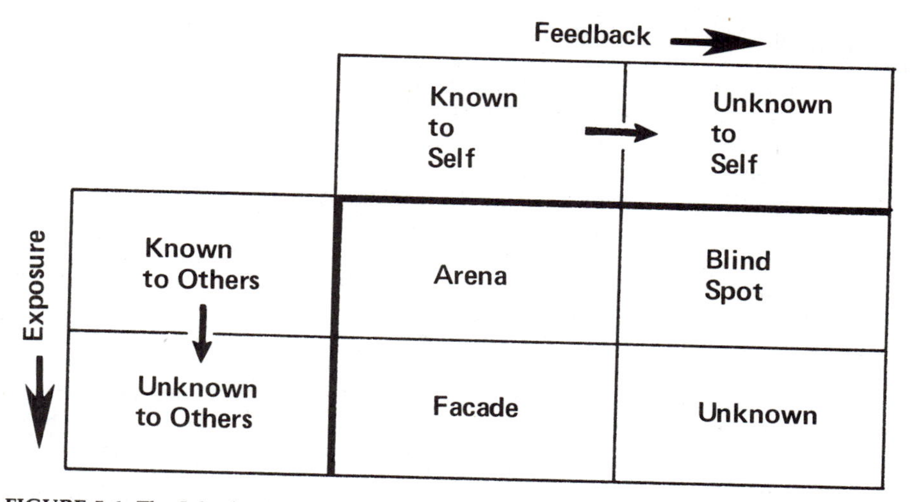

FIGURE 5-6. The Johari window.

stages plus three more. These are, in ascending order, sensory-anal, muscular-anal, locomotive-genital, latency, puberty and adolescence, young adulthood, adulthood, maturity. The squares organized from bottom left diagonally up to top right present the challenges for each stage. These are trust versus mistrust, autonomy versus shame and doubt, initiative versus guilt, industry versus inferiority, identity versus identity confusion, intimacy versus isolation, generativity versus stagnation, and integrity versus despair. Achievements made through the successful interaction of stage phenomena and challenges are presented in ascending order on the right side of the grid. Each new stage builds on the growth achieved in earlier stages. Erikson suggests that the diagonal arrangement of challenges intends conceptually both sequence and variation in tempo and intensity.

Erikson represents the first state as *sensory-anal* and the challenge as basic *trust versus mistrust.* The achievement he postulates as *hope.* The second stage is *muscular-anal;* the challenge is *autonomy versus shame and doubt;* the achievement is *will.* The third stage is *locomotive-genital;* the challenge is *initiative versus guilt;* the achievement is *purpose.* And so we can proceed through the life cycle of eight stages, challenges in psychosocial development, and achievements or outcomes derived from successful growth and development. We can use this model in understanding patient behavior and planning treatment.

A patient who is really dependent, as Maria T. was initially, demonstrates marked social regression as well as physical dependence. Such a patient relies upon the environment for physical and social support for survival. The severely disabled individual *must* trust that basic needs will be provided. In Maria's circumstances, a mild language problem added to the magnitude of trust necessary on her part. We need to help a patient who is functioning at the *basic trust* level to achieve the *hope* necessary to proceed on through the *autonomy* and *initiative* stages in order to achieve success in rehabilitation. Treatment plans must work with the patient where the patient is, not where the therapist thinks the patient ought to be.

In the patient's weakness there is power. The weakness and dependence occur in an environment in which people are highly sensitized to the needs of patients and responsive to them. As staff members orient themselves to accommodate the patient's needs, they grow as individuals and as a group. Just as a family can bring up a baby only as the baby brings up its family, so too the health care staff can "bring up" its patient only as the patient controls and brings up the staff. Clearly, some patients are much better skilled than others at this basic level.

By observing patient behavior, a therapist can identify which of Erikson's stages best characterizes the interaction. The therapist can then infer additional information about the patient's social development, independence, and needs at this time. Treatment program and setting can be structured more specifically for the individual when the therapist understands the stage that is dominantly active and those that may succeed it. Adult patients may travel very swiftly from a regressed status through several of the stages if their physical conditions improve quickly. Just as a child becomes frustrated, then angry, when growth spurts seem thwarted by vigilant and protective parents, so too the adult patient becomes frustrated and angry when individuals or "the system" seems to impede progress or interfere with goal attainment.

The model of stages can also be used in observing therapist behavior, one's own, or that of others; for example, a therapist with three years of experience who is functioning competently may try to initiate new programs or request more responsibility in one form or another. This therapist is probably displaying the dynamics of evolving leadership and authority characteristic of Erikson's stage of generativity versus stagnation. These initiatives should be nurtured and supported with reasonable structure and guidance. If the therapist encounters resistance or rejection, we would expect this to result in frustration and anger. If so, the pressure of these developmental tasks may redirect energy into less constructive activities or lead to a search for another position elsewhere that provides the growth opportunities.

The word "needs" has been used several times in this discussion, and it bears elaboration before we go further. Various psychologists have discussed *needs* in numerous creative ways, identifying a few or close to a hundred different needs. But Abraham Maslow[15] has discussed how needs lead to motivation. Figure 5-7 provides a handy visual tool to help us anchor it in memory. The underlying premise in his theory is that the individual will have accomplished satisfactorily the major portion of one level of needs before advancing to tackle the tasks at the next level up. In other words, essential needs must be met and satisfied at one level before the individual is able to direct energies toward the needs and consequent tasks at the next level. I have left the top of the triangle unfinished to reflect Maslow's eventual conclusion that this last level never can be fully satisfied, but always operates to generate further motivation.

We can see how this model of behavior can be applied to the patient-therapist system in the case of a patient named Ann H. At first meeting, the dire nature of her circumstances is striking.

Ann H. is 34 years old, married, and has one son, age 6. Two years ago, she had a modified mastectomy on the left side without follow-up chemotherapy or radiation. She had no limitations in function and re-

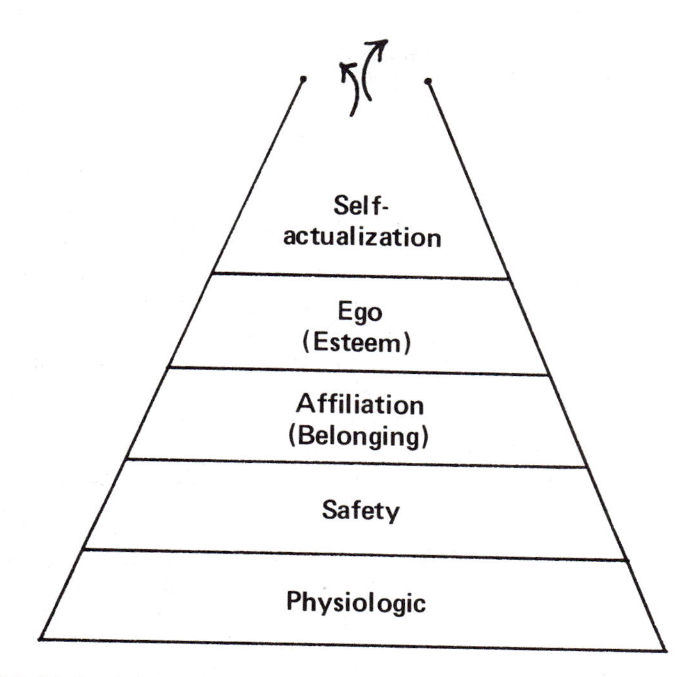

FIGURE 5-7. Maslow's hierarchy of needs.

turned to her position as supervisor of teachers for persons with learning disabilities. Recent hospitalization was for surgery, radiation, and chemotherapy for control of multiple metastases to the brain and subarachnoid space throughout the length of the spinal canal.

Referral for physical therapy home care services identified the treatment goal as maintaining level of function and increasing strength. Initial assessment identified the patient as generally very weak, with pronounced weakness on the left with poor to trace grades. She was alert and intelligent, with no apparent impairment in speech or thought processes. She was totally dependent upon others for her care at the time *(physiologic needs)*. However, she expressed expectations of returning to work in 3 months. Beyond everyone's expectations, Ann achieved the strength she needed to ambulate with a quad cane with moderate assistance and to rise from a chair. Her strong family support system provided the necessary struts to ensure physical safety *(safety needs)* and satisfied her need to be a part of the family *(belonging needs)*. She valued the time she had with her son, engaging in a variety of activities that they could accomplish together while seated. His many hugs each day rewarded her efforts to be with him and satisfied her need to be a part of his life *(ego or esteem needs)*.

With continued but slow improvement, Ann began to reassess her goal of returning to work as the beginning of the school year confronted her. Facing the facts produced depression, but this patient still *needed* to deal with the circumstances constructively. She had the internal personal strength to face the realities, evaluate the data available from the physical therapist, make the needed decisions, and take the required actions *(self-actualization).* The therapist had a dual function: (1) to support the support system the family provided, and (2) to guide the patient safely from one activity to the next within the range of accomplishment. Ann must surely have been a self-actualizing person prior to her illness. The physical limitations imposed by her serious illness took her back through the levels of *need* to physiologic. Her treatment and psychic strength took her back up to self-actualizing again. The success with which she accomplished this was in part due to her family support system, in part due to a therapist who could meet the patient on the ground the patient presented, and in part due to the high level of internal motivation of the patient herself.

Not all patients have the personal maturity, "integrity" in Erikson's scheme, to handle problems in this manner. Physical therapists often find it necessary to stimulate a patient to participate in treatment through the strong bonds of their relationship when the patient lacks the internal motivation necessary to initiate effort. This method can succeed for a time, but it cannot have a lasting effect when the therapist is not there to provide the stimulus. The patient will return to hospital room or home and "forget" to do the follow-up activities as instructed—unless, somehow, the relationship and its motivation have been internalized. One critical clinical responsibility is deciding when to discontinue treatment for a patient who may have good potential but lacks the internal motivation to invest the effort.

The therapist can observe the behavior of self and other staff to identify the motivating forces that provide energy for activities in a manner similar to the observation of Ann H. For example, when *ego* needs are not met, a therapist might behave in a manner to draw attention to self or be unable to take responsibilities seriously or be unwilling to be the naturally appropriate authority or leader. These tools may be useful for you in *planning* your behavior and structuring treatment settings to meet the physical *and* social maturation needs of your patient.

Let us turn now to the interaction of the therapist with the profession, where the same principle applies but the situation is less clear. All realize the significant contribution patient-therapist interactions have made in the maturation of therapists into more mature professionals, but obviously they do not operate alone. The academic setting begins the process and carries it along a bit. We turn now to examine some of the other factors.

The full-time responsibility of professional practice usually includes (1) identification with a peer group. Its explicit and implicit norms for behavior help to (2) clarify the role of the professional. Ongoing patient contact gives constant rehearsal in the role.[16-18] Physical therapists (3) take responsibility for patient care. One result of this role-training is clear. What is not so clear is whether they learn to *take* responsibility *for* the profession.

Follow along with me as we "shadow" a new graduate and try to determine the critical steps on the route to taking responsibility for the profession. When Ellen R. graduated with a bachelor of science degree in physical therapy, her first job was in a midsized urban hospital near the university that she had attended. The patient population was not her first preference, but the supervisor seemed to be effective, and she could easily reach a larger city where "everything was happening." The supervisor encouraged Ellen to make contact with floor personnel and head nurses to discuss treatment goals for patients, plan in-service programs, and develop new treatment techniques. The supervisor also invited Ellen to join her at the APTA district meetings and urged participation in committee activities, and Ellen followed her advice. When Ellen moved to a distant city three years later, the supervisor supplied her with several names of therapists to contact regarding Association activities and employment information. Ellen subsequently renewed her active involvement at the district level, and later at the state level.

Note the thread that runs through Ellen's story. *Enabling* her professional socialization was a task and goal her supervisor took seriously and worked on actively. This process of individuals gathering together in a group has three stages: inclusion, individualization, and responsibility taking, each of which will be discussed briefly in terms of impetuses, anxieties, and consequences.[19]

Stage One: Inclusion. The initiative must come from the peer group, in this case the professional representing the group, to try to include the new person. Then the person must respond positively within a reasonable period of time, become part of the group, and ultimately feel accepted. Characteristic anxieties among group members include concern about the impact the new person will have on the group and on themselves personally. The new person may question whether or not he or she is really wanted or wants to be part of this group at all. Too much effort on the part of group members can lead to smothering, which the new person may reject. If he or she stays, the new person may be hampered in development. Too little inclusion effort by the group may lead to feelings of exclusion for the new person.

Stage Two: Individualization. The impetus required here is a group climate that encourages persons to *risk new behaviors,* which leads to developing individuality. As the new person, along with others, tries various expressions of personhood, the group must affirm the individual, the efforts made, and perhaps even the activity. For the group, characteristic anxieties focus on how much disagreement the group can handle. For the individual, the focus is, "Can I be myself and still belong?" The consequences fall in two directions. Too much individualization can lead to rebellion, domination, and destruction of meaningful group life. Too little effort invested in individualization leads to conformity and unthinking followership.

Stage Three: Responsibility Taking. The impetus at this level is encouragement from the group members to offer leadership in various ways. When the individual responds, offering a form of leadership appropriate to the needs of the group, the group then must be supportive. Characteristic anxieties for group members focus on whether this is the right person to do the job that needs to be done. For the individual, the focus of anxiety is whether the leadership offered will be accepted. The consequence of pushing leadership beyond the group's felt needs is irresponsible behavior, which leads to alienation. Holding back personal resources to avoid rejection leads to inappropriate dependence and loss to the group of important resources.

Each of us can help our colleagues to grow into responsible professionals, helping them to experience a deeper inclusion that enables them to grow in their selfhood and in professional practice so that they can invest that growth in responsibility for our profession. The role models of academia and clinic are very important in the formative years of academic preparation that lead to entry into the profession. The "rites of passage" are memorable to us all. The patients contribute in significant ways to the maturation process of the new therapist. The potential for an amputated process at this point is very high. Consider for a moment the personal growth agenda of the average physical therapist graduate, aged 21 or 22 years. He or she has only recently emerged from late adolescence into young adulthood, with a relatively settled body image, a self-concept with unanswered questions, and sexuality issues not all under control. To this we add a generous dose of professional ethics, jargon, techniques and emerging skills, and expectations for adult behavior. The amazing thing to me is how well these young people manage to accept responsibility and how well we older ones did in our youth. It takes personal strength and social maturity to enter a group of strangers and attempt to become a participating member of the group. It would seem that we are not asking too much of them. Perhaps we need only ask more of ourselves in facilitating the process.

We have come a long way, and we have further to go. How responsible are you *for* the growth of your new colleagues and your profession?

SUMMARY

Decision making and responsibility were examined through a discussion of interactions among patient, therapist, and profession in a systems approach. Two additional conceptual tools from behavioral science were described and applied to the clinical practice of physical therapists.

The role-identification process for the physical therapist was briefly outlined to initiate a discussion of taking responsibility for the profession. Professional socialization was examined within a group process framework of three stages: inclusion, individualization, and responsibility taking. This section concluded with an implicit mandate for all of us to take responsibility for the growth of the profession and to contribute to the growth of our colleagues.

REFERENCES

1. MILLER, GA: *The magical number seven, plus or minus two: Some limits on our capacity for processing information.* Psychol Rev 63:81–97, 1956.
2. BROADBENT, DE: *Perception and Communication.* Pergamon Press, London, 1958.
3. KESNER, R: *A neural system analysis of memory storage and retrieval.* Psychol Bull 80:177–203, 1973.
4. CRAIK, F: *Human memory.* Annu Rev Psychol 30:63–102, 1979.
5. ATKINSON, RC AND SHIFFRIN, RM: *The control of short term memory.* Sci Am 225(2):82–89, 1971.
6. SHIFFRIN, RM AND SCHNEIDER, W: *Controlled and automatic human information processing. II. Perceptual learning, automatic attending, and a general theory.* Psychol Rev 84:127–190, 1977.
7. NORMAN, DA: *What have the animal experiments taught us about human memory?* In DEUTSCH, JA (ED): *The Physiological Basis of Memory.* Academic Press, New York, 1973.
8. SCOVILLE, WB AND MILNER, B: *Loss of recent memory after bilateral hippocampal lesions.* J Neurol Neurosurg Psychiatry 20:11–21, 1957.
9. CHOMSKY, N: *Aspects of the Theory of Syntax.* MIT Press, Cambridge, 1965.
10. FESTINGER, L: *Cognitive dissonance.* Sci Am 207(4):93–102, 1962.
11. BANDLER, R AND GRINDER, J: *Frogs into Princes: Neurolinguistic Programming.* Real People Press, Utah, 1979.
12. LEWIN, K: *Field Theory in Social Science.* Harper & Row, New York, 1951.
13. LUFT, J: *Of Human Interaction.* National Press Books, Palo Alto, 1961.
14. ERIKSON, EH: *Identity: Youth and Crisis.* WW Norton, New York, 1968.

15. Maslow, AH: *Motivation and Personality.* Harper & Brothers, New York, 1954.
16. Rosow, I: *Forms and functions of adult socialization.* Social Forces 44:35–45, 1965.
17. Cottrell, L: *Adjustment of the individual to his age and sex roles.* Am Sociol Rev 7:617–620, 1942.
18. Goode, W: *Norm commitment and conformity to role status obligations.* Am J Sociol 66:246–258, 1960.
19. Ramsden, W: *Basic dynamics of interpersonal relations.* In McNell, B, Ramsden, W, and Waynick, L: *Understanding and Improving Your Human Interaction.* US Army Chaplin Board, Fort Monmouth, NJ, 1982.

Chapter 6

CLINICAL DECISION MAKING: ASSESSMENT AND PLANNING FOR TREATMENT OF PATIENTS WITH PRIMARY CARDIOPULMONARY PATHOLOGY

RAYMOND L. BLESSEY, M.A., P.T.

A major purpose of this chapter is to provide an overview of the background information needed to formulate an effective and appropriate plan for the evaluation and treatment of patients with cardiopulmonary pathology. Thus, the chapter includes a brief review of the etiology of coronary artery disease, coronary anatomy and pathophysiology, the natural history of coronary disease, basic principles of exercise physiology, and the pathophysiology of congestive heart failure.

The chapter is also intended to stimulate considerable thought on assessment-based patient treatment. Therefore, the chapter includes some discussion on the various philosophies currently utilized in treating the patient with cardiopulmonary impairment, and it provides the reader with several specific suggestions for the components of, and sequence for, patient evaluation.

Finally, the two case studies appearing in this chapter are designed to illustrate:

1. the clinical relevance of the previously listed areas of background knowledge
2. the major clinical concerns that should help the clinician formulate a specific evaluation plan
3. the type of data base needed for clinical decision making
4. the development of an assessment-based treatment plan
5. the need for a health care team in the treatment of patients with cardiopulmonary disease.

ETIOLOGY OF CORONARY ARTERY DISEASE

The exact etiology of coronary artery disease remains somewhat of a mystery to scientists. Yet, the results of the prospective epidemiologic studies that were started in 1949 in Framingham, Massachusetts, and have continued to this date have allowed clinicians to identify individuals who are at an increased risk of developing coronary atherosclerosis.[1-3] The Framingham statistics indicate that hypertension, cigarette smoking, elevated serum cholesterol or triglycerides, diabetes, sedentary lifestyle, family history of coronary disease, age, and male sex are all factors that, singly or in combination, increase the likelihood of developing coronary atherosclerosis, and are, therefore, referred to as risk factors. In reviewing this list of risk factors, it becomes obvious that most are factors that relate to lifestyle and are, therefore, potentially modifiable. Studies by Rosenman[4] and Jenkins[5] suggest that what they have identified as the Type A personality is also associated with an increased likelihood of developing coronary disease. Type A persons are those who are excessively time-oriented, impatient, rigid, and set unrealistic goals for themselves.

Recent studies, primarily involving the Framingham population, have indicated that the mechanisms of cholesterol transport in the serum are more predictive of coronary disease than the total serum cholesterol by itself.[6-9] Cholesterol binds primarily with two major classes of plasma proteins to form either low-density lipoprotein (LDL) or high-density lipoprotein (HDL). The risk of developing coronary disease increases significantly with either elevated serum levels of LDL or abnormally low serum levels of HDL.

Based on the findings cited above, coronary disease is a multifactorial illness. Each additional risk factor exponentially increases an individual's likelihood of developing the disease. In addition, there is evidence that the persistence of the major risk factors such as hypertension, cigarette smoking, and abnormal lipoprotein levels in individuals with known coronary disease is associated with an increased likelihood of both progression of the disease and development of a second coronary event.[10-13] Finally, hyperlipidemia and hypertension have been associated with the development of vein graft atherosclerosis.[14,15]

How do these risk factors actually relate to the specific mechanisms of atherogenesis? There are researchers all over the world attempting to explain the relationship between the risk factors and the underlying mechanisms of atherosclerosis. What is known as a result of both human and animal studies is that the process of atherosclerosis begins when the inner lining of the artery, the intima, is injured sufficiently to alter the permeability to certain plasma proteins. Factors such as cigarette smoking and hypertension have been shown to result in intimal injury, which then allows LDL cholesterol, the major component of the atherosclerotic plaque, to enter the media and interact with a number of substances. Research also indicates that another basic mechanism of atherogenesis is the proliferation of arterial smooth muscle cells, which appears to be stimulated by certain peptides released by platelets agglutinated to the intimal surface. Many of the major risk factors have been shown to increase the tendency for platelets to agglutinate.[16-19] There is, therefore, mounting evidence relating most of the risk factors to the basic mechanisms of atherogenesis.

CORONARY ANATOMY AND PATHOPHYSIOLOGY

The exact distribution and areas of perfusion of the coronary arteries vary with each individual. However, autopsy studies have demonstrated certain patterns of coronary perfusion that predominate. The left coronary system consists of the left main artery, which bifurcates to form the left anterior descending artery and the circumflex artery. The left coronary system is critical because it supplies up to 70 percent of the left ventricular muscle mass, including the entire anterior wall, interventricular septum, the superior wall, and, at times, portions of the posterior wall. In addition, it supplies other key structures, such as portions of the papillary muscle and right and left bundle branches, and the AV node. The right coronary artery has a reciprocal relationship with the circumflex artery and perfuses the inferior and often the posterior surface of the left ventricle, the majority of the right ventricular muscle mass, and the postero-inferior aspects of the interventricular septum. It also provides blood supply to the sinus node in the majority of cases, the AV node, and portions of the right and left bundle branches. Understanding the distribution of each of the major coronary arteries is an important step toward appreciating the clinical consequences of either a high-grade obstruction or complete occlusion of any one or a combination of these arteries.

Coronary blood flow is dependent upon two factors: the net driving pressure and the vascular resistance of the coronary system. Since the coronary arteries fill primarily during diastole, the driving pressure is the systemic diastolic pressure. The left ventricular end-diastolic pressure (LVEDP) in the normal individual is only 5 to 10 mm Hg, and, therefore, in the person with normal coronary and left ventricular function, the *net* driving pressure is essentially the systemic diastolic pressure. The vascular resistance of the coronary system is proportional to the tone of smooth muscle fibers in the arteries and the length of the arteries. Arteriosclerotic plaques or occlusions result in decreased coronary flow due to a number of mechanisms that are either directly or indirectly related to the lesions. If the occlusion is of sufficient length or severity (in terms of luminal narrowing), the driving pressure beyond the lesion is reduced significantly, and, therefore, flow is limited. Once the flow across a lesion creates myocardial ischemia, the compliance in the left ventricle decreases as a result of incomplete myocardial relaxation, and the LVEDP increases, which further decreases the net driving pressure.

Coronary blood flow or supply is autoregulated as a result of both neural and chemical influences and varies with the determinants of myocardial oxygen demand, which are heart rate, systemic systolic blood pressure, myocardial wall tension, and rate of pressure generation in the left ventricle. Coronary lesions that result in 70 to 80 percent luminal narrowing significantly reduce flow capacity, especially as the myocardial oxygen demand increases as a result of increased heart rate, systolic blood pressure, and wall tension. Diffuse lesions of less than 70 percent narrowing and sequential lesions can also be hemodynamically significant. In addition, there is evidence that spasm of one or more of the coronary arteries (either with or without a fixed coronary lesion) can cause myocardial ischemia.

In patients with hemodynamically significant lesions and/or with a tendency toward coronary spasm, there are a number of clinical signs and symptoms that can occur when myocardial ischemia occurs. Approximately 50 to 60 percent of patients with coronary disease experience angina pectoris as a manifestation of ischemia. The classic description of angina pectoris is retrosternal pressure or heaviness that can also involve referred discomfort to the neck, jaw, upper extremities, and midscapular region. The key point is, however, that the precipitating factors are similar among patients; that is, when the myocardial oxygen demand exceeds the coronary flow capacity as a result of increases in heart rate, systolic blood pressure, and left ventricular wall tension, the patient experiences anginal symptoms. Emotional upset, exertion, and eating are the most common clinical precipitating factors due to their effect on myocardial oxygen demand. Angina pectoris at rest is often a premonitory symptom of impending myocardial infarction and, therefore, is an obvious contraindication to exercise testing or treatment. Patients with angina pectoris due to coronary spasm have a variant form of symptoms in that they can experience angina at any time, and their symptoms are not necessarily provoked by emotional upset, exercise, or eating. The primary goal of medical therapy designed to control angina symptoms is either to reduce myocardial oxygen demand by lowering the heart rate, systolic blood pressure, and wall tension (using nitrates and/or beta-adrenergic blockers) or to increase coronary flow (using calcium-entry blocking agents).

The classic electrocardiographic changes that can occur with exercise as myocardial ischemia develops include a shift (depression or elevation) in the ST segment and an increase in the R wave amplitude and frequent and complex ventricular or supraventricular arrhythmias. The two major hemodynamic indicators of myocardial ischemia are exercise hypotension (decrease in systolic pressure with increase in workload) as a result of ischemic left ventricular dysfunction, and inappropriate exercise bradycardia.

THE NATURAL HISTORY OF CORONARY ARTERY DISEASE

Although coronary artery disease tends to be a progressive disease process, the prognosis for a given patient depends upon the number of coronary arteries with hemodynamically significant lesions and the degree of left ventricular dysfunction.[20] Patients with left main coronary disease or triple vessel disease (significant lesions in all three major coronary vessels) have a much lower survival rate compared with patients with either double or single vessel disease. Patients with poor ventricular function and/or with a ventricular aneurysm have a poor prognosis compared with those with normal or near normal left ventricular hemodynamics. In fact, recent data from Mock and associates[21] indicate that left ventricular function is a more important predictor of survival than the number of diseased vessels. Awareness of the clinical subset of a patient (i.e., single vessel disease versus multivessel disease, or good ventricular function versus left ventricular aneurysm) is essential in designing an appropriate evaluation and treatment plan. As mentioned earlier, persistence of the key risk factors also influences the prognosis of the patient within a given subset, as does the maximal exercise capacity demonstrated on a symptom-limited exercise test.[22]

Coronary artery bypass surgery is the treatment of choice for patients with either main coronary disease or triple vessel disease accompanied by signs and symptoms of ischemic dysfunction during exercise testing. The aim of the surgery is to eliminate or relieve angina and improve the prognosis of the patient. Patients with single or double vessel disease are generally treated with medical therapy designed to control angina, arrhythmias, hypertension, and so forth. Recently, certain patients with one or two discrete proximal coronary lesions have been treated with angioplasty in an attempt to mechanically reduce the size of the lesion. Ideally, risk factor reduction is part of the overall treatment plan for both the medically and surgically managed patient.

OVERVIEW OF TREATMENT APPROACHES

There are basically two approaches utilized by clinicians working with coronary patients. One is a preprogrammed treatment protocol that is carried out on all patients in a similar manner despite the disparity in their degree of disease and ventricular function. This approach follows a predetermined sequence of activities that commonly is not preceded by any type of extensive evaluation. The major determining factor for progression through this predetermined sequence of treatment is the number of days post-event (post–myocardial-infarction or post–bypass-surgery).

The other, more appropriate, approach to patient treatment is based on individual assessment of each patient. The clinician formulates both a preliminary and a definitive assessment based on a logical sequence of evaluation tasks. The primary preliminary evaluation tasks (Table 6-1) include the chart review, physical examination, and patient interview, with the major concerns being: (1) awareness of the primary diagnosis, (2) identification of the proper clinical subset, (3) awareness of medical therapy, (4) identifica-

TABLE 6-1. Major Concerns and Evaluation Tasks Involved with Individualized Assessment of the Coronary Patient

	MAJOR CONCERNS	EVALUATION TASKS
PRELIMINARY ASSESSMENT	Primary diagnosis Clinical subset Complicated vs uncomplicated Symptoms—etiology Medical therapy Mental status Patient goals Additional significant medical problems Stable vs unstable angina Indications vs contraindications for mobilizing Monitoring needs	Chart—medical Record review Physical exam Patient interview
FINAL ASSESSMENT	Additional vessels involved single vs multivessel disease Good or poor ventricular function Candidate for treatment	Graduated activities/ Exercise tasks ADL monitor Monitored ambulation Exercise test Monitored exercise therapy sessions Monitored job simulations

tion of other potentially significant medical problems, and (5) awareness of either indications or contraindications to mobilizing the patient. The definitive evaluation tasks involve progressing the patient through a series of activities that are graduated in terms of their physiologic demands. The major questions at this point are as follows: (1) Does the patient demonstrate signs and symptoms of myocardial ischemia? (2) Does the patient have good or poor ventricular function? (3) Is the patient a candidate for therapy? The decision to progress the patient to the next phase of the evaluation is based on the appropriateness of the patient's cardiovascular responses at each given level of the evaluation. The final outcome of the individual assessment approach is a treatment program that is based on evaluation results rather than a predetermined sequence.

CASE HISTORY 1

J.R., a 65-year-old salesman, noted onset of retrosternal pressure on exertion associated with forearm and wrist pain in February 1979. The symptoms were initially brought on by vigorous walking and rapid stair climbing, but within a 3-week period they progressed to the point that slow ambulation or mild activity provoked the chest and upper-extremity discomfort. The patient did not have a history of rest pain. He was referred for exercise testing to rule out coronary artery disease. The patient demonstrated electrocardiographic changes and symptoms consistent with myocardial ischemia on the exercise test. In fact, the combination of the onset of ST segment depression and angina at a low workload and low pressure-rate product (systolic blood pressure times heart rate), along with poor exercise tolerance, suggested severe coronary artery disease. Because of the progressive nature of the patient's symptoms and the abnormal exercise test, the patient was referred for cardiac catheterization to determine the severity of the disease. The cardiac catheterization results were as follows:

Left main coronary artery: 40 to 50 percent narrowing.
Left anterior descending artery: 95 percent narrowing at its origin (prior to the first septal perforator), with additional multiple lesions of up to 50 percent in the proximal portion of the artery.
Anterior diagonal artery: 65 percent narrowing at its origin.
Circumflex artery: 75 percent narrowing at its origin.
Right coronary artery: no significant lesions.
Left ventricle: normal in size, with some anteroapical and inferoapical hypokinesis.

Based on the angiographic evidence of severe disease in the left coronary system including involvement of the left main coronary artery, the patient's easily provoked clinical symptoms, which were becoming progressively more unstable, and his poor performance on the exercise test, he was referred for bypass surgery in late February 1979. The patient had triple bypass surgery involving a sequential graft to the left anterior descending artery and the diagonal artery and a single graft to the obtuse marginal branch of the circumflex artery.

Entry Level: Referral for cardiac rehabilitation 3 days post-surgery.
Evaluation Purposes:

1. Establish a data base.
2. Carry out a preliminary assessment, and proceed to more definitive evaluation tasks if appropriate.
3. Establish a treatment plan.

PRELIMINARY EVALUATION AND ASSESSMENT

Medical Chart Review

Prior Medical History: As above. In addition, patient has had a left nephrectomy secondary to a renal tumor. No history of orthopaedic, neurologic, or pulmonary disease or impairment.

Present Illness: Coronary artery disease. Status: post–triple-bypass surgery, as described above.

Personal and Social: Patient is married and has two adult siblings. Patient works as an industrial chemical salesman. History of sedentary leisure activities, and no previous involvement in an aerobic exercise program.

Family History: Positive for hypertension and coronary artery disease; father died of a myocardial infarction at 63 years of age.

REVIEW OF SYSTEMS: Essentially unremarkable.

Physical Examination

ROM: Within normal limits with exception of 10 to 15 degrees limitation of shoulder flexion (limited due to sternal incision pain).

Strength: Good strength in both lower extremities (no obvious foot structure abnormalities). Limited strength testing of upper extremities due to recent surgery.

Sensation: Decreased along medial aspect of mid to distal portion of left lower extremity (vein donor site).

Chest Wall Exam: Parasternal and subclavian pain and tenderness aggravated by palpation, deep inspiration, and trunk movements.

Auscultation: Lungs: clear, no wheezing, rales, or rhonchi. Heart: S_4, no S_3, murmur, or friction rub heard. No bruits noted at carotid or femoral arteries.

Weight and Height: 148 pounds; 5 feet 8 inches.

Blood Pressure:

Supine: right arm, 106/70; left, 100/68; HR 102.
Sitting: right arm, 104/72; left, 100/70; HR 106.
Standing: right arm, 90/60; left, 88/56; HR 112.

Peripheral Pulses: 2^+ to $3^+/4^+$ throughout.

Note: 1^+ pretibial and ankle edema in left lower extremity.

PATIENT INTERVIEW

Symptoms: Patient denies retrosternal discomfort or arm and wrist discomfort since surgery. No paroxysmal nocturnal dyspnea, nocturnal cough, orthopnea. Denies deep chest discomfort with position change, cough, or deep inspiration. Chief complaint: incisional discomfort at the sternum and along vein graft and donor sites. Also complained of fatigue.

Risk Factor Profile:

1. Positive family history as noted.
2. History of hypertension for 8 to 10 years.
3. Cigarette smoker: 1 to 1½ packs per day for 30 years.
4. Sedentary lifestyle.
5. Negative history for hyperlipidemia and diabetes. HDL/LDL cholesterol unknown.
6. Stress related to both occupational and family life.

Personal Goals:

1. Return to work.
2. Travel.
3. Become more active, if possible.

Knowledge/Understanding of Primary Problem: Poor; related his problem to recent stress on job.

RESULTS OF SPECIAL TESTS

Twelve-lead ECG: Sinus tachycardia; otherwise, within normal limits.
Blood Studies: Hct, 33; Hb, 10.8; cardiac enzymes, WNL; arterial blood gases, WNL.
Echocardiogram: Within normal limits.
24-Hour Rhythm Trend Analysis: Brief salvos of supraventricular tachycardia at rates of 140 to 150 beats per minute. Rare PVCs.
Pulmonary Function Tests: Vital capacity 68 percent of predicted. FEV_1/VC, 82 percent.

PRELIMINARY ASSESSMENT

Sixty-five-year-old man, 3 days post–triple-bypass surgery with an uncomplicated hospital course thus far (no evidence of CHF, perioperative infarction, pericarditis, complicated ventricular arrhythmias). Primary symptoms are related to chest wall discomfort. Medical therapy should not influence cardiovascular responses to exercise. Patient is alert and cooperative but somewhat depressed, yet has established realistic and appropriate goals for himself. Additional medical problems in history that warrant ongoing evaluation include hypertension and kidney function. Patient is essentially stable, and there are no major contraindications for mobilization. The problems at this time include: (1) prolonged inactivity—72 hours; (2) decreased hematocrit and hemoglobin, which probably accounts for sinus tachycardia and fatigue; (3) asymptomatic orthostatic hypotension; (4) evidence of supraventricular arrhythmias; (5) incisional pain; (6) pulmonary dysfunction; (7) lack of knowledge regarding disease process, treatment objectives and rationale, and so forth; (8) significant risk factor profile; and (9) depression.

TREATMENT PLAN AND GOALS

Based on the preliminary assessment results, the patient is ready to mobilize. However, the patient's activity level should be progressed depending on the appropriateness of the cardiovascular signs and symptoms observed during a sequence of activities that are graduated in terms of their physiologic demands (Table 6-2).

The short-term goals for this patient relate specifically to the problems

TABLE 6-2. Evaluation and Program Planning Scheme for the Subacute Patient

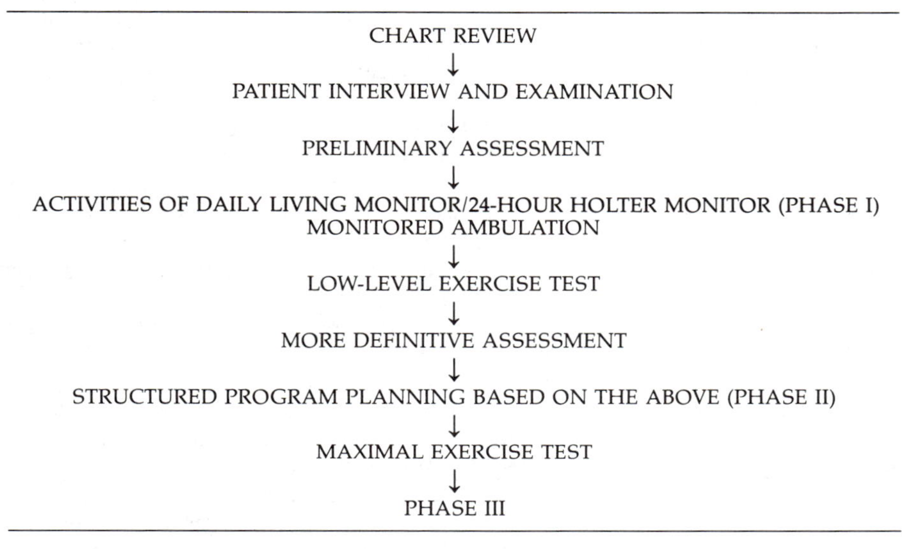

identified during the preliminary assessment and include: (1) Prevent complications of prolonged inactivity such as postural hypotension, decreased pulmonary function, decreased exercise tolerance, and so forth. (2) Educate the patient and spouse regarding the short- and long-term goals of the program, specifically as they relate to the patient's goals of returning to work and becoming more active. (3) Provide an environment to evaluate cardiovascular signs and symptoms during progressive activity, with special attention being paid to blood pressure and heart rate and rhythm responses.

The time of hospitalization post-myocardial infarction and post-bypass surgery has been significantly shortened in the last 5 years, and as a result, the emphasis for patient involvement is on evaluation of the appropriateness of progressive activity and discharge. Thus, there is little time for treatment, as such. Therefore, the majority of time during the inpatient phase of care for this patient should be spent monitoring his responses to activities of daily living, to ambulation, and to moderate physiologic demands imposed by the low-level exercise test.

The remainder of the physical therapy treatment program should include active trunk and upper-extremity exercises, bronchial hygiene and deep-breathing exercises (coordinated with respiratory therapy), and individual informal patient and spouse education.

Assuming the patient responds appropriately to the inpatient, monitored activities and his clinical course remains stable, the emphasis of the next phase of the program (early outpatient phase) is on exercise therapy designed to improve exercise endurance and capacity and to decrease the post-event period of disability. Ideally, this phase of the program should be initiated within 24 to 48 hours after discharge and should be conducted in an environment in which provisions are made for objectively assessing the patient's responses to aerobic exercise while, at the same time, evaluating the effectiveness of the medical therapy in controlling arrhythmias, and so forth. The intensity of the exercise program will depend on the results of the low-level exercise test. In the case of J.R., the patient achieved a maximal heart rate of 125 beats per minute after walking for 9 minutes on the treadmill, and there were no abnormalities noted. Therefore, an exercise intensity (walking speed on the treadmill) was selected that would enable the patient to achieve a heart rate that was 90 to 95 percent of the maximum achieved on the low-level test (125 beats per minute). The patient would then be encouraged to maintain the necessary walking speed for at least 10 to 15 minutes initially, with the goal of eventually progressing to 30 to 40 minutes. When it was indicated (based on results of monitored exercise sessions), the patient would be encouraged to carry out a similar program at home so that the aerobic exercise could be performed at least 3 to 4 times per week.

The importance of providing an environment where the cardiovascular signs and symptoms during exercise can be carefully monitored during this phase of rehabilitation is underscored in this case. Despite the fact that this patient had a very benign post-surgery hospital course and appropriate responses to the first few monitored exercise sessions, within 2 weeks after discharge he reported exertional symptoms (wrist and neck pain) with home activities. These symptoms were reproduced during supervised exercise and were relieved promptly by rest and nitroglycerin. These findings were reported to the patient's physician and a repeat exercise test was ordered, which was abnormal. A repeat angiogram revealed complete occlusion of both the left anterior descending and diagonal grafts, and the patient underwent a second bypass surgery. Currently, the patient is asymptomatic and is in an ongoing exercise and risk factor reduction program and is doing well.

OXYGEN TRANSPORT SYSTEM AND PHYSICAL WORK CAPACITY

The ability to perform physical work or exercise is highly dependent upon aerobic metabolism (metabolism in the presence of oxygen) in the working muscle. Aerobic metabolism yields approximately 18 times the amount of adenosine triphosphate (basic energy source for muscle contraction) compared to anaerobic metabolism. In addition, 80 to 90 percent of the energy for sustained activity (greater than 2 to 3 minutes of continuous exercise) is derived from aerobic metabolism. In essence, then, the body's ability to transport and utilize oxygen is what determines an individual's physical work capacity. The oxygen transport system has three major components: (1) pulmonary system, (2) cardiovascular system, and (3) skeletal muscle.

The pulmonary system's primary functions during exercise are to maintain adequate arterial oxygen content (which is an essential determinant of oxygen transport capacity) and to prevent excessive build-up of carbon dioxide, a by-product of energy metabolism. As the total body demand for oxygen increases due to the increased intensity of exercise, the normal pulmonary system adapts by increasing the volume of air processed in the lungs per unit of time (liters per minute) as a result of increased breathing frequency and depth of breathing (Table 6-3). The maximum minute ventilation is, in fact, correlated with the maximal capacity for oxygen consumption. Obstructive or restrictive lung disease potentially can impair the

TABLE 6-3. Pulmonary Adaptations to Moderate and Maximal Levels of Aerobic Exercise Compared with Resting Values

	REST	MODERATE EXERCISE	MAXIMAL EXERCISE
Oxygen Uptake (liters/min)	0.250–0.300	2.0–3.0	3.5–4.5
Minute Ventilation (liters/min)	5–6	50–70	110–120
Breathing Frequency (breaths/min)	8–10	25–35	40–50
Tidal Volume (ml)	500–600	1500–2000	1800–2200

patient's physical work capacity by: (1) limiting the ability to increase the depth of breathing and breathing frequency of a patient, with the net effect of significantly reducing the maximum minute ventilation, and/or (2) as a result of ventilation and perfusion abnormalities, preventing the lungs from maintaining adequate arterial oxygen content.

The central component of the cardiovascular system, the heart, adapts to increased demands for total body oxygen by increasing the volume of oxygenated blood transported per unit of time (cardiac output) as a result of increases in the stroke volume and heart rate (Table 6-4). Maximum oxygen consumption is directly proportional to maximum cardiac output. The patient with coronary artery disease potentially has an impaired oxygen transport capacity secondary to limitations in maximal cardiac output as a result of poor left ventricular function or exertional angina. In addition, coronary patients are often treated with medications (beta-adrenergic blocking agents) that potentially limit stroke volume and maximum heart rate. Therefore, these patients have a reduced capacity for increased cardiac output and, thus, oxygen transport.

The peripheral circulation adapts to increased demands for oxygen transport by producing a 3- to 3.5-fold increase in oxygen transported in the blood to the peripheral muscle per unit of time as a result of redistribution in cardiac output. The peripheral muscle that normally recieves 20 to 25 percent of the cardiac output at rest can receive as much as 80 to 85 percent of the output during exercise. This relative shift in cardiac output is a result of blood being shunted primarily from the gastrointestinal tract and kidneys to the working muscle. Patients who develop hemodynamically significant lesions in the peripheral arteries of the lower extremities often have a decreased work capacity due to limiting symptoms (claudication) that result from exercise-induced ischemia in the skeletal muscle.

TABLE 6-4. Cardiac Adaptations to Moderate and Severe Levels of Aerobic Exercise Compared with Resting Values

	REST	MODERATE EXERCISE	MAXIMAL EXERCISE
Oxygen Uptake (liters/min)	0.2–0.3	2.5–3.5	5
Cardiac Output (liters/min)	4–6	18–22	30
Heart Rate (bpm)	60–70	130–140	200
Stroke Volume (ml)	80–100	110–130	130

The concentration of oxidative enzymes and the degree of capillarization in the skeletal muscle are also important determinants of oxygen transport and utilization capacity and, therefore, significantly influence the physical work capacity.

Exercise testing is useful in evaluating the patient's maximal exercise or oxygen transport capacity. It is possible, through the use of either invasive procedures (such as analysis of exercise arterial blood gases) or noninvasive procedures (such as expired gas analysis or radionuclide studies), to assess the capacity of the various components of the oxygen transport system and to determine the major limiting factors for a given patient. In addition, exercise testing can be used to evaluate the effects of drugs, surgery, or exercise therapy on the oxygen transport capacity of the patient.

CONGESTIVE HEART FAILURE—INFLUENCE OF CARDIAC AND PULMONARY DYSFUNCTION

By definition, congestive heart failure occurs when the cardiac output is inadequate relative to the total body metabolic demands. Congestive failure, by this definition, can conceivably occur at rest or at various levels of activity. Congestive failure at rest is an obvious contraindication to exercise therapy and, therefore, must be recognized by the clinician if, in fact, evaluation procedures and treatment are to be carried out appropriately in the more severely involved cardiac or pulmonary patient.

Patients with coronary artery disease predominantly develop left ventricular failure due principally to either chronic ischemic dysfunction or to a large myocardial infarction with residual poor ventricular function. Hypertension or chronic arrhythmias, such as poorly controlled atrial fibrillation, are often aggravating factors. The left ventricle attempts to meet the demands for increased cardiac output by hypertrophy, then chamber dilitation, and, usually, increased sympathetic nervous system activity. Unfortunately, in the patient with a large myocardial infarction or chronic ischemia, the compensatory mechanism eventually leads to decompensation secondary to excessive filling pressures that result in increased left atrial pressures and then pulmonary congestion. The pulmonary congestion involves interstitial and alveolar edema and accounts for the classic symptoms of left ventricular failure, which include dyspnea, exertional or nocturnal cough, orthopnea, and paroxysmal nocturnal dyspnea. Right ventricular failure can then occur as a sequela to left ventricular failure and can result in clinical signs of peripheral venous congestion such as neck vein distention, hepatomegaly, or peripheral edema (pitting edema in lower extremities).

Patients with advanced stages of obstructive or restrictive pulmonary disease can develop primary right ventricular failure or cor pulmonale as a result of increased workload on the right ventricle secondary to increased pulmonary artery pressures. The pathophysiology of right ventricular failure is the same as that described for left ventricular failure. The clinical signs were discussed above.

It is essential for the clinician dealing with patients who have a primary or secondary diagnosis of cardiac or pulmonary disease to be able to detect right or left ventricular decompensation early and to establish a protocol for ongoing evaluation of these patients based on the clinical signs and symptoms.

CASE HISTORY 2

A.B., a 46-year-old former foundry worker, was well until October 1976, at which time he began having chest pain and what he felt to be flu-like symptoms. The patient did not seek medical attention at the time. However, because the chest pain persisted intermittently for approximately 2 weeks, the patient was urged by a friend to see a cardiologist. At that time, there was evidence of a recent myocardial infarction, and the patient was hospitalized. The patient had an uneventful course during this admission but continued to have chest pain after discharge. As a result, the patient was referred for exercise testing to further evaluate the extent of coronary disease. The treadmill test results were abnormal in that the patient demonstrated poor exercise capacity and exercise hypotension (a fall of 34 mm Hg in systolic blood pressure during exercise), along with ECG changes and symptoms consistent with ischemia and complex arrhythmias. Due to the exercise test findings, the patient was referred for cardiac catheterization, with the following results:

Left main coronary artery: normal.
Left anterior descending artery: completely occluded at the level of the first septal perforator.
Circumflex artery: 50 percent narrowing at the midpoint.
Right coronary artery: normal.
Left ventricle: enlarged, with areas of anterior, superior, and inferior hypokinesis; ejection fraction, 40 percent.

Following the angiogram, the patient was discharged and referred for cardiac rehabilitation.

Entry Level: Outpatient referral for cardiac rehabilitation in a patient approximately 2 months post-infarction.
Evaluation Purposes:
1. Obtain data base.
2. Perform both preliminary and definitive evaluation.
3. Establish treatment plan.

PRELIMINARY EVALUATION AND ASSESSMENT

Medical Chart Review

Prior Medical History: As above. Patient never hospitalized prior to October 1976.
Present Illness: Essentially single vessel coronary artery disease.
Medications: Nitroglycerin, propranolol, quinidine.
Chief Complaint: Severely limiting dyspnea on exertion; exertional chest pain.
Personal and Social: Married twice; six siblings; high degree of stress and anxiety at home; former foundry worker. No strong leisure-time activities. No history of involvement in aerobic exercise program.

Family History: Positive for coronary disease; mother with MI at age 60.

PHYSICAL EXAMINATION

Strength/ROM: Within normal limits; no leg length discrepancy or major structural abnormalities.
Sensation: Within normal limits.
Chest Wall Exam: Negative.
Auscultation: Lungs: breath sounds decreased bilaterally; expiratory wheezing at both bases. Heart: S_3
Weight and Height: 136 pounds; 5 feet 8 inches.
Blood Pressure:
Supine: right arm, 124/70; left, 100/60.
Sitting: right arm, 126/72; left, 102/60.
Standing: right arm, 136/74; left, 106/64.
Peripheral Pulses: $3^+/4^+$; no bruits.
Edema: None.

PATIENT INTERVIEW

Symptoms: Patient reported severe dyspnea after 3 to 4 blocks of rapid walking. Also reported chest discomfort and burning at times with exertion. Positive history for paroxysmal nocturnal dyspnea and chest discomfort.
Risk Factor Profile:
1. Smoker: 54 year history.
2. Labile hypertension.
3. Stress.
4. Sedentary lifestyle.
5. Negative for hyperlipidemia (HDL/LDL unknown).

Personal Goals:
1. Unsure about returning to work.
2. Wants to feel better.

Knowledge/Understanding of Primary Illness: Poor.

RESULTS OF SPECIAL TESTS

Twelve-lead ECG: Sinus bradycardia; old anteroseptal myocardial infarction.
Lipids: Cholesterol, 233; HDL, 46; chol/HDL ratio, 5:1; triglycerides, 165mg/dl.
Chest X-Ray: Cardiomegaly.
Echocardiogram: Diffusely hypocontractile left ventricle.
Pulmonary Function Tests: Vital capacity 95 percent of predicted. FEV_1/VC, 50 percent. Maximal expiratory flow rates, 208 liters/min prior to bronchodilators; 436 liters/min post-bronchodilators.

PRELIMINARY ASSESSMENT

The overall goal of the preliminary assessment is to determine whether the initiation of cardiac rehabilitation is indicated or contraindicated based on the patient's medical and psychosocial problems. The list below summarizes A.B.'s problems based on the results of the medical chart review and patient interview and examination:

Problems

Medical

1. Evidence of compromised left ventricular function at rest (generalized hypokinesis, reduced ejection fraction as determined by catheterization).
2. Evidence of compromised left ventricular function during exercise (hypoadaptive systolic blood pressure, poor exercise tolerance).
3. Possible congestive heart failure, based on clinical findings such as S_3, history of paroxysmal nocturnal dyspnea, and enlarged heart on roentgenogram.
4. Obstructive lung disease, as evidenced by pulmonary function tests and clinical findings such as expiratory wheezing.
5. Clinical history of limiting dyspnea on exertion—3 to 4 block tolerance.
6. Exertional chest discomfort typical of angina pectoris, nocturnal chest discomfort—variant angina versus unstable angina, or preinfarction angina versus noncardiac origin.
7. Coronary risk factors, including smoking, hypertension by history, and hyperlipidemia (elevated triglycerides and cholesterol; abnormal cholesterol/HDL ratio).

Psychosocial

1. Family problems: tension.
2. Vocational status unclear. High likelihood of need for retraining.
3. Limited patient goals, probably secondary to lack of understanding and awareness of underlying medical problems complicated by language barrier (patient's primary language is Spanish).

The primary concerns or potential contraindications to initiating any further activity or structured exercise therapy are as follows: (1) nocturnal chest discomfort, possibly indicative of unstable angina, and (2) clinical signs and symptoms suggestive of decompensation or congestive heart failure. Further discussion of nocturnal symptoms with the patient and his physician and results of a trial of nitroglycerin essentially ruled out unstable or variant angina as the underlying cause. Also, there was no overwhelming clinical evidence of decompensated congestive heart failure; thus, the patient was considered a candidate for post-myocardial infarction rehabilitation.

TREATMENT PLAN

The patient's problem list suggests a need for intervention from a variety of health care professionals including physician, physical therapist, occupational and/or vocational rehabilitation counselor, medical social worker, and nutritionist.

The physical therapy treatment goals for this patient should include at least the following: (1) provide environment for ongoing evaluation of exertional chest discomfort and dyspnea, as well as blood pressure and heart rate and rhythm responses to activity; (2) increase patient's physical work capacity and endurance to provide greater physiologic reserve for vocational and leisure-time activities; (3) risk factor reduction, specifically improved blood pressure and lipid levels (triglycerides and HDL cholesterol); (4) reduction in exertional chest discomfort; (5) patient education in areas of program goals and management of home exercise program and etiology of disease; and (6) family/spouse education in above areas.

The emphasis of the exercise therapy program should be on aerobic exercise if, in fact, the above goals are to be accomplished. Aerobic exercise involves large muscle activity that is rhythmic and sustained. The other variables that need to be considered in designing the therapeutic exercise program for this patient include intensity (workload, i.e., walking speed or measured resistance on bicycle, as examples), duration of each exercise session, and frequency in terms of number of exercise sessions performed per week. Ideally, the intensity of exercise should be sufficient to elevate the heart rate to at least 65 to 70 percent of the patient's maximal rate achieved on a symptom-limited exercise test. For obvious reasons, when establishing the proper exercise intensity, the therapist needs to consider several variables, including the patient's clinical status, activity history, musculoskeletal status, and ischemic signs and symptoms (angina, hypotension, arrhythmias). For this patient, the primary factors to consider regarding establishing a therapeutic exercise intensity are exertional dyspnea and chest discomfort. Therefore, the patient's exercise intensity initially may be set at a level that provokes mild symptoms, especially if these symptoms occur at a heart rate below 65 to 70 percent of the patient's maximal rate. Ideally, the patient will be gradually progressed to the point where he can exercise at an adequate intensity for at least 20 to 30 minutes per session at least three to four times per week. Studies have indicated that this type of exercise program results in improved exercise capacity, reduction of risk factors, and, often, reduction in exertional symptoms. The rate at which the exercise intensity and duration are adjusted will depend on the clinical status of the patient and the appropriateness of the patient's cardiovascular signs and symptoms observed during the monitored exercise sessions. Each monitored session is, in effect, an "exercise test," the results of which enable the therapist to reassess and re-establish the therapeutic exercise plan.

The success of the rehabilitation program for this patient goes beyond designing the appropriate therapeutic exercise program. The patient needs to establish some realistic goals, and there is considerable need for education of the patient, his wife, and his siblings. Family support is essential for the achievement of the goals of risk-factor reduction and long-term compliance with the exercise, diet, and medical therapy programs.

The successful rehabilitation of this patient also depends on the involvement of a "team" of health care professionals in his total program. Below is a brief summary of the potential role of the various team members in solving the "problems" identified in the initial evaluation of the patient.

Team Member	Problem	Intervention
Medical Social Worker	Family problems: tension	Identify source of tension/stress; counsel to relieve or reduce tension. Aid with applying for interim financial aid during disability period.

Dietician/Nutritionist	Coronary risk factors: hypertension, elevated serum lipids	Educate patient and wife regarding importance of diet in altering certain risk factors; provide suggestions for alternative in diet plans. Provide ongoing follow-up based on results of serial food diaries, lipid studies, and so forth.
Occupational Therapist Vocational Counselor	Need for job retraining	Test for interest and skills in alternative vocation. Resource to direct patient to formal job retraining, if needed.

SUMMARY

The clinician interested in formulating an assessment-based treatment plan must have a thorough understanding of the etiology and pathophysiology of the various cardiopulmonary disease processes and the potential impact cardiopulmonary pathology can have on adaptations to exercise. This knowledge base will allow the therapist to develop a thorough evaluation plan, make appropriate assessments based on evaluation results, and design a treatment program that will provide maximum benefit to the patient.

The initial evaluation plan, involving a thorough review of the medical record and patient examination and review, should be designed to allow the therapist to gather information in at least four areas:

1. the severity of the primary cardiopulmonary disease
2. the presence of additional significant medical and/or socioeconomic problems
3. the medical therapy currently being given to the patient
4. the patient's short-term and long-range goals.

The above information should then allow the therapist to make at least a preliminary assessment of either the indications or the contraindications for treatment. Provided it is indicated, a more definitive assessment of the patient's candidacy for treatment can be made by taking the patient through a series of activities that are graduated in terms of their physiologic demands and by carefully documenting the appropriateness of the patient's cardiopulmonary adaptations to these activities.

The specific treatment goals are based on the problems identified in both the preliminary and definitive portions of the evaluation. This allows the therapist to individualize the treatment program and, therefore, to maximize the effectiveness of therapy. Ideally, the treatment goals of the physical therapist are coordinated with the members of the health care team involved with the total care of the patient.

REFERENCES

1. DAWBER, TR, ET AL: *An approach to longitudinal studies in a community: The Framingham Study.* Ann NY Acad Sci 107:539, 1963.
2. GORDON, T AND KANNEL, WB: *Predisposition to atherosclerosis in the head, heart and legs: The Framingham Study.* JAMA 221:661, 1972.
3. KANNEL, WB: *Some lessons in cardiovascular epidemiology from Framingham.* Am J Cardiol 37:269, 1976.
4. ROSENMAN, RH, ET AL: *Coronary heart disease in the Western Collaborative Group Study: Final follow up experience of 8½ years.* JAMA 233:872, 1975.
5. JENKINS, CD, ET AL: *Prediction of clinical coronary heart disease by a test for the coronary-prone behavior pattern.* N Engl J Med 290:1271, 1974.
6. GORDON, T, ET AL: *High density lipoproteins as a protective factor against CHD.* Am J Med 62:707, 1977.
7. GOFMAN, JW, ET AL: *Ischemic heart disease, atherosclerosis and longevity.* Circulation 34:679, 1966.
8. KANNEL, WB, ET AL: *Serum cholesterol lipoproteins and risk of coronary heart disease: The Framingham Study.* Ann Intern Med 24:1, 1971.
9. ALBRINK, MJ, ET AL: *Serum lipids, hypertension and coronary artery disease.* Am J Med 31:4, 1961.
10. HYPERTENSION DETECTION AND FOLLOW-UP COOPERATIVE GROUP: *5 year findings of the Hypertension Detection and Follow-Up Program. I. Reduction in mortality of persons with high blood pressure including mild hypertension.* JAMA 242:2562, 1979.
11. SANMARCO, ME, ET AL: *Smoking and high density lipoproteins and coronary change in two and three vessel disease (abstr).* Am J Cardiol 41:423, 1978.
12. MILLER, H, ET AL: *Tromso heart study: HDL and coronary artery disease—A prospective case control study.* Lancet 2:965, 1977.
13. KAVANAGH, T, ET AL: *Prognostic Indexes in post-infarction exercise rehabilitation candidates.* Am J Cardiol 44:1230, 1979.
14. PULAC, RT, ET AL: *Risk factors related to progressive narrowing in aortocoronary vein grafts studied 1 and 5 years after surgery.* Circulation (Suppl I) 66:1–40, 1982.
15. LAWRIE, GH, ET AL: *Vein graft patency and intimal proliferation after aortocoronary bypass: Early and long-term angiopathologic correlations.* Am J Cardiol 38:856, 1976.
16. FORBISZEWSKI, R AND WOROWSKI, K: *Enhancement of platelet aggregation and adhesiveness by beta lipoproteins.* Journal of Atherosclerosis Research 8:988, 1968.
17. CORVALHO, AC, ET AL: *Platelet function in hyperlipoproteinemia.* N Eng J Med 290:434, 1974.
18. SULLIVAN, JM, ET AL: *Studies of platelet adhesiveness, glucose tolerance and serum lipoprotein patterns in patients with coronary artery disease.* Am J Med Sci 264:475, 1972.
19. MUSTARD, JF AND MURPHY, CA: *Effect of smoking on blood coagulation and platelet survival in man.* Br Med J 1:846, 1963.
20. PROUDFIT, WL: *Natural history of obstructive coronary artery disease: Ten year study of 601 nonsurgical cases.* Prog Cardiovasc Dis 21:53, 1978.
21. MOCK, MB, ET AL: *Survival of medically treated patients in the Coronary Artery Surgery Study (CASS) Registry.* Circulation 66:562, 1982.
22. MCNEER, JF, ET AL: *The role of the exercise test in the evaluation of patients for ischemic heart disease.* Circulation 57:64, 1978.

BIBLIOGRAPHY

ASTRAND, PO AND RODAHL, K: *Textbook of Work Physiology.* McGraw-Hill, New York, 1970, pp 277–315.

SOKOLOW, M AND MCILROY, MB (EDS): *Clinical Cardiology.* Lange Medical Publications, Canada, 1979, pp 295–339.

Chapter 7

CLINICAL DECISION MAKING: CARDIOPULMONARY REHABILITATION

Scot Irwin, M.A., R.P.T.

The purpose of this chapter is to discuss the decision-making processes involved in a physical therapist's approach to the specific clinical problems of a patient with chronic obstructive pulmonary disease (COPD). It is not within the purview of this chapter to present all aspects of chest physical therapy, but simply the rationale and treatment plan for an individual patient's case.

To appreciate some aspects of the decision-making process, several basic scientific concepts need to be reviewed. These concepts include: (1) the pathomechanics of gas movement and exchange, (2) arterial blood gas response to exercise, and (3) the effect of decreased oxygen tension on right ventricular heart function. A brief review of these concepts is developed here, but the reader is encouraged to review this information in more detail by consulting the bibliography at the end of this chapter.

PATHOMECHANICS OF GAS MOVEMENT AND EXCHANGE

Normal respiration involves a complex process of gaseous exchange between the external environment (atmosphere) and the internal environment (lungs and blood). This process varies according to interrelationships between oxygen consumption demands, ventilatory mechanics, and ventilation/perfusion ratio within the lung. Oxygen consumption demands result from the needs of the body tissues to perform their normal functions. These demands increase as higher rates of function are required. One of the primary causes of increased oxygen consumption is exercise. Patients with COPD have poor oxygen consumption reserves due, in part, to the fact that a great percentage of the oxygen they consume is used up by the work of breathing. The work of breathing increases or decreases according to the ventilatory mechanics utilized by the patient.

Normal pulmonary ventilation, the process of moving air in and out of the lungs, is depicted mathematically by the formula, $\dot{V}_E = \dot{V}_T \times f$, where $\dot{V}_E$ equals minute volume of air expired, $\dot{V}_T$ equals tidal volume, and f is the frequency of breaths taken. Actual gaseous exchange, though, occurs at the alveolar level. Alveolar ventilation is not the same as pulmonary ventilation because not all the air we breathe reaches our alveoli. The difference between alveolar ventilation and pulmonary ventilation is called dead-space ventilation. Mathematically, this is expressed as $\dot{V}_D = \dot{V}_E - \dot{V}_A$, where $\dot{V}_D$ is the minute volume of dead-space, $\dot{V}_A$ is the minute volume of alveolar ventilation, and $\dot{V}_E$ is the minute volume of air expired. Dead-space ventilation can result from both anatomic and physiologic causes. Anatomic dead-space results from air moving in and out of our conducting airways (mouth, trachea, bronchi, bronchioles). Physiologic dead-space is created when air reaches an alveolus that is not perfused; thus, no gas exchange occurs. The latter is a common phenomenon in patients with obstructive pulmonary disease. The combination of decreased ventilation capacity and an elevated dead-space exchange in the patient with chronic obstructive pulmonary disease has an extremely adverse effect on gas movement and exchange. Thus, any factor that increases the difficulty of ventilation will worsen the problem.

Patients with COPD are often confronted with two additional pathomechanical factors that decrease their ability to ventilate: (1) obstruction to airflow, and (2) poor ventilatory mechanics. Congestion, bronchial secretions, and bronchospasm directly obstruct airflow. Abnormal secretions can cause an increase in airflow turbulence, and this means that a greater amount of muscular work is required to create ventilation. Bronchospasm has the same effect, but often to a greater extent. The second pathomechanical problem, poor ventilatory mechanics, is the result of a rigid chest wall and hyperexpanded lung. Patients with COPD have a restrictive component to their disease. They have rigid, fixed chest walls and flattened diaphragms. These anatomic abnormalities are accommodated by the use of accessory respiratory muscles. The result is an increase in the work of breathing. Thus, a combination of obstructed airflow and restricted ventilatory mechanics makes the oxygen consumption demands of respiration much higher at rest and exponentially higher with increased oxygen consumption requirements.

The final pathomechanical problem, ventilation/perfusion defects, is directly involved with gas exchange. Normally, ventilation and perfusion of the lungs result in a fairly uniform match. Although different zones of the lung have varied ventilation to perfusion ratios, the net effect is uniform. In patients with pulmonary disease, mismatches of ventilation to perfusion are common. Areas of the lung that are well ventilated may be poorly perfused, and areas that are well perfused may receive little or no ventilation. This mismatching phenomenon can result in venous blood passing through the lung without contacting fresh air. Thus, venous blood mixes with arterial blood in the left atrium and ventricle, creating marked changes in arterial blood gas concentrations.

The pathomechanics of gas movement and exchange are interrelated. Increased oxygen demands require increased ventilation, which is met by poor ventilatory mechanics, obstructions to airflow, and mismatching of ventilated lung with perfused lung. The result is patients with severe limitations in their exercise capacity and oxygen consumption reserves. At times, this reserve is so impaired that assisted ventilation through mechanical methods is necessary to meet the respiration requirements for life.

ARTERIAL BLOOD GAS RESPONSE TO EXERCISE

The normal blood gas response to exertion is to have arterial PO_2 remain unchanged or rise slightly and arterial PCO_2 fall slightly. Such is not the case for the patient with obstructive pulmonary disease (Fig. 7-1). The patient in Figure 7-1 exhibits a dramatic fall in arterial PO_2 during exercise and a small rise in arterial PCO_2. This abnormal response occurs because of an inability to increase alveolar ventilation to match the increased cardiac output (perfusion) going to the lung. Concurrent with this mismatch is the increased oxygen consumption costs of breathing. What is the significance of this low arterial PO_2? A decreased arterial PO_2 has a cause-and-effect relationship with pulmonary arterial vasoconstriction. As arterial PO_2 falls, and thus venous PO_2 decreases, the pulmonary arterial vasculature constricts. An increased resistance to blood flow into the lung results in an elevated pulmonary arte-

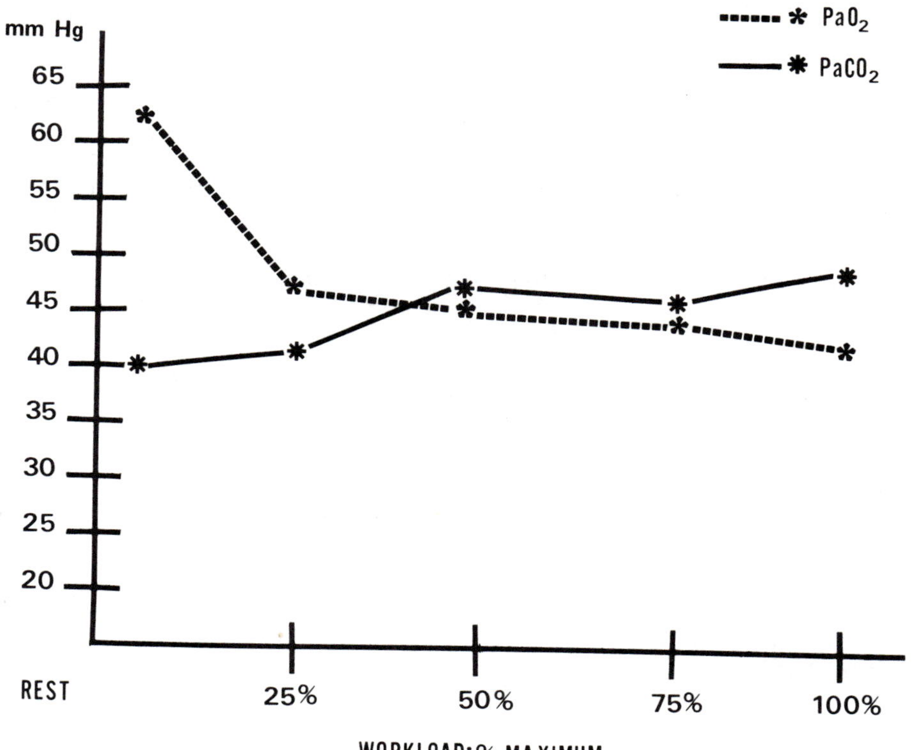

FIGURE 7-1. Oxygen and carbon dioxide responses to exercise in a patient with severe chronic obstructive pulmonary disease. Demonstrates marked hypoxia with minimal hypercapnia that worsens during exercise.

rial pressure, which, in turn, may cause elevated diastolic and systolic pressures in the right ventricle. If this elevated pressure persists, chronic changes in the right ventricle will result. Initially, right ventricular and atrial hypertrophy occur and can be detected by changes in the 12-lead electrocardiogram. As time goes on, signs of right ventricular failure, including venous distension, dependent edema, and sudden weight changes, begin to appear. Chronically low arterial PO_2 has numerous detrimental effects on other organs of the body. Thus, it is very important to carefully and regularly assess the arterial PO_2 of patients at rest and during activity to avoid the chronic effects of this disorder.

With these concepts in mind, decisions made about patient treatment during the following patient case example should be clear. The presentation is divided into three phases: acute, subacute, and rehabilitative. Each phase is subdivided into data, assessment (decision making), and treatment.

CASE STUDY 1

MEDICAL CHART REVIEW

The patient is a 47-year-old woman. She was admitted to the intensive care unit on June 25, 1980, with a diagnosis of COPD and respiratory failure. Her chief complaints were shortness of breath, exhaustion, and congestion.

Data

ECG: Right ventricular hypertrophy, right atrial enlargement; BP, 160/100; RHR, 120.

Chest X-ray: Admission: severe hyperinflation without infiltrate. 5 days post-admission: severe hyperinflation with blunting of the left costophrenic angle.

Medications: Theo-Dur, Bronkosol, HydroDIURIL, erythromycin.

Admission Blood Gases:	PO_2, 66	HCO_3, 45
on IMV_2 V_1 *700*	PCO_2, 84	O_2Sat, 71%
25% oxygen	pH, 7.34	Vol%, 12.4

PHYSICAL EXAMINATION

Weight: 85 pounds, dropping to 69 pounds as a low.

Strength: Fair to fair plus lower-extremity strength. Fair to fair plus to Good upper extremities. ROM, within normal limits.

Sputum: Dark green, thick, copious.

Temperature: Spiking to 103°F.

Breath Sounds: Coarse, bubbly rales throughout; right worse than left.

Dyspnea: 3+ at rest.

Cough Function: Poor.

Chest Mobility: Restricted.

Breathing Pattern: Primarily an accessory-muscle breather.

3+ ankle edema.

PHYSICAL THERAPY EVALUATION

Initial Assessment

A 47-year-old woman with severe respiratory limitations. There are several items that were identified through the physical therapy evaluation that are amenable to therapeutic measures. The patient exhibited decreased musculoskeletal strength, abnormal sputum, poor sputum clearance, poor cough function, restricted chest mobility, and abnormal gas exchange. Her dyspnea level, at rest, off the ventilator was 3+. The description of our dyspnea scale is as follows:

- 1+ unable to complete an average sentence without taking a breath
- 2+ can speak only in short phrases, three to four words at a time
- 3+ can speak only one word at a time
- 4+ unable to speak; respiratory rate is 40 or greater.

How are each of these pieces of information useful in assessing and treating the pulmonary patient?

ECG: Right ventricular hypertrophy and right atrial enlargement indicate a chronic process with a probable history of prolonged hypoxia. The observation also should alert the therapist to look for atrial arrhythmias and signs of right ventricular failure. The absence of left ventricular hypertrophy or any history of myocardial infarction is a positive finding that indicates the patient has less chance of exhibiting signs of left-sided failure. This fact leads one to believe that the patient's coarse rales are not due to left-sided ventricular failure. Heart function will alter the patient's chance of progression during any exercise activity, thus placing restrictions on the therapist's potential treatment program.

CHEST X-RAY: Hyperinflation is common in patients with COPD. The blunting of the left costophrenic angle found 5 days after admission is significant because it may indicate the primary area of infiltrate or congestion. The chest X-ray can assist the therapist in concentrating bronchial drainage treatment.

MEDICATIONS: Many medications have fairly common side effects. Most bronchodilators have systemic effects that may cause marked elevation in resting heart rate. Excess doses of bronchodilators can create muscle tremors and sensations of anxiety. These may cause the patient to hyperventilate, which, in turn, can lead to respiratory crisis in patients with severe COPD.

The other medications are erythromycin and HydroDIURIL, an antibiotic and a diuretic, respectively. HydroDIURIL is used as an antihypertensive.

VENTILATOR DATA IMV$_2$ V$_1$ 700: This notation means that the patient requires mechanical assistance of two breaths per minute at a volume of 700 ml in order to live. As these values are adjusted, it gives the therapist an indication of the patient's status. You will note that 2 months later the patient required an IMV of 8 and a volume of 800 ml. This indicates an increased dependence upon mechanical assistance and was necessitated by a need to obtain some measure of normal gas exchange to allow her to initiate higher activity levels.

ARTERIAL BLOOD GASES (ABGs): ABGs can indicate the patient's status and are useful values that assist in determining when patients can be progressed. (A full description of blood gases can be found in the text by Shapiro.) Other items in the data base are explained in the text.

GOALS

The decision-making process is dependent upon achievable goals. In the acute stage, the physical therapy goals are to: (1) improve muscle strength, (2) increase clearance of bronchial secretions, (3) improve chest wall mobility, (4) improve cough function, and (5) decrease dyspnea at rest.

INITIAL TREATMENT PROGRAM

The physical therapy treatment program consisted of bronchial drainage through percussion, postural positioning, shaking and chest wall stretching, and active and active-resistive range of motion to all extremities.

PROGRAM PROGRESSION—SUBACUTE

Two months later, the patient remains on a ventilator with a tracheostomy, an intermittent minute volume rate of 8, and a delivered volume of 800 ml with 25 percent oxygen. Physical therapy evaluation is basically unchanged, except that sputum production is decreased and cough function has improved. Her arterial blood gases are as follows: PO_2, 79; PCO_2, 41; pH, 7.48; HCO_3, 31; O_2Sat, 96%; Vol%, 16.6.

How do these arterial blood gas values affect a physical therapy treatment program?

In this patient, it is apparent that she is better oxygenated, has normalized her PCO_2 acid-base balance, and has improved the total oxygen content in her blood. These findings strongly indicate that the patient is better prepared to engage in increased amounts of activity.

For this patient, additional physical therapy procedures were introduced. The patient was exercised upright in a room chair using a Restorator (Fig. 7-2). This equipment allows for increases in duration and workload. Gradually, the patient's tolerance to upright activities and her lower-extremity strength improved to the point that ambulation was possible. In order to accommodate the patient's ventilator dependence and weak lower extremities, the patient walked with the assistance of a wheeled walker (Fig. 7-3) and ambulated from her room ventilator to a ventilator set up 100 feet from her room. As her tolerance for ambulation improved, the distance to the ventilator was lengthened.

The physical therapy treatment program, nursing care, respiratory therapy treatments, and medical therapeutics eventually prevailed, and the patient was weaned off of her ventilator. Her tracheostomy was removed, and a stoma plug was inserted. Four months after admission, she was discharged with the following data base: (1) arterial blood gases in room air:

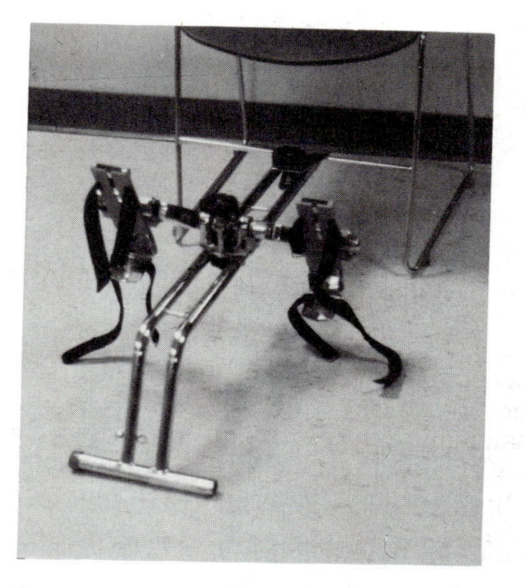

FIGURE 7-2. A mobile lower-extremity exercise unit, Restorator. This unit can be attached to a chair and used in the patient's room.

PO_2, 66; PCO_2, 63; pH, 7.37; O_2Sat, 92%; HCO_3, 37; Vol%, 13.3; (2) ambulatory for short distances—300 to 500 feet; (3) capable of performing all self-care activities; (4) a wheelchair requirement for long-distance activities (shopping); and (5) continues to produce small amounts of thick, white sputum.

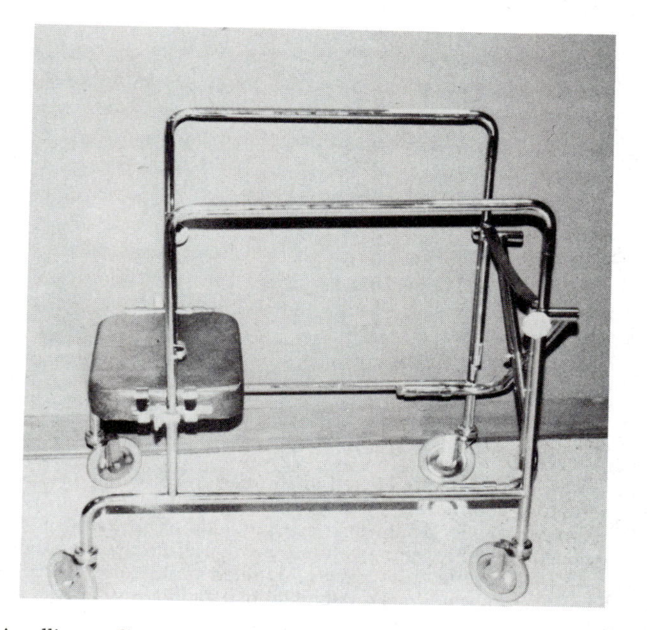

FIGURE 7-3. A rolling walker with a fold-down seat. Allows for ease of interval training in severely debilitated patients.

OUTPATIENT PULMONARY REHABILITATION

Additional data obtained: vital capacity 1000 ml; forced expiratory volume in 1 sec, 490 ml. All additional pulmonary function data can be found in Table 7-1.

Goals

PATIENT GOALS: (1) independence from oxygen, (2) the ability to care for her 10-year-old son, and (3) return to some type of gainful employment.

PROGRAM GOALS: (1) increase lower-extremity strength and endurance (total independence in self-care activities, shopping); and (2) prevent readmission by: (a) maintaining clear lungs, (b) instructing the patient and family in bronchial hygiene, and (c) constant assessment of the patient's status in order to alert the physician to timely intervention with medications, oxygen, or other therapies.

The pulmonary function data (see Table 7-1) documented that the patient has essentially no tidal volume reserve, which means that with any increase in oxygen consumption demand, the patient does not have the abil-

TABLE 7-1. Pulmonary Function Report

Patient Name:	**Age:** 47	**Height (in):** 65
Doctor Name:	**Sex:** F	**Weight (lb):** 116
Patient ID: 9418622	**Date:** 5/15/81	**Room No.:** OP

SPIROMETRY FROM RUN 2		MEASURED	PREDICTED	% PREDICTED
FVC (L)		1.00	3.50	29 ***
$FEV_{.5}$ (L)		0.35	2.17	16 ***
$FEV_{.5}$/FVC		0.35	0.68	51 ***
FEV_1 (L)		0.49	2.68	18 ***
FEV_1/FVC		0.49	0.76	64 ***
FEV_3 (L)		0.78	3.40	23 ***
FEV_3/FVC		0.78	0.97	80
FEF 25–75%	(L/SEC)	0.24	3.04	8 ***
FEF 75–85%	(L/SEC)	0.09	0.96	9 ***
FEF 50%	(L/SEC)	0.31	4.73	7 ***
FEF 200–1200	(L/SEC)	0.01	5.20	0 ***
V(EXT)/FVC		8.0		
FET 100%	(SEC)	6.5		
PEFR	(L/SEC)	1.18	6.18	19 ***
FIF 50%	(L/SEC)	2.35		
FEF_{50}/FIF_{50}		0.13	1	
PIFR	(L/SEC)	2.43		

Interpretation

Spirometry and Flow Volume Loop: Forced vital capacity is severely reduced (1 liter). One second forced expiratory volume (FEV_1) is severely reduced (490 cc). FEV_1/FVC ratio is severely reduced. Flow volume loop shows severe limitation of expiratory flow rates. Inspiratory flow rates are adequate for low lung volumes being utilized. Flow volume loop is consistent with severe obstructive pulmonary disease. Limited ventilatory reserve. Absolute value of FEV_1 of less than 500 cc indicates marked limitation of ventilatory capacity and is associated with a poor short- and long-term prognosis.

*** Outside normal range.

ity to increase ventilation except through increased respiratory rate. An increased respiratory rate in this patient really means an increase in dead-space ventilation. The ultimate outcome of these limitations should be a gross mismatch between ventilation and perfusion, which is only worsened by the increased perfusion occurring during exertion. All of these deductions should be part of the therapist's decision-making process, which then may lead to careful education of the patient and family about the importance of oxygen use.

Outpatient Program

1. Exercise training using ambulation.
2. Patient and family education.
3. Preventive bronchial hygiene.

The patient's exercise program initially consisted of intervals of ambulation three times a week with a wheeled walker and oxygen of 2 liters per minute. Initially, each walking interval was 5 minutes. As the patient progressed and her dyspnea level for the same interval duration of ambulation decreased, the duration of each interval was lengthened, and the number of intervals was decreased. Progression went as follows:

Weeks 1 to 3: four intervals, 4 to 6 minutes each, limited by dyspnea. Patient required assisted manual breathing at the end of each interval during the first 2 months (Fig. 7-4).

Weeks 3 to 6: two to three intervals, 8 to 15 minutes each.

Weeks 6 to 8: two intervals, 20 minutes each. At this point, the patient began ambulating about 1/2 mile in 30 minutes, three times a week in the hospital and two additional times a week at home.

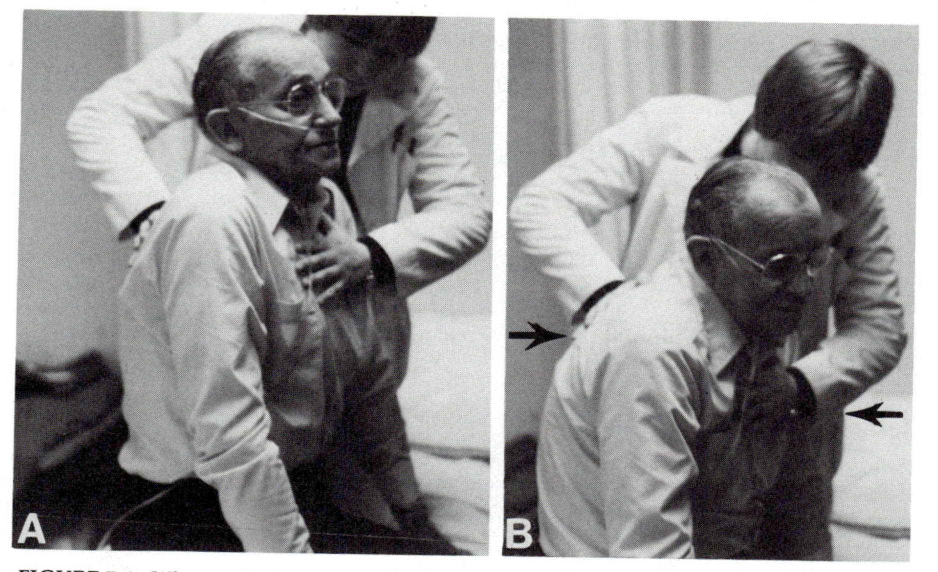

FIGURE 7-4. When patients are severely dyspneic, assisted expiration, performed manually, brings them under control rapidly. *(A)* Assisted inspiration. *(B)* Assisted expiration.

TABLE 7-2. Pulmonary Treadmill Protocol

SPEED	GRADE	TIME	METS
1.3	3%	2 min	2
1.6	5%	2 min	3
1.7	10%	3 min	4
2.0	10%	3 min	5
2.2	11%	3 min	6
2.3	14%	3 min	7
2.3	15%	3 min	8
2.7	16%	3 min	9
2.8	17%	3 min	10

Patient and family education is directed toward prevention of contact with bronchial irritants. They are instructed to avoid crowds, babies, extreme changes in temperatures, and irritants (e.g., sprays, powders, cleaners).

Her son was instructed in percussion, postural positioning and shaking. The frequency of bronchial drainage has decreased to one time a day. The patient is minimally productive, with no change in the color of her sputum.

At this time, the patient's progression is restricted by the therapist's limited knowledge about how well-oxygenated the patient would remain if higher levels of exercise training were attempted. The patient has also requested that she no longer use oxygen. Additional data were needed and were obtained from an exercise test with arterial blood sampling.

The exercise test protocol is found in Table 7-2. The results can be seen in Table 7-3. The patient completed 5 minutes and 20 seconds and was lim-

TABLE 7-3. Exercise Arterial Blood Gas Results

RA/F_{IO2}	TIME	POSITION	pH	Po_2	Pco_2	%Sat	HCO_3
1 L02/min	10:45 am	Sitting	7.41	91	39	97	25
RA	11:00 am	Sitting	7.43	63	42	93	28
RA	2 min exercise	Ambulate	7.43	47	45	84	30
RA	2 min exercise	Ambulate	7.40	45	46	81	29
RA	Peak exercise	Ambulate	7.38	43	48	77	28
1 L02/min	3 min post-exercise	Sitting	7.38	89	45	97	26

Exercise Study:

The patient was exercised using a low-level pulmonary protocol. The patient completed 5 minutes and 20 seconds of the pulmonary protocol. Limiting factors included cyanosis, dyspnea, and leg fatigue.

Interpretation:

Hemodynamic Data: Resting heart rate: 105; peak heart rate: 135. The patient maintained sinus rhythm throughout the study. Resting blood pressure: 150/100; blood pressure at peak exercise: 182/112, which dropped to 122/100 after a 5-minute rest period after exercise was completed.

Electrocardiographic Data: Sinus rhythm was maintained throughout study. There were no ST-T wave changes consistent with myocardial ischemia noted during this study.

ited by 4+ dyspnea. This patient's exercise arterial data indicate that she remains in need of supplemental oxygen during any activity. The first stage of this test requires about 2 mets of work. Many self-care activities are about 2 mets of work. If the therapist is going to progress this patient's exercise tolerance, careful attention must be paid to oxygen supplementation. Even moderate levels of hypoxia can cause more stress on the right ventricle, as described earlier in this chapter.

This patient eventually achieved the following exercise tolerance: 1.3 to 1.5 miles in 45 to 50 minutes with oxygen supplement of 1½ liters per minute. Functionally, she is capable of caring for herself and her son at all levels. She does not work but conceivably could carry out part-time secretarial functions if she had the skills.

Thus, we have, on an ongoing basis, evaluated, assessed, and treated a patient with severe COPD through an acute episode of respiratory failure to complete independence and a relatively high level of function. It should be clearly understood that physical therapy intervention alone cannot begin to explain all of this patient's improvements. As with any patient, a team approach with multidisciplinary intervention is required to achieve the desired goals. Finally, the patient is an individual, and all individuals have differences in their medical data bases, physical therapy evaluations, assessments, psychosocial situations, and motivations that require a varied, adaptable, and functional treatment approach based on decision-making processes founded in the basic sciences.

CASE STUDY 2

The patient is a 55-year-old editor of a small newspaper who had his initial myocardial infarction in July 1976. After his infarction, the patient experienced frequent episodes of chest pain that required large quantities of medications to control. The patient was referred to the outpatient cardiac rehabilitation program 2 years after his heart attack. Following an exercise test and cardiac catheterization (found in Tables 7-4 and 7-5, respectively), he entered into the program.

ENTRY LEVEL: Outpatient referral for cardiac rehabilitation in a patient who was functionally limited to short-distance ambulation due to the onset of angina.

EVALUATION PURPOSES: (1) to obtain initial data base, (2) to assess patient's level of function and motivation, and (3) to establish treatment program.

PRELIMINARY DATA BASE

Medical Chart Review

Prior Medical History: Infero-apical infarction July 1976. Patient was never hospitalized prior to that time.

Present Illness: Severe functionally limiting angina in a patient with two-vessel coronary disease and moderate hemodynamic impairment.

TABLE 7-4. Exercise Test Results, Test 1

Date: 4/17/78 **Age:** 55
Protocol: High Level Bruce Protocol
Medications: Inderal, Isordil, Lasix

Completed: 6 minutes (2.5 mph 12% grade)
Limited by: Level two angina
Resting HR: 52. *Max HR:* 96. *Resting BP:* 140/100. *Max BP:* 150/100.
BP response: Flat systolic BP response with mild diastolic hypertension throughout the test
Chest pain: Initial chest burning began at Stage II minute one, worsened to level two by peak exercise; resolved gradually post-exercise
ST segment: Negative test for ischemic ST changes to a HR of 96
Heart sounds: Normal pre-exercise, S_4 post-exercise
Arrhythmias: 1 supraventricular arrhythmia post-exercise
Physical work capacity: Poor functional aerobic impairment 30% below predicted for a sedentary male

Medications: Nitroglycerin (as needed); Inderal 60 mg, q.i.d.; Isordil; Lasix 40 mg daily.
Chief Complaint: Angina, feeling of fatigue, taking medications.
Personal and Social: Married, two children, very compulsive, aggressive personality, former paratrooper. Editor of a World War II paratrooper magazine. Has attempted a walking program on his own.
Family History: Positive for coronary artery disease. Father died suddenly at age 59; mother had diabetes and died of a heart attack at age 66.

Physical Examination

Strength/ROM: Within normal limits.
Sensation: Within normal limits.
Chest Wall Exam: Palpable tenderness to the left lower rib cage, lateral to the sternum and medial to the fourth intercostal space.
Auscultation: Lungs clear; heart sounds normal.
Weight and Height: 155 pounds; 5 feet 7 inches.
Blood Pressure:

	R arm	*L arm*
supine	140/100	140/100
standing	142/102	144/102

Peripheral Pulses: Normal.
Edema: None.

Patient Interview

Patient is very skeptical that anything can be done for him. He has tried exercising and has stopped smoking, but he continues to have angina. He gets angina with minimal levels of exertion, including slow walking in cold temperatures, sexual intercourse, and walking up slight inclines or stairs. Patient's problems include: (1) angina, (2) high doses of medications, (3) poor understanding of exercise methods and disease processes, (4) fair ventricular function, and (5) persistent hypertension. Clinical decisions are

TABLE 7-5. Cardiac Catheterization Results (Brief)

Hemodynamic Data

Ventricular Function: Hypokinetic movement of the antero-apical and inferior walls
Left Ventricular End-Diastolic Pressure (LVEDP): 14 mm Hg (normal, 0–12 mm Hg)
Left Ventricular End-Diastolic Volume (LVEDV): 139 m^2 (normal, 70 m^2)
Ejection Fraction SV/EDV: 46%

Coronary Anatomy

Right Dominant System
Right Coronary: 75% stenosis at its midportion, and significant stenosis of the posterior descending branch
Left Anterior Descending: 80–90% stenosis of the proximal third with diffuse distal disease
Circumflex: Normal

directed to achieving the patient's goals and to alleviating problems. The program is continually revised as the patient's responses change.

GOALS

Treatment goals are to: (1) educate the patient in proper, safe methods of exercise; (2) educate the patient and his family in the processes of his disease; (3) reduce his angina, and show him how to control his angina; (4) increase exercise tolerance; (5) decrease medications; and (6) decrease hypertension.

PROGRAM

Patient was started on an exercise training program, using aerobic exercise. He was instructed in how to monitor his own heart rate and symptoms. Specifically, we instructed him in how to grade his angina on a scale of levels 1 to 4. This scale is as follows:

level one (L_1): initial perception of discomfort
level two (L_2): intensification of the discomfort in the same place, or a spreading of the discomfort to another area (arms, neck, jaw, and so forth)
level three (L_3): the discomfort is so bad that you stop anything you are doing immediately
level four (L_4): the discomfort associated with a myocardial infarction.

His exercise program consisted of walking at 2.5 mph to a heart rate of 84 and a blood pressure of 160/86 for 30 minutes. He experienced mild level one angina and some calf discomfort. Prior to this peak exercise period, he warmed up with some mild calisthenics and a slow walk. He carried out this program three times a week in the hospital and two times a week at home. The intensity of exercise was not determined by his heart rate response, but rather by his symptoms, which, in turn, gave both of us an initial heart rate guideline for carrying out his home program. Although many textbooks and articles profess that a target heart rate can be obtained from an exercise test, such is rarely the case. The method of work application in an exercise test is not the same as a prolonged bout of exercise. Thus, exercise intensity must be individually determined during the initial weeks of training and based on the patient's exercise responses and data base.

This patient was instructed to exercise to his angina threshold, to level one angina but not beyond. This approach resulted in the following improvements after 4 months. Patient walked at 3.5 mph 6 percent grade for 35 to 45 minutes at a heart rate of 96 and a blood pressure of 150/90. He continued to experience level one angina but also began to experience a walk-through phenomenon. A walk-through phenomenon is occasionally experienced by patients with angina. They exercise to the level of their angina, and even though their workload, heart rate, and blood pressure do not change, their angina goes away. As this program progressed, the patient was instructed about his disease and his risk factors. He initiated a self-designed fat-free diet and compulsively adhered to it.

After 5 months, his Inderal was reduced from 60 mg to 40 mg q.i.d., and his exercise training program was revised. He continued to exercise twice a week at the hospital and three times a week at home. His new program was to walk-jog at 4 mph for 45 minutes, to a heart rate of 108 and a blood pressure of 186/96. He continued to experience occasional episodes of angina. At this point, he injured his left calf at home and was unable to continue his progression.

Six months later, his injury is fully recovered and his Inderal is reduced to 20 mg q.i.d. His exercise program has progressed to walk-jog at 4 mph for 45 minutes to a heart rate of 114 and a blood pressure of 150/80 without angina. He continued to exercise under supervision one to two times a week, and the other three to four times a week at home.

By May 1979, a year after his initial program, he was taken off all his medications, and a repeat exercise test was conducted (Table 7-6). He continued to be followed for nearly another 6 months. His final exercise program consisted of jogging continuously 3.5 to 4 miles in 40 to 45 minutes five to seven times a week, with a peak heart rate 144 to 150, blood pressure 142/82, and no angina. By this time, he weighed 142 pounds and had achieved all

TABLE 7-6. Exercise Test Results, Test 2

Date: 5/30/79
Protocol: High Level Bruce Protocol
Medications: None

Completed: 9 minutes (3.4 mph 14% grade)
Limited by: Fatigue
Resting HR: 56. *Max HR:* 145. *Resting BP:* 130/86. *Max BP:* 158/86.
BP response: Normal response
Chest pain: None
ST segment: Positive test for ischemia, initial ST changes began in Stage I minute 3; maximum ST depression at peak exercise; 2.5–3 mm depression in (V_5) 1.5 mm (V_6); baseline at 9 minutes post-exercise
Heart sounds: S_4 post-exercise
Arrhythmias: None
Physical work capacity: Good to excellent; functional aerobic impairment 8% below predicted for a sedentary male

his goals. His follow-up did not end at this point; he continued to be involved with the program through a bimonthly meeting at a local junior college, where he exercised with other patients and staff of the rehabilitation program.

Thus, this patient was assessed, treated, and continually reassessed and progressed as tolerated until his goals were achieved. The reader should realize that this is an extraordinary patient. He blended the appropriate compliance, intelligence, and motivation into a program that directed him toward his goals. All of these components, along with appropriate clinical decision making based on continuous assessments, are required to achieve success.

SUMMARY

Patient-care decisions need to be predicated upon certain basic elements, which include, but are not limited to, continuous, accurate assessments, basic scientific knowledge of human physiology, and careful coordination of the treatment program with the patient, the patient's family, and other numerous members of the health care team. Assessment of the patient's responses to physical therapy is an objective, continuous process and the foundation for any revisions of goals or modes of treatment. All patient-care decisions should be founded upon these individual assessments, and the resulting treatment program should reflect integration of the patient's data base with well-supported scientific principles.

BIBLIOGRAPHY

ASTRAND, PO AND KAARE, R: *Textbook of Work Physiology*, ed 2. McGraw-Hill, New York, 1977.

CAMPBELL, EJM, ET AL: *Simple methods of estimating oxygen and efficiency of muscles of breathing.* J Appl Physiol 11:303, 1957.

DEMPSEY, JA AND REED, CE (EDS): *Muscular Exercise and the Lung*. University of Wisconsin Press, Madison, 1977.

HEDLEY-WHYTE, J, ET AL: *Applied Physiology of Respiratory Care.* Little, Brown & Co., Boston, 1976.

MASON, DT (ED): *Congestive Heart Failure.* Yorke Medical Books, Dun-Donnelley Pub. Corp, New York, 1976.

MOUNTCASTLE, VB (ED): *Medical Physiology*, ed 14. CV Mosby, St. Louis, 1980.

SHAPIRO, BA, ET AL: *Clinical Application of Blood Gases*, ed 2. Year Book Medical Publishers, Chicago, 1977.

Chapter 8

CLINICAL DECISION MAKING AMONG NEUROLOGIC PATIENTS: SPINAL CORD INJURY

CAROL E. COOGLER, Sc.D., P.T.

In this chapter, clinical problem solving will be approached through evaluation and treatment of a cervical spinal cord injured patient. To facilitate problem solving with a spinal cord injured patient, the relationship of the neural and bony elements of a cervical injury will be presented. The process to be used for clinical problem solving will be based on clinical decision analysis, which was discussed in Chapter 1. A brief review of the clinical decision-analysis process will be presented. Finally, you will be given the opportunity to practice decision analysis by evaluating and editing a decision tree that is based on an evaluation problem encountered with an acute cervical spinal cord injured individual.

ANATOMIC INFORMATION

To facilitate an understanding of how a specific bony injury to the vertebral column can produce precise neurologic symptoms, a brief review of the anatomic relationship of the vertebrae and the spinal cord follows.[1] There are seven cervical vertebrae and eight pairs of cervical nerve roots. The C-1 roots lie between the occiput and the C-1 vertebra; the rest of the cervical roots exit from the foramina at the disk spaces above the vertebra for which they are named. The relationships of the spinal cord, nerve roots, and the vertebrae are shown in Figure 8-1.

Another important anatomic point to remember is that the vertebral bodies are located anteriorly, and the spinous processes are located posteriorly, as noted in Figures 8-1 and 8-2. Locate the body of the vertebra in Figure 8-2 to orient yourself to the anterior-posterior anatomic positions. The spinal cord is located just posterior to the vertebral body. The alpha and

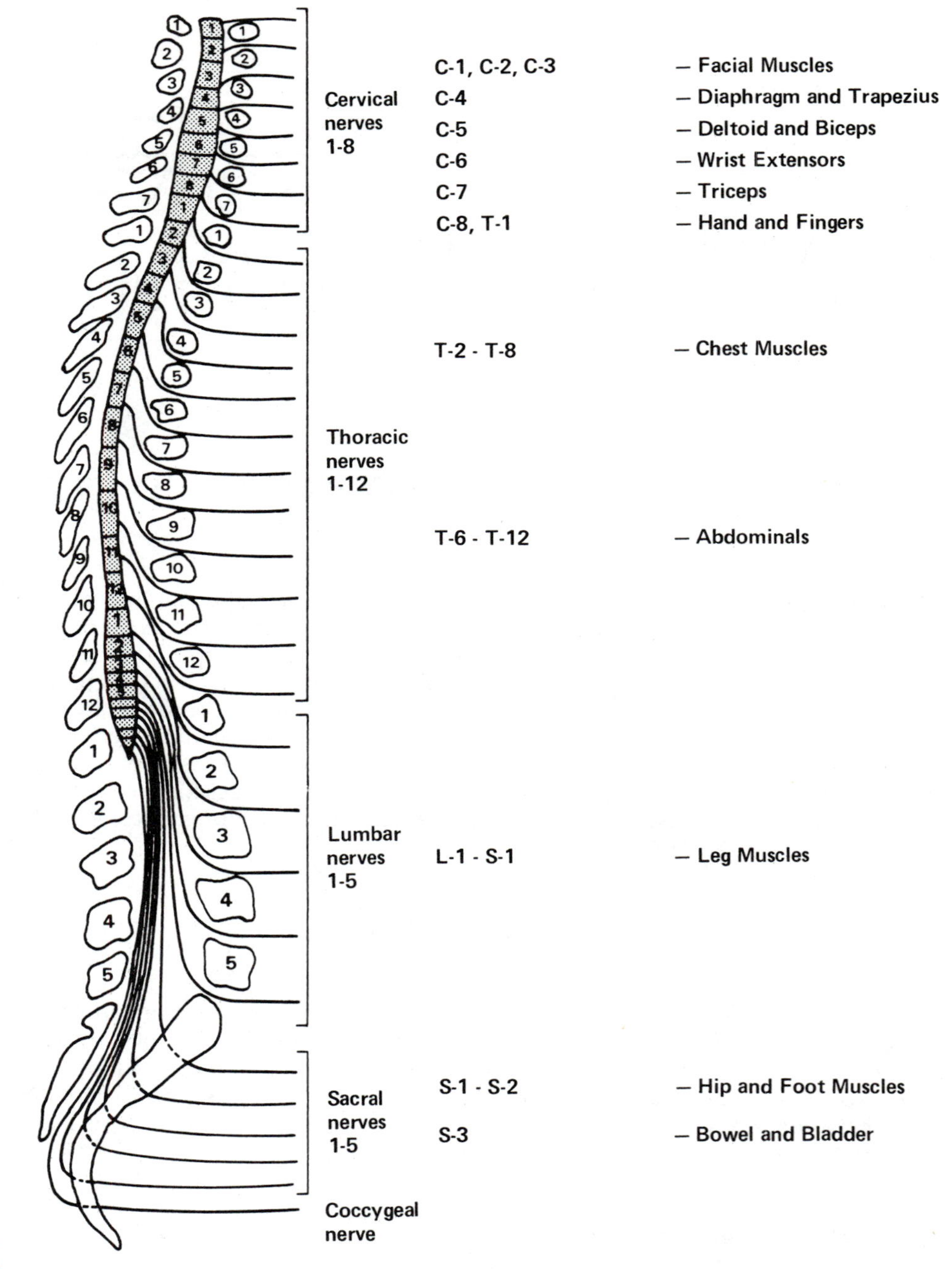

FIGURE 8-1. Diagram of position and segments of the spinal cord with reference to bodies and spinal processes of vertebrae, vertebral column, and spinal cord innervation of key muscles.

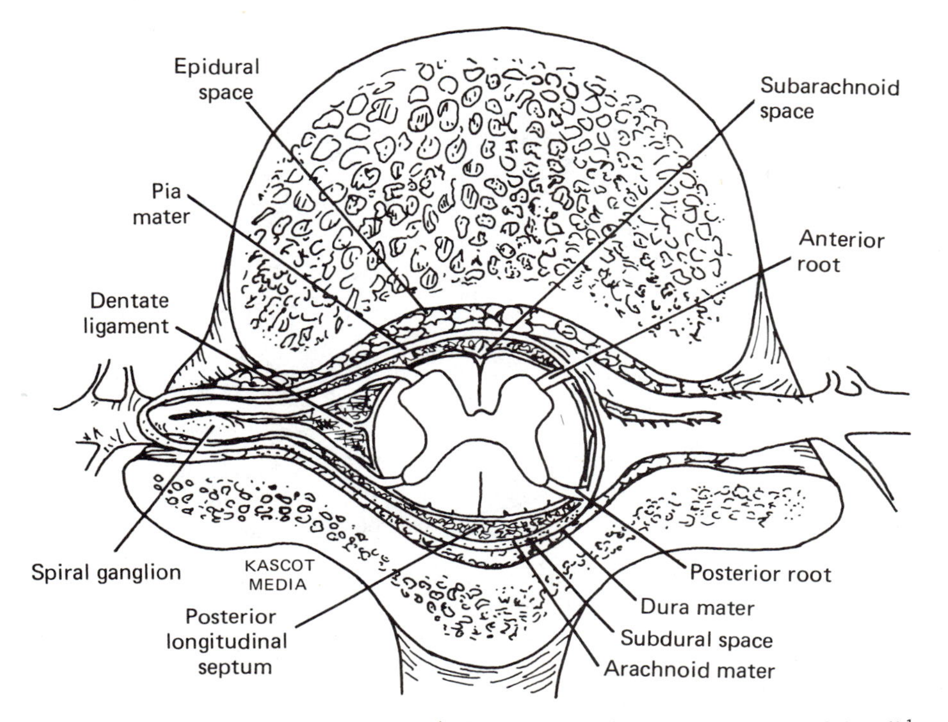

FIGURE 8-2. Diagram of a transverse section of the spinal cord and vertebra. (From Calenoff,[1] with permission.)

gamma motor neurons are located in the anterior horns of the gray matter of the spinal cord.

Knowledge of spinal cord neuroanatomy can produce a more complete understanding of the syndromes seen in the various bony lesions of the vertebral column. Figure 8-3 shows the laminations of several spinal cord tracts. The posterior funiculus, which carries proprioception, deep sensation, and vibration, is divided into the medial and lateral divisions. The medially located fasciculus gracilis contains ascending fibers that enter the cord at the sacral, lumbar, and lower thoracic levels; the fasciculus cuneatus contains fibers that enter above T-6 up to C-1. The lateral spinothalamic tract carries pain and temperature; the ventral spinothalamic tract contains touch fibers. The spinothalamic tracts and the lateral corticospinal tracts are laminated, so the cervical fibers are located medially and the sacral fibers are lateral. The motor neurons, as well as the descending motor fibers, demonstrate anatomic laminations. The lamination of fiber tracts and motor neurons often is the basis for the prediction of neurologic deficits based on bony vertebral injuries.

The neurologic assessment of the spinal cord injured individual includes an evaluation of various levels of reflexes. Spinal-level reflexes are those that occur at the spinal level without any requirement of input from higher centers. The monosynaptic stretch reflex, which results from a tendon tap, is an example of a spinal-level reflex. The tonic vibration reflex (TVR), elicited by vibration of a muscle, is an example of a polysynaptic

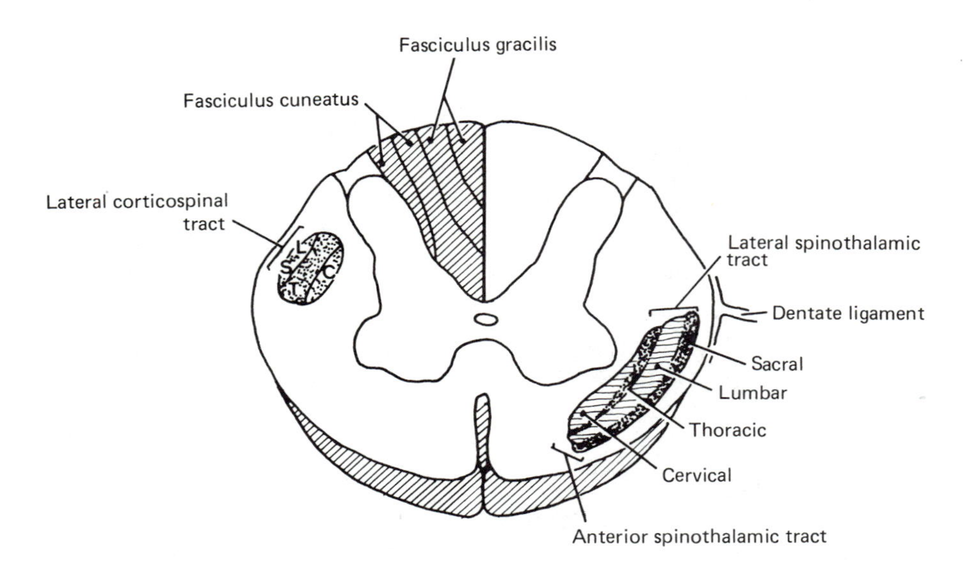

FIGURE 8-3. Laminations of the posterior column, the spinothalamic tract, and the corticospinal tract. (From Calenoff,[1] with permission.)

stretch reflex, which is dependent on input from higher centers. Pathways for both of these types of reflex arcs can be seen in Figure 8-4.

Since spinal-level reflexes are not dependent on input from higher centers, they are present below the level of injury most of the time. Two exceptions to this frequent observation occur when the patient is in spinal shock or

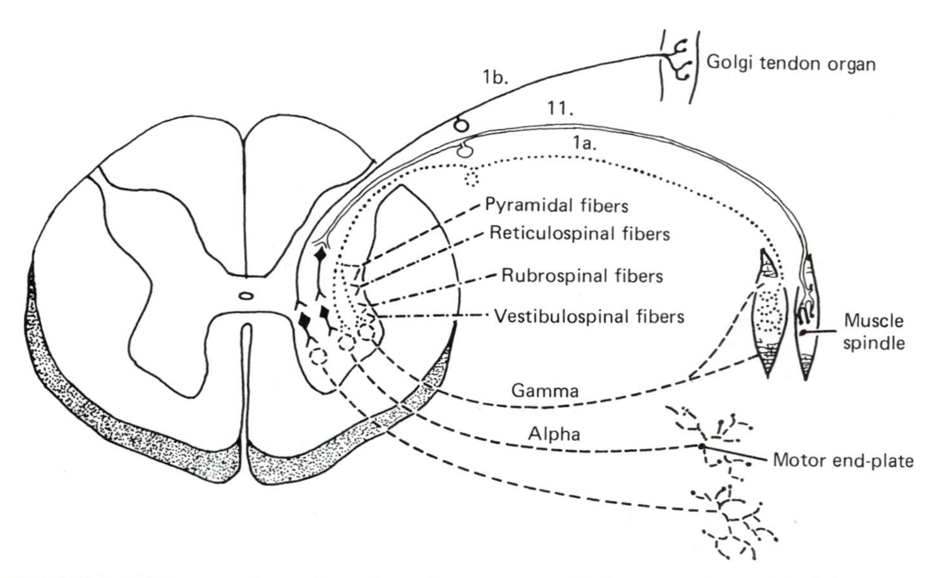

FIGURE 8-4. Diagram of muscle and tendon receptors, their connections with alpha and gamma motor neurons, the monosynaptic, bisynaptic, and polysynaptic types of reflex arcs. (From Calenoff,[1] with permission.)

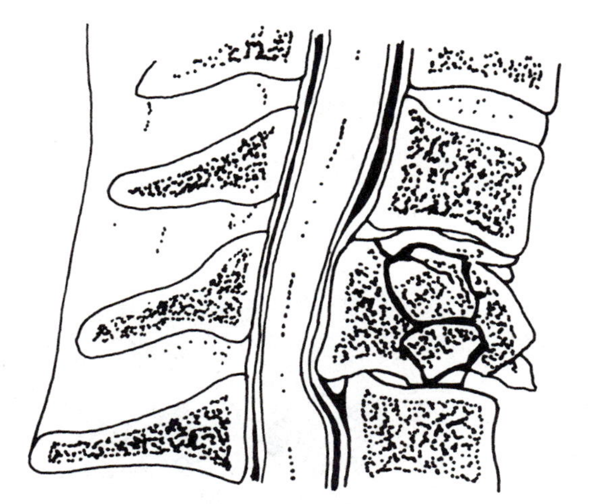

FIGURE 8-5. Diagram of a compression-force injury to the cervical vertebra producing a vertebral body fracture with posterior movement of the body. (From Calenoff,[1] with permission.)

when a nerve root has been injured. Spinal shock is the cessation of all reflex activity below the level of a spinal cord injury.[2] Spinal shock may last from hours to weeks, but generally, the most distal reflex activity begins to return after 24 hours.[3] The bulbocavernosus reflex is part of the physician's examination and is positive if pressure to the glans penis or the glans clitoridis produces a retraction of the bulbous urethra.[3,4] If this reflex is negative, there will be no reflex activity below the injury site. If the bulbocavernosus reflex is positive, but there is no voluntary motor function or sensory innervation (especially in the perianal area), one cannot generally expect future improvement in spinal cord transmission across the injured area or any further return of motor function, except for the improvement of one nerve root level distal to the injury.[2,3] The nerve roots exiting from the spinal cord at the level of the fracture may also be damaged; since nerve roots are peripheral, they may regenerate. A patient who has a complete spinal cord injury and no voluntary motor or sensory function below the injury after spinal shock has ended can expect function to improve by one nerve root.[2,3]

Various forces can produce specific types of vertebral injuries causing spinal cord injury. Most spinal cord injuries result from indirect forces to the vertebrae rather than from direct blows.[1] The areas between the C-4 and the C-7 vertebrae appear to be the most frequent sites of injury in the cervical area.[1] Therefore, these areas are the most susceptible to indirect forces. Blows or forces to the head and upper trunk might be expected to produce injuries in the C-4 to C-7 areas. Flexion is the most common force acting on the vertebral column to produce spinal cord injury.[1] The fulcrum for the cervical movement during a flexion force is the anterior portion of the vertebral body. Such a force can result in an anterior wedging of the vertebral body, a posterior ligamentous tear, and a fracture of the posterior elements.[1,5] Flexion forces rarely occur without compression forces, and the compression forces add another facet to the injury. Compression forces can be great enough to explode the disk into the vertebral body, producing a fracture of the body of the vertebra,[1] as seen in Figure 8-5. There is a specific cervical bursting type of fracture that can result from flexion and compression forces to the head called a "teardrop" fracture. The name results from an anterior-inferior chip of the body of the vertebra that is dislodged and appears similar to a teardrop[1] (Fig. 8-6). The teardrop fracture is a fracture-dislocation of the vertebral body with posterior displacement of the body into the spinal canal. Often, there are accompanying fractures of the posterior bony structures and tearing of the ligamentous supports.[1]

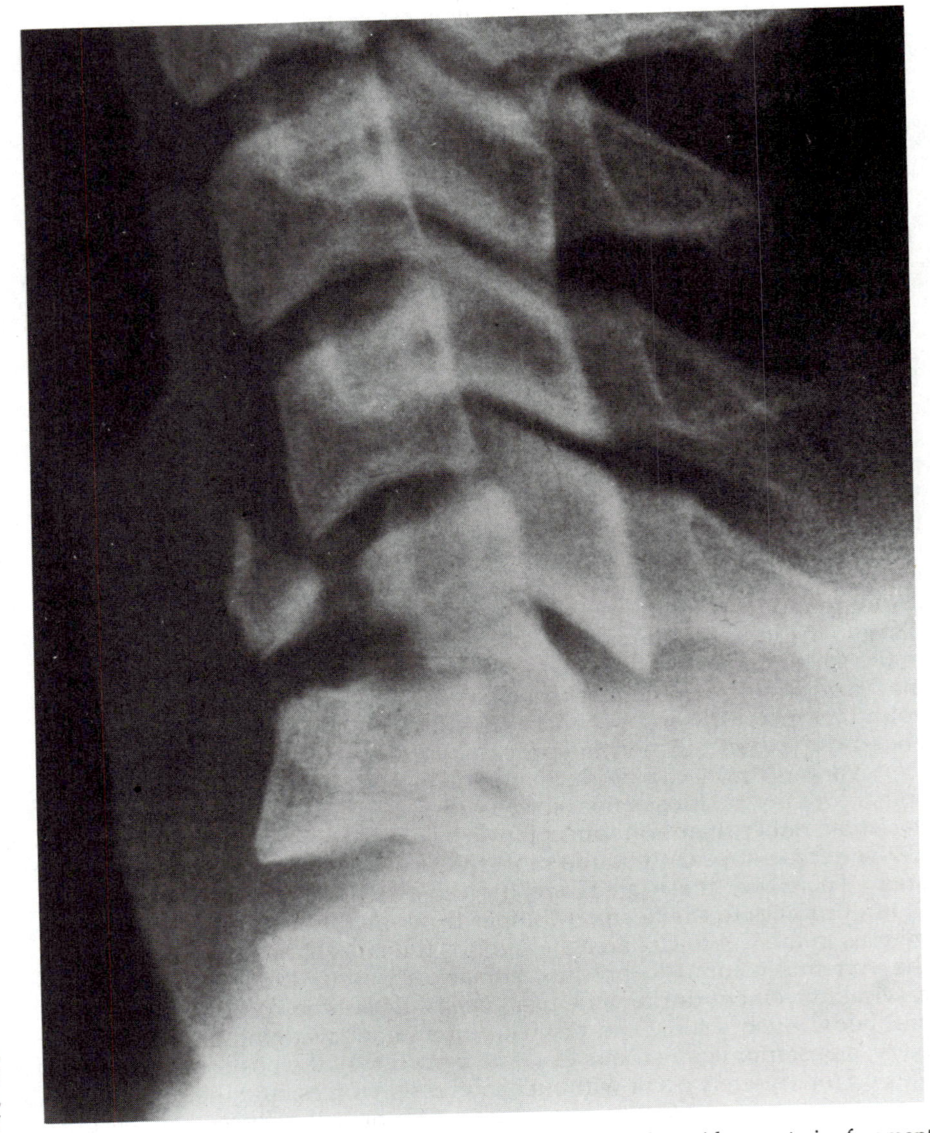

FIGURE 8-6. Lateral view of a "teardrop" fracture of C-5 vertebra with an anterior fragment and posterior displacement of C-5 on C-6. (From Calenoff,[1] with permission.)

A posterior movement of the vertebra will place pressure on the anterior component of the spinal cord and produce a motor deficit from either damage to the motor neurons or damage to the anterior spinal artery.[3,5] The posterior section of the spinal cord is usually spared in this type of injury because it is located away from the injury site. Proprioception, deep pressure, and vibratory sensations should endure.

The spinothalamic tracts, which carry pain, temperature, and touch, are located between the injured and intact areas of the spinal cord. Therefore, these tracts may demonstrate varying degrees of involvement. The specific symptoms of impaired or lost motor function, impaired pain, touch, or temperature, and intact proprioception below the level of a spinal cord injury are referred to as anterior cord syndrome.[1-3,5] Information about the bony injury can allow predictions about the neurologic expectations in a spinal cord injured individual. Neurologic predictions are often useful in planning the initial patient evaluation session.

SPINAL CORD INJURY EVALUATION

Thus far, we have looked at the anatomic and neuroanatomic relationships of the vertebrae and the spinal cord and the effects of compression and flexion forces on these structures. We have hypothesized the type of clinical picture we could see in a patient who has been exposed to these cervical forces. However, hypothetical clinical results do not produce accurate rehabilitation or treatment goals. As physical therapists, we have very special and specific evaluation skills that will allow us to gain an accurate clinical picture of the patient and therefore produce more realistic and accurate goals.

What information is needed to plan the patient's therapeutic rehabilitation goals? These goals are defined as the patient's level of function at the time of dismissal. So you will need information that will allow you to determine if the patient will be independent or dependent in functions such as transfers, ambulation, dressing, eating, bowel and bladder care, driving, and so forth. You will also need to place a time limit on dismissal; for example, independent in all wheelchair functions in 3 months. Patient data that often allow setting the rehabilitation goals during the first week of treatment are as follows: (1) completeness or incompleteness of the spinal cord injury, and (2) the level of the spinal cord injury. These data may be obtained by performing a motor and a sensory evaluation. Figure 8-1 shows key muscles innervated at specific spinal cord levels. A very gross manual muscle test should permit a determination of the injury level and the completeness of an injury.

The same type of gross sensory exam can be used to determine level and completeness of sensory innervation. A dermatome chart (Fig. 8-7) demonstrates that key sensory areas are innervated at specific spinal cord levels.

The level of injury is determined at the lowest normally functioning nerve root segment.[1-3] The term "normally functioning" has a very specific meaning in seeking the lowest nerve root segment. On the manual muscle test, it means that a muscle is operating at a Fair+ or 3+ manual muscle test grade. Looking at Figures 8-1 and 8-7, you will see that the wrist extensors and the skin over the radial aspect of the forearm, thumb, and index finger

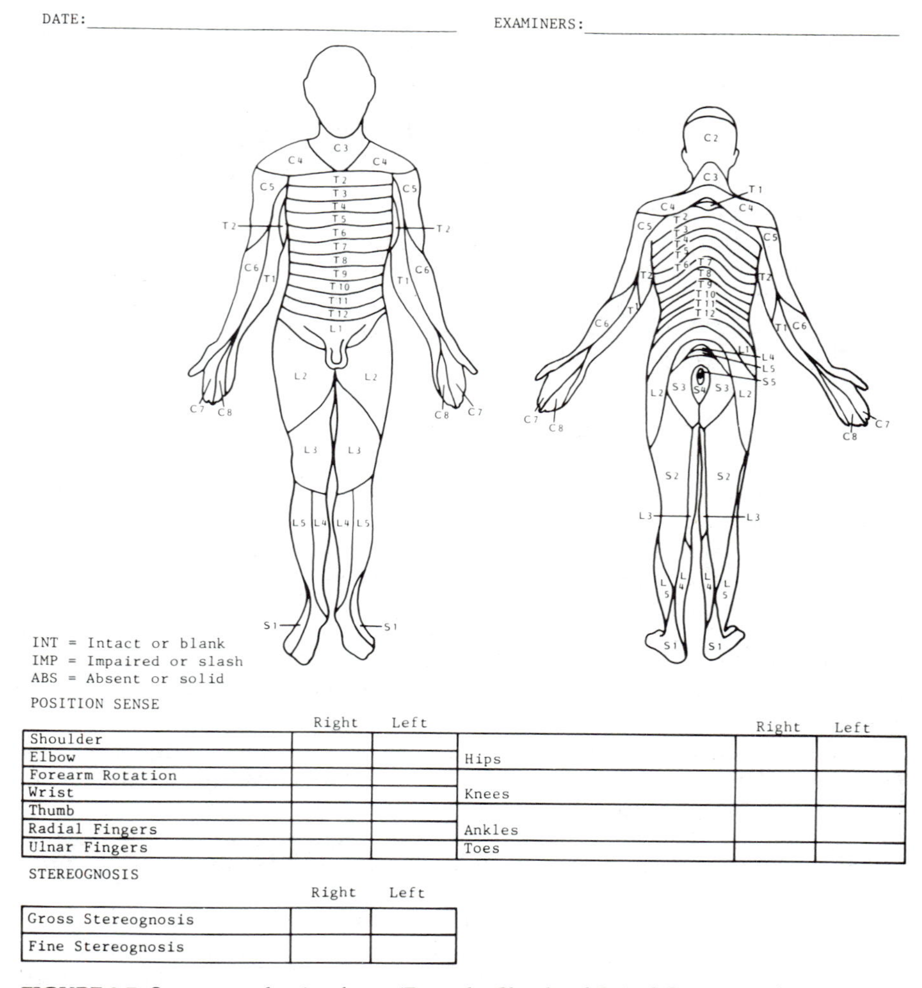

SENSORY EVALUATION

DATE: ______________________ EXAMINERS: ______________________

INT = Intact or blank
IMP = Impaired or slash
ABS = Absent or solid

POSITION SENSE

	Right	Left
Shoulder		
Elbow		
Forearm Rotation		
Wrist		
Thumb		
Radial Fingers		
Ulnar Fingers		

	Right	Left
Hips		
Knees		
Ankles		
Toes		

STEREOGNOSIS

	Right	Left
Gross Stereognosis		
Fine Stereognosis		

FIGURE 8-7. Sensory evaluation form. (From the Shepherd Spinal Center,[6] with permission.)

are innervated at the C-6 level. If an individual has the C-6 nerve root functioning and no motor or sensory function below that level, then the evaluation yields: C-6 functional level, complete. If the individual had spotty sensation or impaired sensation and muscle grades of less than 3+ below the C-6 level, the classification is changed to C-6 functional level, incomplete. Incomplete spinal cord injured individuals may present varied motor and sensory involvements and may be incomplete sensory with a complete motor involvement. Incomplete injuries may demonstrate the incompleteness in the sacral level of innervation first, which means that one could do a very rapid evaluation to determine completeness of injury. In determining the completeness of a spinal cord injury, the toe flexors and the perianal sensation

TABLE 8–1. Potential of the Spinal Cord Injured Patient*

FUNCTIONAL LEVEL	MUSCLES PRESENT	EQUIPMENT	FUNCTION (exceptions to all)
C-1, C-2, C-3	Facial	Mouth-control wheelchair with respirator. Hydraulic lift. Environmental Control System.	Dependent
C-4	Upper trapezius	Mouth-control wheelchair, hydraulic lift, static wrist splint. Environmental Control System.	Dependent
C-5	Deltoid, biceps	Electric cable or rachet brace, motorized wheelchair, hydraulic lift(?). Tub or shower chair.	Self-feeding, light grooming, some communications skills. Weight shifts and transfer assisted(?).
C-6	Wrist extensors	Wrist-driven flexor hinge hand brace, wheelchair, sliding board, tub or shower chair.	Independent in feeding and grooming, communication skills, weight shifts. Wheeling chair, may be able to dress and transfer, may drive.
C-7	Triceps, wrist flexors, possible finger flexors(?), extensors	Possible flexor hinge or finger devices or may not need brace. Wheelchair, tub chair.	Usually independent in self-care and transfers, or may need minimal assist. Drives.
C-8	Flexors, extensors, thumb muscles, maybe intrinsics minus hand	Usually none for upper extremity. May need opponens. Wheelchair, tub chair.	Independent wheelchair and ADL.
T-1–L-1	Upper extremity and various levels of trunk muscles	Wheelchair, possible tub chair, possible long leg braces and crutches.	Independent in wheelchair and ADL. Nonfunctional ambulation.
Below L-2	Various levels of lower extremity muscles	Wheelchair, crutches, long leg or short leg braces.	Independent in wheelchair and possible independent ambulator.

*Adapted from the motor function chart of the Shepherd Spinal Center.[6]

are evaluated first due to their sacral spinal level innervation (Figs. 8-1 and 8-7).

Experience has produced some rather specific rehabilitation goals for the various functional levels of complete spinal cord injuries[1,2,6] (Table 8-1). These goals or expectations are changing with evolving computer and electronic sophistication. The goals in Table 8-1 will apply to most individuals, except those with ample funds or those involved in experimental projects. These goals do not always apply to incomplete spinal cord injuries since 3+ grade muscles could be present in the toe or foot with little present in the hip and trunk, thus producing a sacral nerve root level involvement without the functional abilities at that level.

Putting a time limit on meeting goals involves many of the variables involved in the rehabilitation of the spinal cord individual. Some of the variables that affect the time involved in rehabilitation are as follows: thrombophlebitis, heterotopic ossification, skin problems, spasticity, respiratory problems, urinary problems, autonomic dysreflexia, funding, educational level of the individual and family, family support, and home environment.

While Table 8-1 allows a prediction of functional goals for the complete spinal cord individual, there are additional variables that can affect the reality of these goals and the time required to meet them. The individual's functional ability is greatly affected by age, weight, height, physical condition, and personality. The incomplete spinal cord individual has even more uncertainties operating since there is no early way to determine the final muscle or sensory picture. The incomplete spinal cord injured individual appears to provide an excellent situation for the clinical decision-analysis–problem-solving approach because of the tenuous nature of this condition.

DECISION ANALYSIS

Decision analysis is a systematic approach to decision making under conditions of uncertainty.[7] As physical therapists, we must constantly make decisions about our patients. Like most of the medical profession, we operate under conditions of uncertainty. The basic steps and processes of the systematic approach and the designated outcomes of decision analysis will be used as the basis for clinical problem solving with a spinal injured individual. Less emphasis will be placed on decision making based on quantifiable data (probabilities) because we lack such data in physical therapy, not because the process is unimportant.

Weinstein and associates[7] described the conditions of uncertainty as arising from four major areas in clinical decision analysis. The first area concerns errors in clinical data, which "may be due to inaccurate recording by the observer, faulty observations or misrepresentation of the data by an instrument or by the patient." Secondly, uncertainties arise from ambiguity of clinical data and variations in interpretation. Not only do each of us differ in our abilities as observers (evaluators), but we also differ in clinical education, experience, and values. These differences lead to alternative interpretations of the data gathered. The third source of uncertainty pertains to the relationship between clinical information and the presence of disease. Clinical signs and symptoms are rarely specific to one disease in all patients. Symptoms and signs may be present or absent for any disease process. Apraxia and

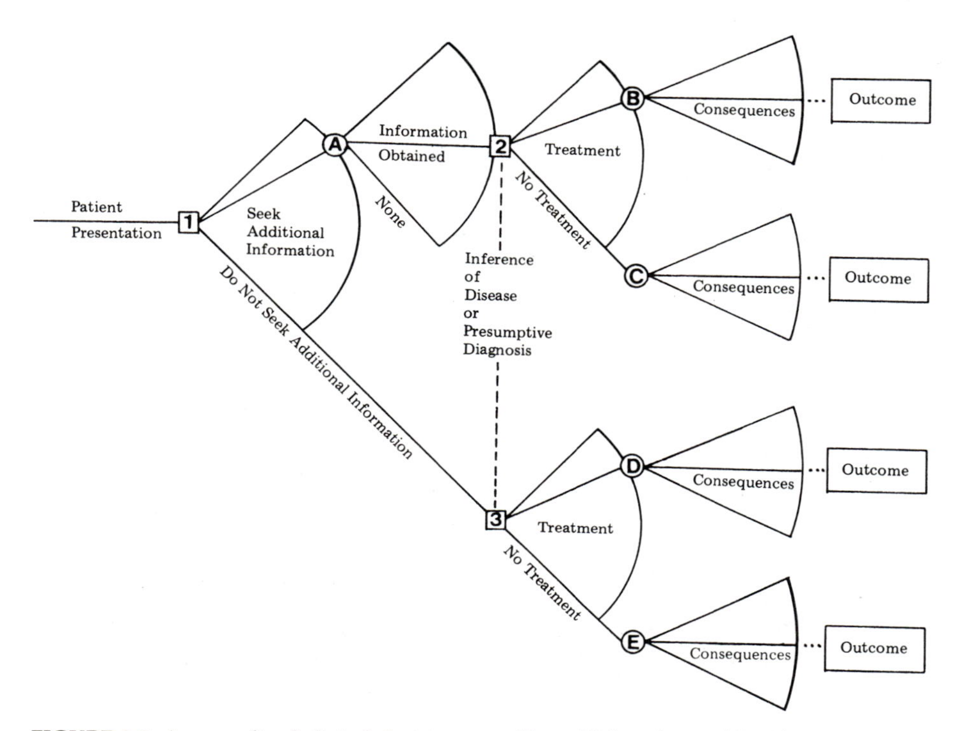

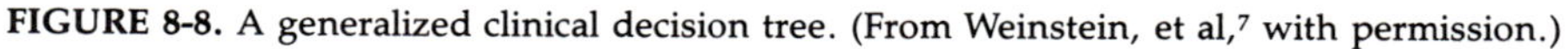

FIGURE 8-8. A generalized clinical decision tree. (From Weinstein, et al,[7] with permission.)

aphasia often occur in individuals who have had a left cerebrovascular accident; however, either or both may be absent. The fourth source of uncertainty is one that is well known to physical therapists—the uncertainty of various treatment effects. There are many variables that affect treatments, from patients of differing physical, social, or value systems to therapists with different experiences, abilities, and values.

Values are always part of decision making, especially when uncertainty exists. In Chapter 1, Watts stressed that the patient's values must play a major role in deciding risks worth taking, since it is the patient's quality of life that is affected by such decisions. One of the specific elements considered in the decision-analysis process is identifying and defining the problem and related factors.[7] These elements involve deciding if there is missing information that can affect subsequent decisions. Looking at alternate treatment options might be involved. This examination requires an evaluation of the clinical states of the patient—not only the present state but possible future and final states. Once the problem has been identified and the limits set, the decision tree can be constructed. A decision tree is a flow diagram that helps us look at sequence and outcome of events.[7] The diagram has two types of nodes:

- The *choice* or *decision node* is a point in time at which the maker can elect one of several alternative courses of action and is designated by a small square.

- The *chance node* is a point in time at which one of several possible events beyond the control of the decision maker may take place and is designated by a small circle.

The choice and chance nodes can be seen in Figure 8-8, which presents a generalized decision tree and its components.

Making a decision tree related to problem solving is an excellent method for analyzing a problem-solving process because it first and foremost requires a specific definition of the problem within a time base. This process requires a list of all possible outcomes of the decision and thus is a great benefit in conditions of uncertainty and for obtaining quantifiable data upon which to base future decisions.

One negative aspect of decision analysis is its time-consuming nature. Physical therapists often have to make far too many decisions to afford the luxury of documenting each of them with a decision tree. Several options to the time problem are as follows: (1) make one decision tree per week; (2) make a decision tree on a specific type of problem every time that it is encountered; and (3) have the therapists in the department make a decision tree on an especially difficult problem each week. The options are many, but practice is needed to internalize the process and make it quicker.

You will be presented with a decision tree that might have been encountered by a physical therapist in her initial evaluation of an acute spinal cord injured individual. The specific case will be presented to you along with the conditions under which the evaluation must be made.

CASE STUDY

INITIAL PATIENT INFORMATION

Bill is a 20-year-old man who sustained a cervical spinal fracture 9 days previously, when he dived into the water after running out from the beach. He said that he dived into a wave and hit his head on a sandbar. He was then floating face down in the water, conscious but unable to turn over and take a breath of air. He subsequently aspirated seawater and lost consciousness. He was taken to a local hospital and placed in Crutchfield tongs. Since the myelogram showed no block, he was left in tongs without surgery. During that time, he was treated for aspiration pneumonia. He was transferred to a spinal center by helicopter and was accompanied by a nurse. Upon arrival at the spinal center, he was examined by the physician, and the following results were found:

Skeletal: ''teardrop'' fracture of the C-5 vertebra
Sensation Level: T-1
    Pin Prick: scrotal = sharp; perianal = R—dull, L—sharp
    Achilles Pressure: +
    Proprioception: intact
Motor Function: lowest functional muscle = wrist extensors
    Lowest muscle present = triceps
    Root level = C-6

Reflexes: Knees = 0, ankles = 1+, Babinski = +, bulbocavernosus = +, anal sphincter = +
Impressions: C-6 incomplete quadriplegia, anterior cord syndrome.

This information was obtained by the physician on the evening of the patient's arrival. The patient was probably fatigued during the evaluation since he had traveled, in skull tong traction, by ambulance from the general hospital to the airport; by helicopter 250 miles; and again, by ambulance from the airport to the spinal center. The therapist was unable to see the patient on the day of his arrival but was to evaluate him the next day. The physician's evaluation would therefore be available to the therapist before she saw the patient.

The therapist knew from the physician's evaluation that Bill was out of spinal shock and was a probable C-6 anterior cord syndrome patient. From the physician's assessment, a typical anterior cord syndrome could be demonstrated because Bill had intact proprioception, motor impairment (complete in this case), and impaired pain and tactile sensation. Is this information sufficient for the therapist to set rehabilitation and treatment goals within a time base? An example of a time-based rehabilitation goal would be independence in transfer and self-care activities in 4 months. If additional or more precise information is needed to set the goals, the therapist must justify the additional time, expense, and hassle caused to the patient. In Chapter 1, Watts described three questions to ask before seeking additional information:

1. Will this information make a difference in how I treat the patient?
2. Is this information necessary to be precise?
3. Can I wait to see if I will need the information?

The information the therapist needs involves determining the accuracy of the physician's muscle evaluation. If motor function is present below the injury level and potential for muscle improvement can be determined, then the rehabilitation goals as well as the treatment are very different. The therapist has decided to seek additional information for the following reasons: (1) the patient was fatigued during the physician's evaluation due to the long trip from the general hospital to the spinal center; (2) incomplete spinal cord injured patients with sensation have difficulty at times initiating muscle contractions without assistance; and (3) the physical therapist has specialized skills and equipment for evaluating motor function.

To determine if the patient's lack of motor function was due to fatigue, the therapist will ask the patient for a voluntary muscle contraction of the toe flexors. The toe flexors were chosen because they have a sacral innervation and should be the first and most obvious muscle present in a patient with an incomplete injury. If the patient is unable to voluntarily produce a muscle contraction, the therapist will apply a vibratory stimulus to the toe flexor muscles with an electric vibrator to hopefully elicit a tonic vibration reflex (TVR). The TVR is a reflex contraction of the muscle that is maintained as long as the muscle is vibrated.[8] This reflex is a stretch reflex that appears to be dependent upon the input from supraspinal centers. If the TVR is present, it might provide evidence that motor pathways are present from supraspinal centers to the spinal motor neurons, thus indicating an incomplete motor involvement. The TVR is maintained by the vibration, and the muscle contraction may be resisted. The patient is asked to contract a muscle and to focus his attention on the "feeling" of that contraction while the therapist elicits then resists responses to vibration in the same muscle. The patient may then regain the ability to produce a voluntary contraction in that muscle. I have observed clinically that sensory incomplete spinal cord injured patients who are unable to initiate voluntary muscle contraction in isolation are often able to do so after using the vibratory stimulus in conjunction with voluntary effort and resistance.

Unfortunately, this method does not provide information on the potential for motor function. Setting therapy rehabilitation goals for an incomplete spinal cord injured individual remains a risky task because the uncertainty is still present. Assessment of the muscular response to treatment, even for just one session, would provide information on the potential for improvement and would allow less uncertainty in goal setting.

In Bill's case, the rehabilitation team's meeting for goal setting is 3 days away, thus allowing time to evaluate his motor completeness and the potential for improvement. The therapist has decided to evaluate the patient for completeness of motor injury and will begin by checking voluntary muscle function. If no voluntary muscle contraction is present below the level of the lesion, then vibration will be used in an attempt to elicit the TVR.

There is one problem with the plan: the possible presence of thrombophlebitis. Many spinal cord injured individuals develop deep venous thrombophlebitis during the first 3 months after injury, and for that reason, venograms are usually a standard admissions procedure at a spinal injury center. The therapist does not know when the venograms will be completed; often, either the test or the results are not available for 2 to 5 days. If the therapist waits for the results of the venograms before using vibration, the treatment, as well as the goals, could be inappropriate. She has no data giving the probabilities of the occurrence of thrombophlebitis in a 20-year-old man with a C-6 spinal cord injury of 9 days. She also has no data about the probabilities of muscle vibration dislodging an existing thrombus. The therapist does have another option for muscle evaluation—electromyography (EMG) biofeedback. By placing surface electrodes over a muscle, it is possible to pick up action potentials from a muscle contraction that is too small to be seen with the eye or palpated.[9] The feedback from the muscle contraction is then displayed visually or auditorally to the therapist and the patient. EMG biofeedback depends on voluntary muscle contraction, and the only assistance to the muscle is through the feedback. The therapist has to make a decision about this evaluation problem.

The problem is defined as follows: How to proceed with a motor evaluation procedure to obtain information needed to set time-based treatment and functional goals for a C-6 spinal cord patient 9 days after injury. The goals need to be set within the next 3 days.

The decision tree for this problem is presented in Figure 8-9. Several of the terms used in Figure 8-9 are unclear and are defined as follows:

wait: wait for the venogram results before vibrating
not wait: go ahead with vibration before the venogram results return
better: improvement in muscle response over what the physician found or over what existed prior to that treatment

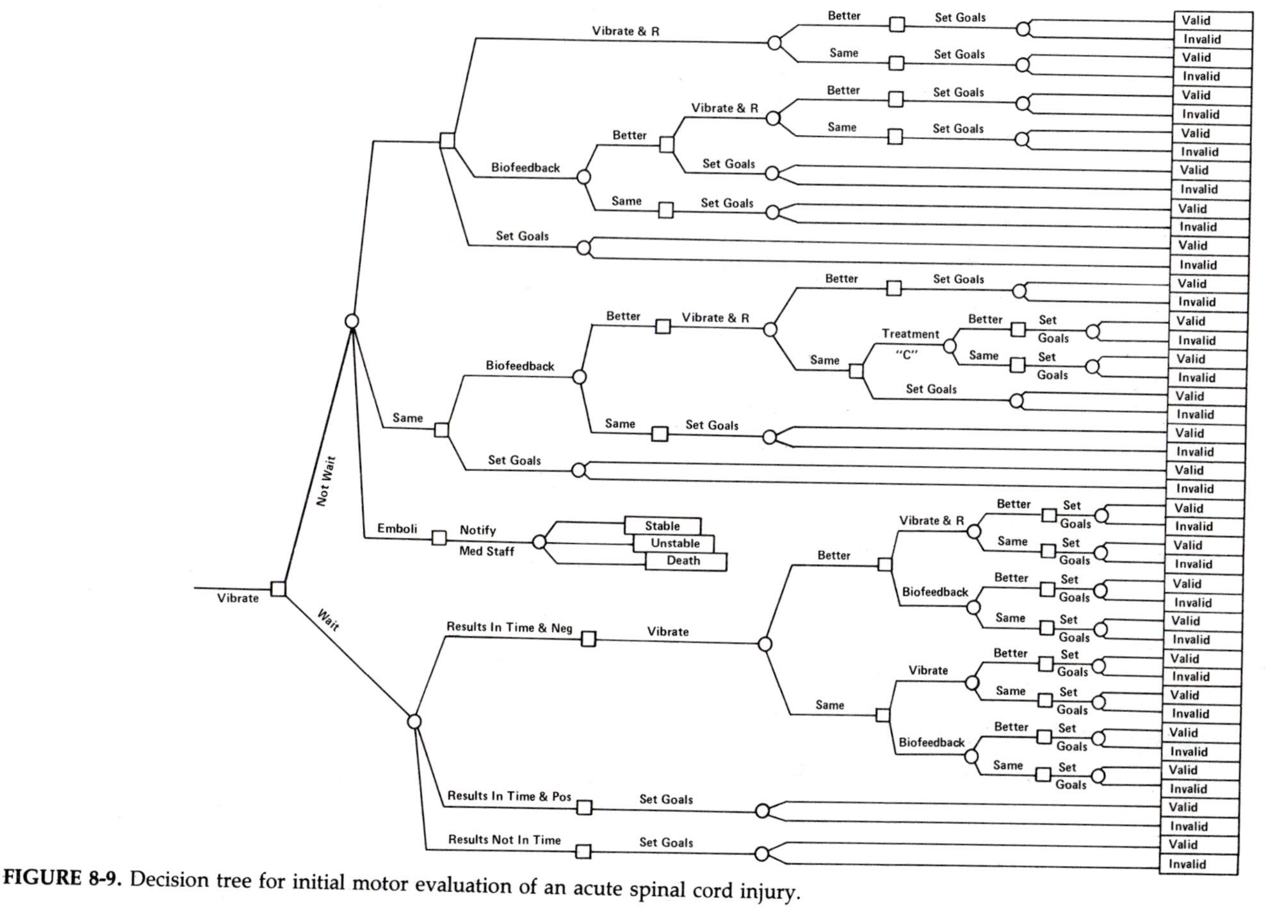

FIGURE 8-9. Decision tree for initial motor evaluation of an acute spinal cord injury.

same: no change in muscle response from what the physician found or from what existed prior to that treatment

biofeedback: use of the portable EMG biofeedback unit to provide visual or auditory feedback to the patient about a voluntary muscle contraction

vibrate: use of electric vibrator to hopefully elicit the TVR

vibrate and R: vibration eliciting a TVR, and resistance given to the muscle contraction

treatment "C": any additional treatment to facilitate or activate the muscle contraction; for example, sensory stimulation or overflow

results in time: results from the venograms returned in time to allow motor evaluation before the goal-setting session

results not in time: the venogram results were not known before the goal-setting session.

You have received information that hopefully will allow you to analyze the decision tree in Figure 8-9. This decision tree represents one thinking process, and you should try to decide which path is the most logical or prune the tree or make additional branches for solving the stated problem.

Two different paths for solving the problem can be ascertained after discussing the case with several therapists. One path is based on the decision not to wait for the venogram results but to vibrate two of the sacral-level innervated muscles, the flexor hallucis longus and the gluteus maximus. The other path is based on the decision to wait for the venogram results before

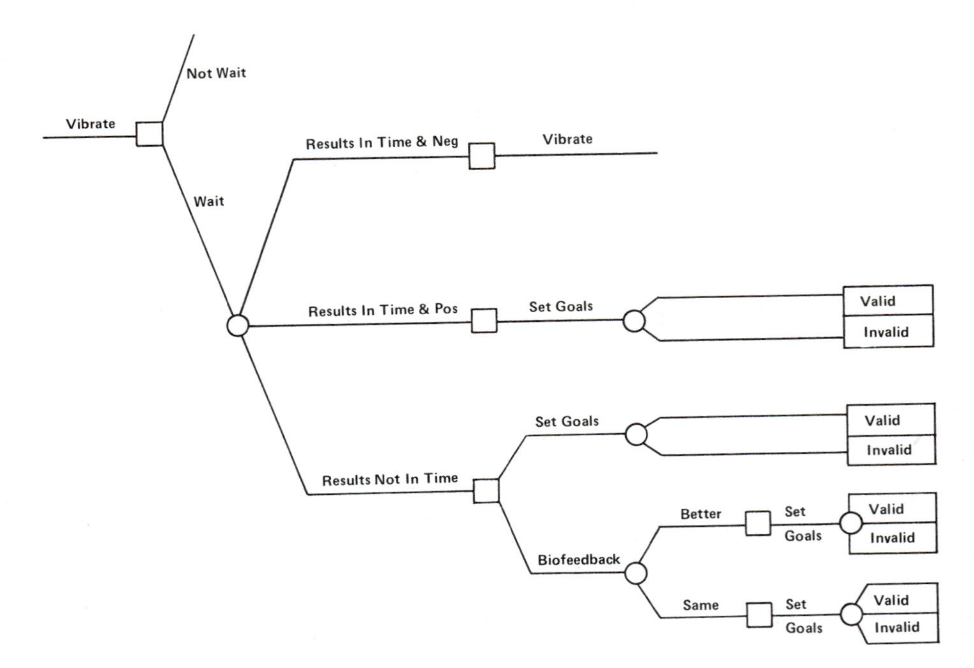

FIGURE 8-10. Additional branch for decision tree for the initial motor evaluation of an acute spinal cord injury.

vibrating. The second decision also assumes that the venogram results might be too late to be of use in the initial goal-setting session, so an additional branch can be added to the decision tree. Rather than just be idle while waiting for the results of the venograms, EMG biofeedback can be implemented (Fig. 8-10). If the venogram results do happen to return "in time," then vibration can still be tried; but if they are "not in time," then the biofeedback might have yielded information that could be of value in setting valid goals.

The additional branch seen in Figure 8-10 is an excellent addition to the tree, and had it been available when the decision was being made about Bill's case, it might have been the decision of choice. The decision not to wait for the venogram was the path taken in Bill's evaluation. The factors that produced this decision were the low incidence of deep venous thrombosis in acute injuries that had occurred at the spinal center at that time and the extreme depression exhibited by the patient.

When the therapist went to evaluate Bill, he was so depressed that he could hardly talk. His voice was shaking, and he was teary. He told her that he had been so happy to come to a spinal center where they would be able to "help" him, but later he had been told that at the spinal center they would be able to teach him to use equipment that would allow him to feed himself again. He had been defining "help" as teaching him to use all of his muscles again, and now he was, for the first time, facing the fact that he might not be able to regain his muscle function. Permanent loss of muscle function is certainly a factor that many or most spinal cord injured individuals have to face; if they do have to face it, then emotional support and guidance must be given. Since Bill was an incomplete injury, special attention must be given to muscle evaluation before he starts the emotional adjustment to permanent paralysis. He either needed the special emotional support and guidance immediately, or he needed to know if he had the possibility for muscle function.

The therapist's evaluation also showed no voluntary muscle function present below the level of injury. The TVR was elicited in the right long flexor of the great toe, in the right gluteus maximus, and in the left gluteus maximus, but not in the left long flexor of the great toe. The therapist went on to evaluate additional muscles and found the TVR present in all of the muscles evaluated in the right lower extremity and in all but the forefoot muscles of the left lower extremity. Voluntary effort and resistance were used in conjunction with vibration. Bill developed the ability to initiate and maintain muscle contractions without vibration. The therapist treated Bill in four different sessions during that first day, and the first manual muscle test was recorded during the second session. The trunk and lower-extremity portion of the first manual muscle test is presented in Figure 8-11 under the date of 3-9-76. Bill's muscle picture, emotional state, and rehabilitation goals had drastically changed.

He not only had most of the trunk and lower-extremity muscles functioning under voluntary control, but they were also demonstrating the ability to improve in just two therapy sessions. During the team meeting, his therapy rehabilitation goals were set for independent ambulation in 4 months time. A quick glance at Figure 8-11 suggests that the goals were met. However, the muscle test does not tell the entire story. Bill demonstrated additional problems that make his case an excellent decision-analysis exer-

MUSCLE EXAMINATION

NAME Bill **BIRTHDATE** 1/6/56

DIAGNOSIS Quadraparesis **ONSET** 2/28/76

4/22/76	3/31/76	3/17/76	3/9/76	Date				Date	3/9/76	3/17/76	3/31/76	4/22/76
RPT	RPT	RPT	RPT	Therapist				Therapist	RPT	RPT	RPT	RPT
				LEFT				RIGHT				
						Facial (check if involved)						
-	-	-	-	St.	C1-3	Sternocleidomastoid	Accessory	St.	-	-	-	-
-	-	-	-	Cl.	C1-3	Sternocleidomastoid		Cl	-	-	-	-
-	-	-	-	C	C1-6	Back Extensors		C	-	-	-	-
4-	3+	3	2	D	T1-T9	Back Extensors		D	2	3-	3+	4
4-	3+	3	2	L	T10-L5	Back Extensors		L	2	3-	3+	4
-	-	-	-		T12-L2	Quadratus			-	-	-	-
4	4	4	3+		C6-8	Latissimus	Thoracodorsal		3+	4	4+	4+
4-	3+	2+	1+		T7-10	Upper Rectus			2	2+	3+	4
↓	↓	↓	↓		T10-L1	Lower Rectus			↓	↓	↓	↓
↓	↓	↓	↓	Med.	T7-10	External Obliques		Med.	↓	↓	↓	↓
↓	↓	↓	↓	Lat.	T7-10	External Obliques		Lat.	↓	↓	↓	↓
↓	↓	↓	↓	Med.	T10-L1	Internal Obliques		Med.	↓	↓	↓	↓
↓	↓	↓	↓	Lat.	T10-L1	Internal Obliques		Lat.	↓	↓	↓	↓
4-	3-	2+	2		L5-S1	Gluteus Maximus	Inf Gluteal		↓	2	3-	4-
3-	↓	↓	1		L4-S1	Gluteus Medius	Sup Gluteal		1	2	3	4-
-	-	-	0		L4-S1	Tensor Fascia Lata	Sup Gluteal		1	-	-	-
3-/4-	2+	2+	0		L1-4	Iliopsoas			0	3	3+	4
2+	-	-	0		L2-4	Sartorius	Femoral		0	1	2+ ½	4-
3-	3	3	1		L2-S1	Hip Adductors	Obturator		1+	3+	4	4+
4	3+	3	1	Ext.	L3-S2	Hip Rotators		Ext.	2	↓	4-	5
4	4-	3	1	Int.	L4-S2	Hip Rotators		Int.	2	↓	4+	4+
4+	3+	2	1		L2-4	Quadriceps	Femoral		1+	2+	3+	↓
4	3+	2+ ½	1	Int.	L4-S2	Hamstrings	Sciatic	Int.	1	2+	4-	↓
4-	3+	2+ ½	0	Out.	L5-S3	Hamstrings	Sciatic	Out.	1	2+	4-	↓
4-	4	3	0	Ly.	S1-2	Triceps Surae	Tibial	Ly.	0	3	4	-

3	-	-	-	St. S1-2	Triceps Surae	Tibial	St.	-	-	-	4-
2+	1+	1+	0	L4-5	Anterior Tibial	Peroneal		0	4-	4	5
4	4-	2+	↓	L5-S2	Posterior Tibial	Tibial		2	3+	4+	↓
4+	4-	2+		L4-5	Peroneals	Peroneal		2	↓	↓	
4	3+	3-		L4-S1	Extensor Digitorum Lonqus	Peroneal		0		4	4
4	3+	2+		L4-S1	Extensor Digitorum Brevis	Peroneal		1+	2	3+	↓
4	3+	3		L4-S2	Extensor Hallucis Proprius	Peroneal		2-	3+	4	5
4+	4+	3+		L4-S2	Flexor Hallucis Longus	Tibial		2	↓	↓	↓
↓	↓	↓		L5-S2	Flexor Digitorum Longus	Tibial		2+ ↓			
				L5-S1	Flexor Digitorum Brevis	Plantar					
				L5-S2	Intrinsics	Plantar		1	-	-	
				L5-S2	Flexor Hallucis Brevis	Plantar		1+	2	3+	

KEY:

5	Normal	Complete range of motion against gravity with full resistance
4	Good	Complete range of motion against gravity with moderate resistance
3	Fair	Complete range of motion against gravity
2	Poor	Complete range of motion with gravity eliminated
1	Trace	Evidence of slight contractility. No joint motion
0	Zero	No evidence of contractility

Plus (+) and minus (-) signs after the letter indicate a more precise grade as: 5-; 4+; 4-; 3+; 3-; 2+; 2-.
Str = strand of muscle. P+ ½ = ½ test range.

Muscle spasm, contracture or weakness may limit range of motion; thus, a grade for range and a grade for resistance as:
3-/4 = Fair minus range with good or medium resistance at that point.

COMMENTS: Right hand used for writing

FIGURE 8-11. Lower-extremity and trunk manual muscle test for a C-6 incomplete spinal cord injury.

cise. Some of the additional decisions encountered during Bill's hospitalization are briefly described in the following paragraphs.

Bill's lower-extremity strength increased so much that it was soon difficult to treat him on the Stryker frame. Movement of and resistance to the lower extremities often would result in a loss of cervical traction. The decision was made to place him in halo traction rather than to allow him to remain in tong traction or to undergo a surgical stabilization. Three to 4 days after being placed in halo traction, Bill was up in a wheelchair, beginning assisted stand pivot transfers and being treated on the mat. His upper-extremity motor function was not returning nearly as rapidly as his lower-extremity function, and he had to move his wheelchair with his lower extremities. While Bill's trunk and lower-extremity muscle grades were improving rapidly, his "coordination" in the use of those muscles was poor. Mat work with a patient in halo traction allows rather limited movement.

Bill appeared to need some form of guided resisted movement for the postural muscles of the trunk and lower extremities. The Swiss Gymnastic Ball is a method used to initiate the postural muscles during movement in an antigravity position. But is this a feasible treatment for an individual in halo traction? The patient has both trunk and lower-extremity muscles, and with two individuals guarding him, he should be safe on the Ball. Therefore, it is a feasible treatment. An additional rationale for the use of the Swiss Gymnastic Ball for an individual in halo traction is to increase vestibular stimulation. Since his injury, Bill had been in tong and halo traction with limited or no head or neck movement. The upper extremities normally function in conjunction with eye, head, and neck movements, two of which no longer exist for a patient in halo traction. Considerable sensory input had been lost because of limited head and neck movements. Little can be done to improve upon the amount of sensory input from the neck proprioceptors while Bill was in halo traction.

Activities on the Swiss Ball such as bouncing, turning, and lateral moves would increase the vestibular input. This increase in vestibular input might serve to increase the "resting excitatory level" of the upper-extremity neuromuscular system and allow extremity function to be more easily elicited. Bill was the first patient in halo traction to be treated on the Swiss Ball at the spinal center, and he did better than expected. His upper-extremity function improved, as did his trunk and lower-extremity "coordination." He was soon ambulating with a forearm crutch. Swiss Ball Gymnastics was not the only treatment that he was receiving, so his improvement could not have resulted from that treatment alone. Bill continued to improve. The halo was ultimately removed, and he was discharged. His strength was not normal at discharge. The muscles in his left hand had 2 (Poor) to 3 (Fair) grades; the muscles in his right hand were mostly 4 (Good), with the exception of the intrinsics, which were at 2 to 3 grades. His lower extremities were much better. All grades were at the 4+ (Good+) to 5 (Normal) level except for the left tibialis anterior, which was 3+ (Fair+). He went home on an exercise program for the summer and returned to college in the fall. He did have to return to the spinal center after starting college because he found that his anterior tibial muscle did not have the endurance needed for college life, and a plastic ankle foot orthosis shoe insert was ordered for his left leg. Bill graduated from college and is currently a successful businessman and happily married.

Had the therapist decided not to vibrate but to use biofeedback as the first choice, the results of Bill's case probably would not have been any different. The decision is different in each case, as could be the results. While decision analysis may be the result of one person's thinking process, this case has shown how a beneficial branch can be added to the decision tree if several people contribute to the thinking process. Involving many therapists in outlining problem solving with decision analysis and decision trees and solving the problems according to the outlined processes would allow more specific documentation of successful and unsuccessful decisions. If this procedure is followed, then probabilities of success for the different methods used in physical therapy could be established. Once the probabilities of various therapy approaches are available, then the patients can play a more active and responsible role for their own health care decisions and outcomes.

Physical therapists are required to make many decisions daily about patient treatments. Many different decision-making methods are used by therapists in problem solving. Unfortunately, many of the decision-making methods do not allow for the uncertainty that exists in patient care, and many of these methods do little to decrease uncertainty for future decision making. In my many years of physical therapy practice, I have made many decisions regarding patient treatments. Many of my decisions resulted in good outcomes, but some resulted in poor outcomes. Since I did not document the decisions and outcomes, they have been of little help to other therapists or to me today. Clinical decision analysis is a method of problem solving in the presence of uncertainty. In Chapter 1, Watts presented a description of this method of problem solving and its rationale. This method requires an explicit definition and delineation of the problem, with a diagram of all possible time-based solutions and outcomes. This method allows for documentation and communication of the outcomes from the decision making. Little documentation exists for the outcomes of many physical therapy treatments; thus, clinical decision analysis appears to be a much needed approach for physical therapists. While decision analysis initially requires more time than most therapists have available for this process, therapists working together using this method of problem solving for specific problems once or twice a week can make an excellent peer-review or in-service session.

Clinical decision analysis is a logical and necessary approach to decision making for physical therapists, and it will benefit our profession.

SUMMARY

Anatomic and rehabilitation information necessary for decision making with spinal cord injury was presented. The basis for clinical decision making was presented, with emphasis on making a decision tree and involving the patient and/or the family in this process. The case history of an acute spinal cord injured young man and the physician's initial evaluation were used for solving a therapy problem by clinical decision analysis. A decision tree was given with possible solutions and outcomes along with an additional branch produced by a group of therapists working together. Some advantages of clinical decision analysis for physical therapists were presented.

REFERENCES

1. Calenoff, L (ed): *Radiology of Spinal Cord Injury.* CV Mosby, St. Louis, 1981.
2. Pierce, DS and Nickle, VM (eds): *Total Care of Spinal Cord Injuries.* Little, Brown & Co, Boston, 1977.
3. Young, RF and Feldman, RA: *Spinal Cord Injuries: Case Studies.* Medical Examination Publishing, Garden City, NY, 1981.
4. *Dorland's Illustrated Medical Dictionary,* ed 23. WB Saunders, Philadelphia, 1960.
5. Donovan, WH and Bedbrook, G: *Comprehensive management of spinal cord injury.* Clin Symp 34:12, 1982.
6. Shepherd Spinal Center, Occupational and Physical Therapy Departments, 2020 Peachtree Road, N.W., Atlanta, Georgia 30309, 1980.
7. Weinstein, MC, et al: *Clinical Decision Analysis.* WB Saunders, Philadelphia, 1980.
8. Bishop, B: *Vibratory stimulation. I. Neurophysiology of motor responses evoked by vibratory stimulation.* Phys Ther 54:1273, 1974.
9. Nacht, M, Wolf, SL, and Coogler, CE: *Use of electromyographic biofeedback during acute phase of spinal cord injury.* Phys Ther 62:290–294, 1982.

Chapter 9

CLINICAL DECISION MAKING AMONG NEUROLOGIC PATIENTS: STROKE

MAUREEN K. HOLDEN, M.M.Sc., R.P.T.

THE DECISION-MAKING PROCESS

Every year in this country, physical therapists treat thousands of patients who have suffered strokes.[1] The number and variety of physical therapy techniques available to treat these patients are quite large and growing at a rapid pace.[2-13] How do we as physical therapists intelligently choose, from among the myriad of techniques available, those that will be the most effective? How can we adapt approaches to meet the needs of our particular patients?

Improving our ability to choose the treatments to maximally benefit our patients requires that we begin to analyze the process used to make these treatment decisions. Without knowledge of the factors that interact to influence our clinical decisions, both our attempts to improve our decisions and the quality of the patient care we provide will be hampered.

Examining my own clinical-judgment process has led me to distill the key components that influence my clinical decision making and to synthesize the components into a working model. I will explain the model and attempt to demonstrate its usefulness by illustrating the application of the model to the case problem of a patient who suffered an embolus to her middle cerebral artery.

The decision-making model is illustrated in the flow chart in Figure 9-1. The key decisions made by the therapist are located in the center of the diagram:

1. elements to evaluate and which methods of evaluation to use
2. assessment of problems and setting of goal priorities
3. method and frequency of treatment
4. measurement of outcome of treatment

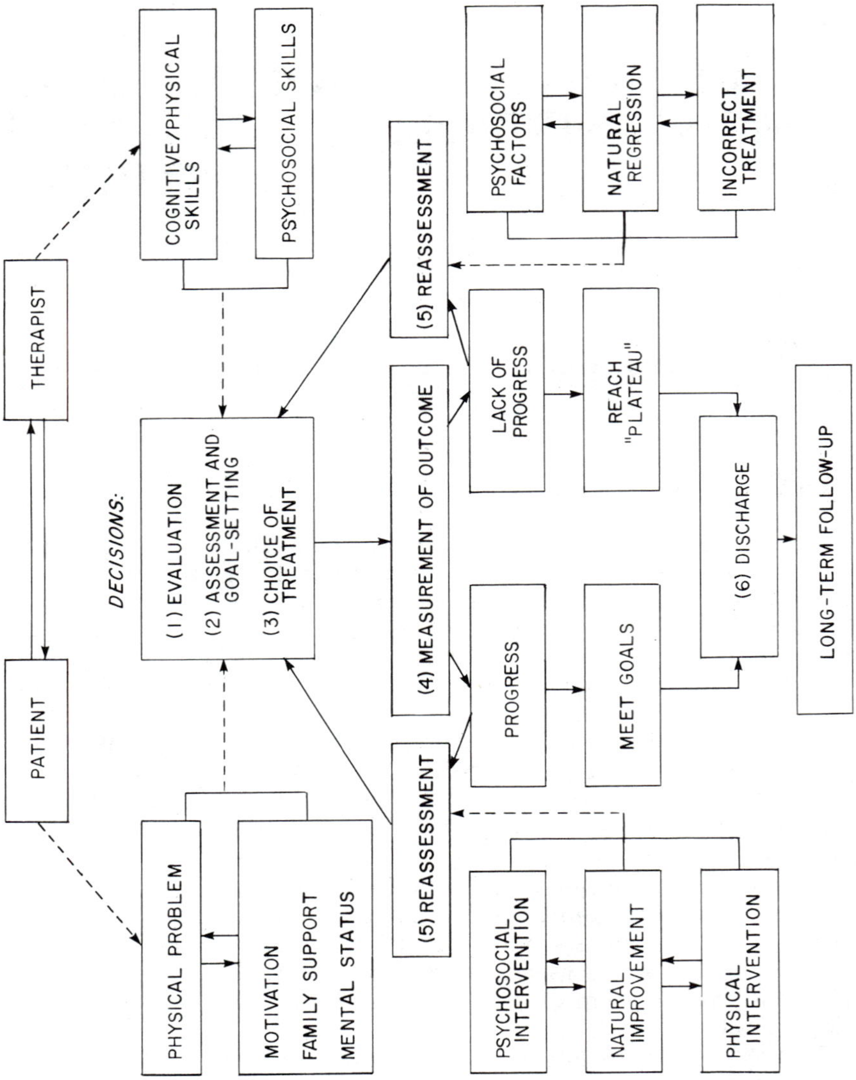

FIGURE 9-1. Flow chart illustrating the decision-making model.

5. criteria to change treatment (reassessment)
6. criteria to discharge patient.

Factors that influence these decisions are shown in the boxes surrounding the decision list. The two main actors in the process are the patient and the therapist.

For the purpose of clarity and emphasis, the factors that influence the patient or therapist in the decision-making process are distilled. For the patient, the essential elements are as follows: (1) physical status, and (2) psychosocial status. The physical status includes all of the general medical problems of the patient, but the major emphasis is on the physical problem for which the patient is seeking physical therapy treatment. Psychosocial status includes the major factors of motivation, family support, and mental status. A recent report by DeJong and Branch[14] revealed that of 17 social/demographic, disability related, and environmental variables, the two most important factors in predicting independent living in stroke patients were marital status and ability to get in and out of a car. This study points out the pitfalls of too narrow a focus on the patient's physical problem (for which we are most skilled to intervene) to the exclusion of other factors in making our treatment decisions and predicting outcomes.

Two key factors in the therapist's decision making are as follows: (1) the therapist's cognitive/physical skills, and (2) the therapist's psychosocial skills. Knowledge of the problem and of ways to treat it are obviously prerequisites to effective decision making. If knowledge of pathophysiology of the disorder or tools available to treat the disorder are limited, the likelihood of errors in judgment increases. The therapist's psychosocial skills can influence the ability to make appropriate decisions as well. If the therapist cannot communicate well with other health professionals who possess information essential to patient management, such as the physician, nurse, social worker, occupational therapist, and speech therapist, or does not listen to the stated goals of the patient and family, incorrect decisions can easily be made. The double line directly between the therapist and the patient serves to emphasize that a direct personal interaction between the two may be an unconscious factor in the decision-making process. For example, Lobitz and Shepard[15] recently illustrated this unconscious influence by describing the effect of patient-therapist psychological "dyads" on treatment outcomes in physical therapy management of spinal cord patients.

How are the cognitive, physical, and psychosocial skills of the physical therapist put to use in the actual decisions identified in the center of the diagram in Figure 9-1? To show this, we must examine the decision points in greater depth. Figure 9-2 illustrates the steps involved in evaluation, assessment and goal setting, and choosing methods of treatment and outcome measurements. If outcome measures are not directly related to the therapy goals and treatment, reassessment and discharge decisions become extremely difficult. Later, the discussion of a case history will show how the skills of the therapist are used to make decisions in each of the steps illustrated in Figure 9-2.

The decisions of whether and how to change treatment result from the process of reassessment, shown in the lower half of Figure 9-1. Once therapy has been initiated, the patient either makes progress toward the goals or does not. In reassessing the patient, the therapist is making judgments

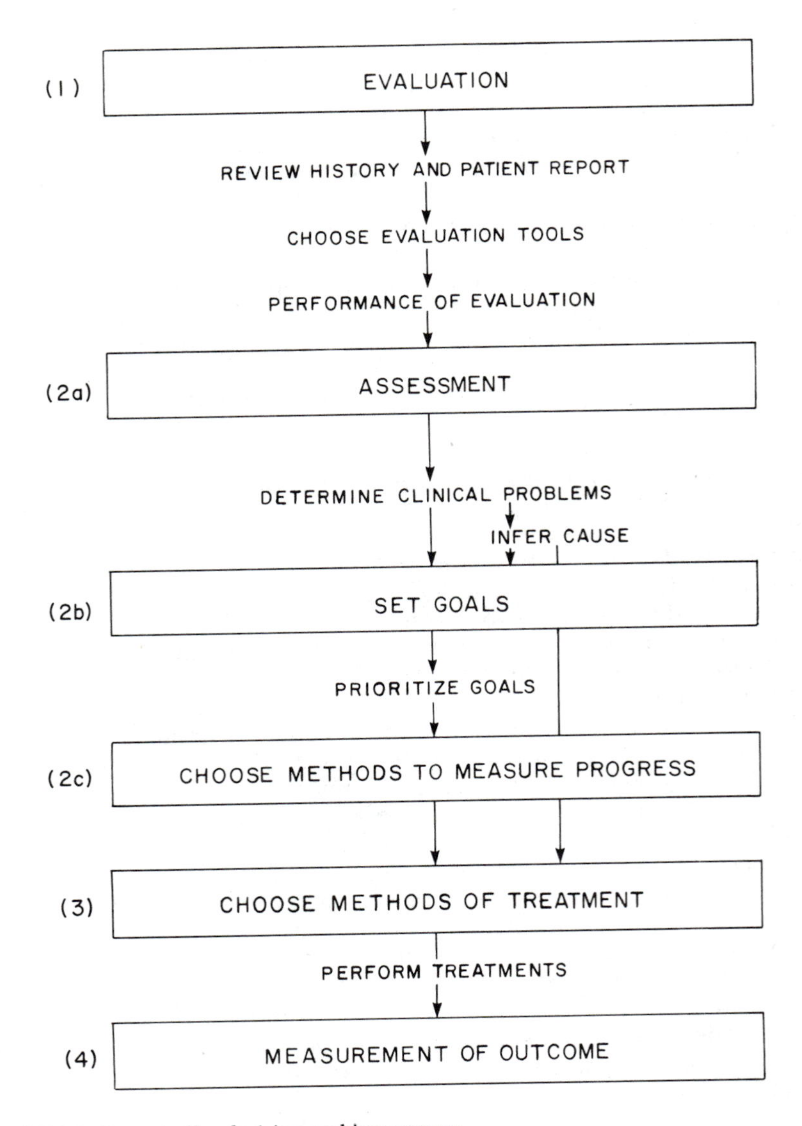

FIGURE 9-2. Steps in the decision-making process.

about the reasons for that progress or lack of progress. The three key elements that can explain the patient's response to treatment are responses due to: (1) intervention, (2) psychosocial factors, (3) natural recovery/regression factors. In reassessment, we take our judgments concerning the cause of the treatment response and cycle again through to decisions in the upper part of the model to refine the goals and methods of treatment to meet the needs of that particular patient.

Ideally, in working with the patient one continues to cycle through the reassessment channel until all of the desired goals have been achieved, or until the patient reaches a ''plateau'' of nonresponse to intervention. If the measured outcomes truly reflect the goals of treatment, then the decision to discharge should be made easier. Long-term follow-up is included in the model because it is essential to identify those patients who would continue to regress without periodic therapy (e.g., in patients for whom a natural regression can be expected, maintaining a "plateau" may really be defined as progress), and because long-term follow-up is essential for determining the long-term benefits of physical therapy intervention.

What may be apparent is that this decision-making model offers a partial explanation for why physical therapists have resisted the development of standardized treatment protocols for defined patient populations (in its extreme form, known as the "cookbook" approach). Therapists with experience and high skill levels recognize that the interaction and influence of the key elements influencing patients' responses to treatment are unique for each particular patient and, thus, dictate an individualized approach to evaluation and treatment planning. Yet, standardization of treatment protocols is a necessary element in the clinical research we sorely need to examine the effectiveness of our techniques. Is there a way to balance these two demands? Physical therapists are not alone in the dilemma of attempting to determine effectiveness of interventions and in trying to apply therapeutic principles of management to individual cases that may differ from the "typical" case. The decision-making model in Figure 9-1 could easily be considered generic for all types of medical/psychological management. Other disciplines have attacked the problem of extracting general principles of management from a collection of unique and individual case problems and have progressed in testing these principles in controlled trials. Physical therapy can do so as well. What is required is a commitment to objectively testing our cherished beliefs (and perhaps learning that some of them are not true), a commitment to recording and sharing our observations so that we may develop a larger knowledge base, and an increased awareness and use of information that is already available and published.

This decision-making model can help us direct our efforts to collect and synthesize our present knowledge and to identify the areas where more knowledge is needed. For example, sound and detailed descriptive data on the natural course of patients' functional status and motor control abilities following various disabling conditions commonly treated by physical therapists would go a long way in helping us to differentiate the effects of the disease/recovery from the effects of our treatment. Maintaining more accurate records of patients' characteristics and their responses to treatment would provide us with the type of data base needed to eventually predict the probability of success with treatment X for patient with Y characteristics; that is, to put a more quantitative grid on the factors that we know influence our decisions but that presently do so in a less-definable fashion.

ANATOMY AND PATHOPHYSIOLOGY OF STROKE

To make decisions about what to note in the patient's history and verbal report and what to evaluate in any particular stroke patient, the therapist needs knowledge of the basic pathophysiology involved and the symptoms that may be expected, especially as related to alterations in motor and functional abilities. Better knowledge of the relationship of pathophysiology to symptoms can assist therapists in making more intelligent decisions about long-term goals, the types of treatment to employ, and the frequency of those treatments.

The purpose of this section is to provide the reader with a brief overview of the general pathophysiology of stroke. For in-depth information on the pathophysiology, the references cited should be consulted.

Stroke is the third most common cause of death in the United States and is a significant cause of disability. Approximately 1 million persons each year are left disabled by stroke. It is the most common and urgent of the adult neurologic disorders, accounting for about 50 percent of neurologic disorders seen in hospitals.[1,16,17]

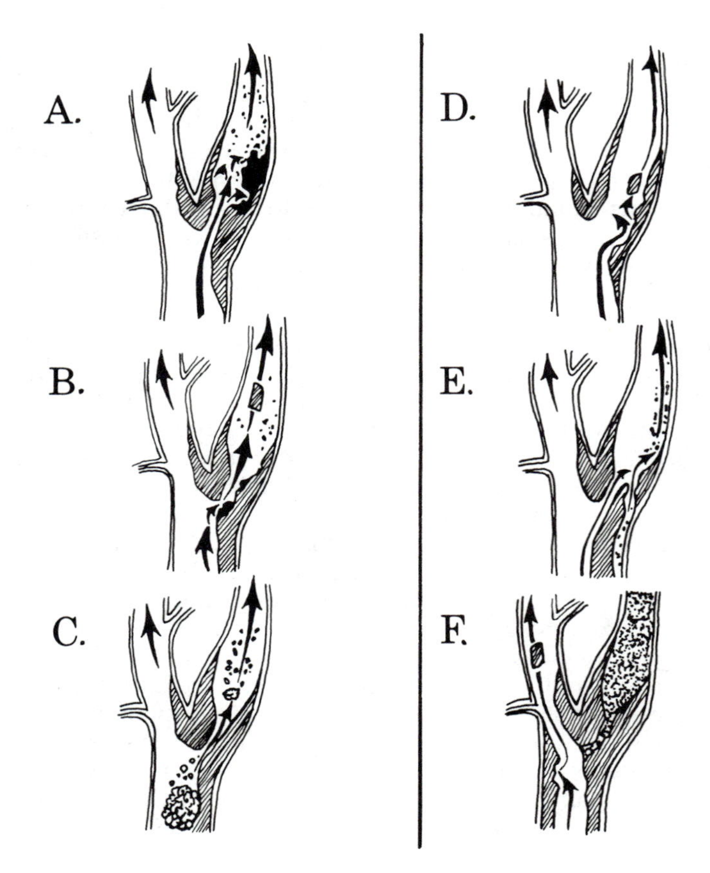

FIGURE 9-3. Schematic of the mechanisms of cerebral and ocular embolization from atheromatous thrombotic lesions at the carotid bifurcation (based on observations during an operation). *(A)* Blood clots in the turbulent eddy flow distal to a zone of tight stenosis in the internal carotid artery. *(B)* Blood clots from intimal crater. *(C)* Blood clots in the eddy current proximal to stenotic lesion. *(D)* Atheromatous intimal fragment. *(E)* Discharge of clotted blood aggregates following intramural hemorrhage and rupture of the intima. *(F)* Embolization to the brain or eye through the external carotid artery, with complete occlusion of the internal carotid artery. (From Wylie and Ehrenfeld,[19] p. 37, with permission.)

Adams and Victor[16] define the term "stroke" as a sudden, nonconvulsive, focal, neurologic deficit resulting from cerebrovascular disease. The pathology involved in stroke may be discussed in terms of (1) the blood vessels themselves, and (2) the effects of the impaired circulation on the brain tissue.

BLOOD VESSELS

Gross pathologic changes occurring in the blood vessels fall into three major categories: thrombosis, embolism, and rupture of a vessel (hemorrhage). The underlying primary disorders that account for these pathologic changes are formation of atherosclerosis, hypertensive arteriosclerotic change, arteritis, aneurysmal dilation, and developmental malformations.[16,17]

Thrombosis

Cerebral thrombosis is a frequent, if not the most common, cause of stroke,[16,17] accounting for 32 percent of strokes in one series studied.[18] Thromboses usually develop as a result of damage to the walls of the vessel[16] or abnormal hemodynamics[19] caused by atheromatous plaques (Fig. 9-3). These plaques tend to form near the bifurcations of major vessels, the most common sites being the internal carotid artery at the level of the carotid sinus and near its transition to the middle cerebral artery, the basilar artery near the junction of the vertebrals, and the main bifurcation of the middle cerebral artery (Fig. 9-4).[16,19,20] It is rare for the cerebral arteries to develop plaques beyond their first major branching.[16] Although plaques may narrow or stenose a vessel, complete occlusion is always the consequence of thrombosis.[16] Although thrombosis is more likely to occur in cases with severe atherosclerosis, it can occur in vessels with few or no atherosclerotic plaques.[16,19] The basic process of atherosclerosis is degeneration of the subendothelial layer of the intima and the innermost fibers of the media, associated with the focal deposition of lipids, that may progress to frank ulceration through the endothelium. Platelets and fibrin adhere to the ulceration and form delicate clots or mural thrombosis. The thrombus may spew emboli into the lumen or progress to occlude the lumen completely.[16,19] Once the lumen is occluded, the thrombus may extend to the next branching point and occlude anastomotic channels.[16,20] Figure 9-3 illustrates these processes.

This pathophysiology explains the usual clinical picture of a thrombotic stroke; that is, slowly evolving (several hours) symptoms that may change and a history of transient ischemic attacks (from emboli released by a thrombus). Infarcts from completed thrombotic strokes are often less severe because the slower occlusion permits the anastomotic circulation to adapt and to substitute for the impaired blood supply caused by the thrombosis.[20] However, the patient's specific clinical symptoms will depend on which vessels are involved, whether emboli are released, and the integrity of anastomotic circulation.[16]

Embolism

Cerebral embolism accounts for approximately one third of all strokes.[16,18] In most cases, the embolic material has broken away from a thrombus within the heart. Less often, the source is intra-arterial, usually the internal carotid

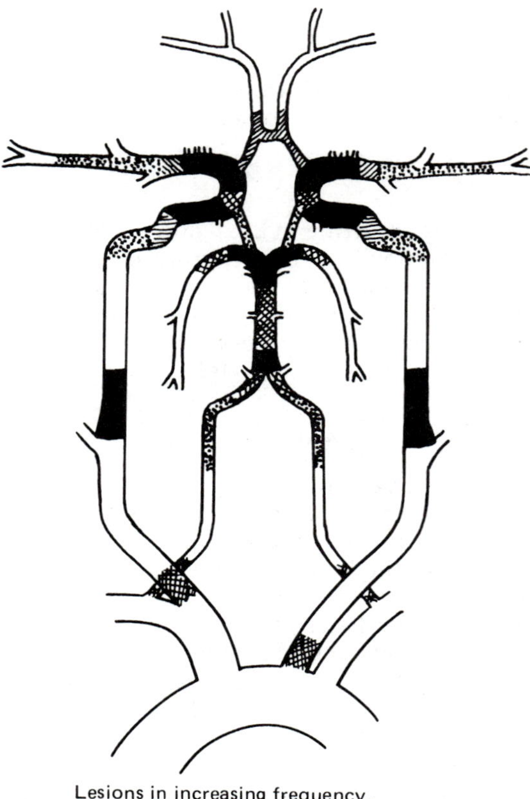

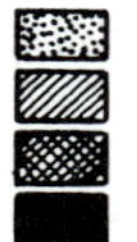

FIGURE 9-4. Diagram demonstrating the frequency and severity of atherosclerotic lesions in the arterial cervicocerebral tree. (From Escourolle and Poirier,[20] p. 87, with permission.)

artery. Since more blood flows through the carotids than the vertebrals (ratio 3 to 1), emboli are more likely to travel in the carotids and thus affect the cerebral hemispheres (which are supplied by the carotids). Anatomically, the middle cerebral artery is a direct continuation of the internal carotid (Fig. 9-5), so emboli traveling in the internal carotid are most likely to lodge in one of its branches.[16,17]

Embolic material may remain stable and plug a lumen solidly or may break up into fragments that enter smaller vessels or may disappear completely. The evolution of a stroke due to cerebral embolism is extremely rapid (several seconds to a minute) and usually is not preceded by any warning episodes.[16,17] Because of the rapidity with which occlusion develops in embolism, there is not much time for collateral circulation to become established. Thus, infarct of tissue distal to the occlusion is more severe than with thrombosis.[16,20] Specific symptoms depend on which vessels are involved and the length of time these vessels remain occluded.[16]

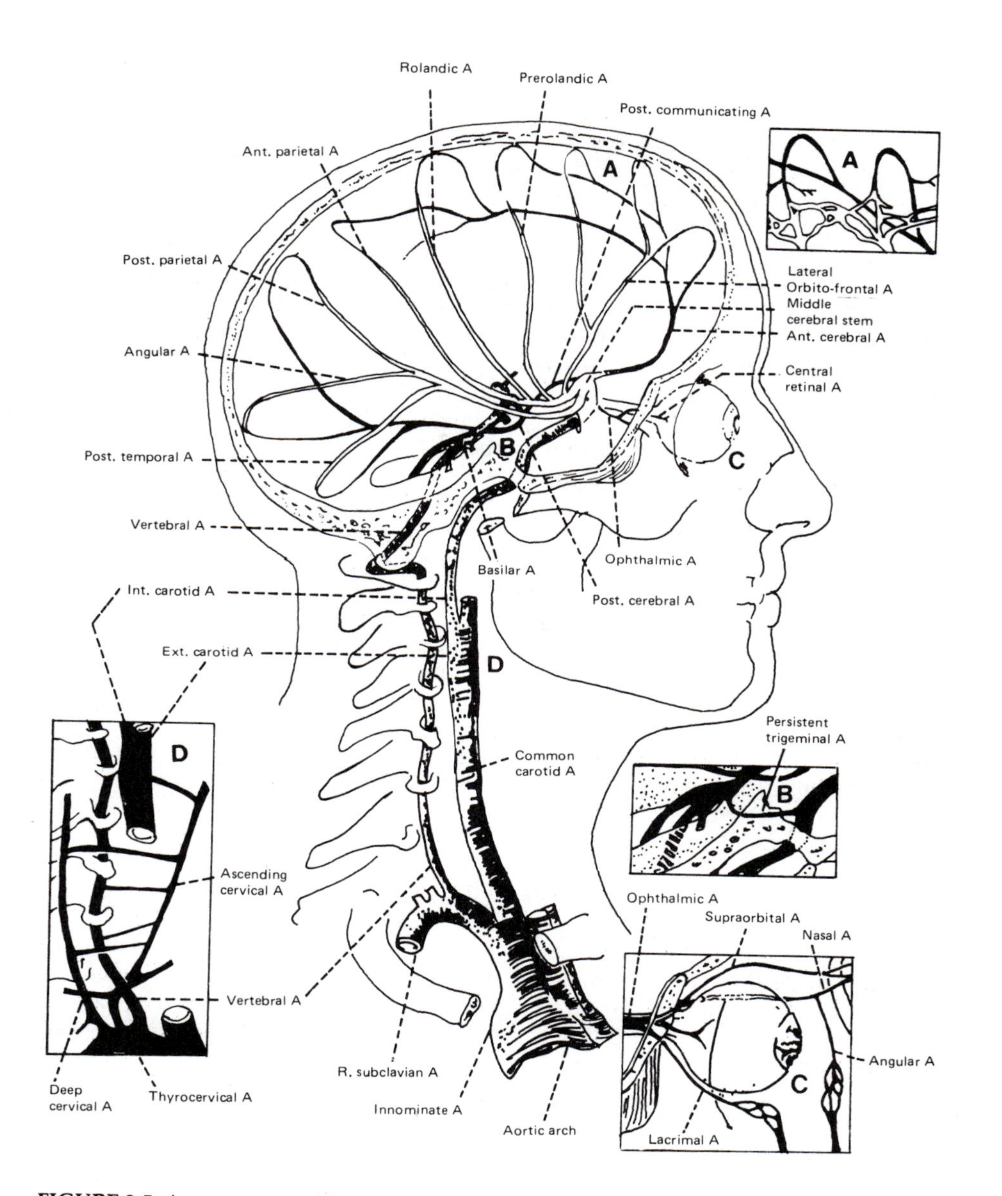

FIGURE 9-5. Arrangement of the major arteries of the right side carrying blood from the heart to the brain. Also shown are collateral vessels that may modify the effects of cerebral ischemia. For example, the posterior communicating artery connects the internal carotid and the posterior cerebral arteries and may provide anastomosis between the carotid and basilar systems. Over the convexity, the subarachnoid interarterial anastomoses linking the middle, anterior, and posterior cerebral arteries are shown, with *inset A* illustrating that these anastomoses are a continuous network of tiny arteries forming a border zone between the major cerebral arterial territories. Occasionally, a persistent trigeminal artery connects the internal carotid and basilar arteries proximal to the circle of Willis, as shown in *inset B.* Anastomoses between the internal and external carotid arteries via the orbit are illustrated in *inset C.* Wholly extracranial anastomoses from muscular branches of the cervical arteries to vertebral and external carotid arteries are indicated by *inset D.* (From Adams and Victor,[16] p. 532, with permission.)

Hemorrhage

Intracranial hemorrhage is the third most common cause of stroke, with hypertensive hemorrhage being the most frequent variety. Hypertensive hemorrhage occurs in the arteries penetrating the brain itself rather than in the vessels of the circle of Willis (unlike aneurysms). Thus, the lesions produced by hemorrhage involve the subcortical white matter much more frequently than do embolic or thrombotic lesions, which are more likely to involve the cerebral cortex. The extravasated blood forms a mass that compresses and displaces brain tissue as the bleeding continues. The most common sites are the putamen and internal capsule (50 percent), other parts of the central white matter, thalamus, cerebellar hemisphere, and pons.[16,17]

There is usually an abrupt onset of the clinical symptoms, which continue to worsen over several hours or even days, depending on the speed of the bleeding. Unlike cerebral thrombosis, there are usually no warning or prodromal signs. With large hemorrhages, the patient becomes comatose almost immediately; but with smaller lesions, the patient may be only mildly confused or stuporous. The prognosis is grim. Seventy-five percent of patients die within 1 to 30 days, usually due to bleeding into the ventricular system, or temporal lobe herniation and midbrain compression. However, if the patient survives (usually those with smaller lesions), the chances for recovery of function are better than in lesions resulting from thrombosis or embolism, because much of the brain tissues have been pushed aside by the hemorrhage rather than having been destroyed by infarction. As the blood is resorbed over a period of several weeks, recovery occurs.[16,17] Some authors disagree with this view and report the prospects for recovery of function as extremely grim.[21]

EFFECTS OF IMPAIRED CIRCULATION ON BRAIN TISSUE

The extent of brain damage caused by these vascular lesions depends on a number of factors, the foremost of which is the degree of integrity of the anastomotic network of the cerebral circulation (see Fig. 9-5).[16,19] The potential for collateral circuits in the major proximal arteries of the brain is great, but the potential for collateral blood flow decreases in the more distal elements of the cerebral vasculature. Thus, dysfunction is more likely to result from obstruction in the middle cerebral artery than from the obstruction of the proximal internal carotid artery.[19] This means that severe stenosis of the internal carotid artery can be present with little functional deficit. Brice, Dawsett, and Lowe[22] have shown that the lumen of the internal carotid artery needed to be reduced to 2.0 sq mm before significant reduction in arterial pressure beyond the constriction occurred.

Other important factors in the amount of brain damage that results from impaired circulation are as follows: the speed of the occlusion; the presence of hypotension, hypoxia, hypocapnia, or hypoglycemia; or alterations in the viscosity or osmolality of the blood.[16,19] Etiologic factors determining cerebral infarcts are summarized in Figure 9-6.

In animal experiments, complete ischemia for more than 3 to 5 minutes produces irreversible cell damage. This cell damage may also be termed necrosis, infarction, cerebral softening, or encephalomalacia.[16,19,23] Chiang and

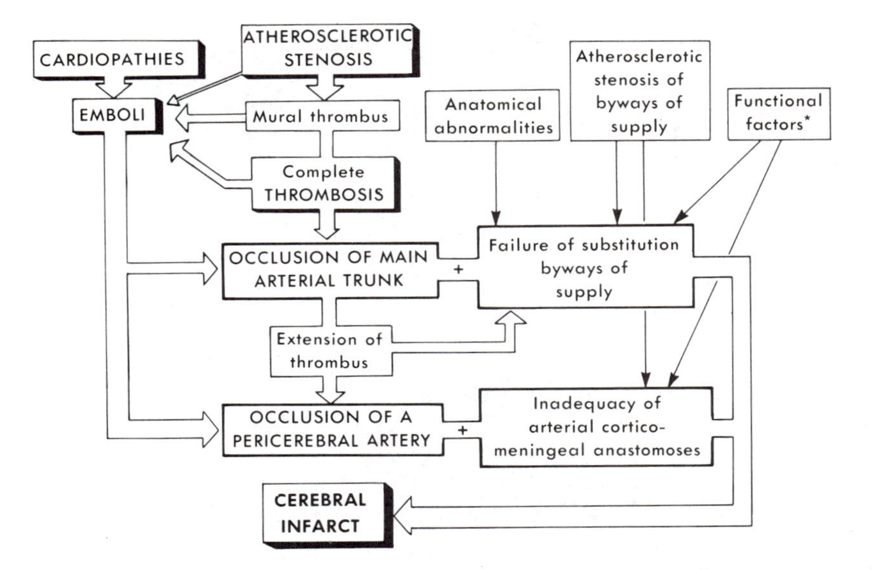

FIGURE 9-6. Etiologic and pathophysiologic factors determining cerebral infarcts. *Functional factors: decrease in caliber of ischemic arteries; drop in blood pressure; loss of autoregulation of arterial caliber. (From Escourolle and Poirier,[20] p. 85, with permission.)

associates[23] produced cerebral ischemia by clamping the aorta in rabbits. After 5 minutes, many areas of the brain failed to reperfuse even though the blood supply level had been restored. They found that the capillaries in the nonperfused areas were obstructed by swelling of the feet of periovascular astrocytes and by bleb formation in the capillary endothelium.

Cerebral infarction (brain cell damage due to ischemia) may be of the pale (anemic), red (hemorrhagic), or mixed type.[16,20,24] In pale infarction, extravasation of erythrocytes into the infarcted tissue is limited; in red infarctions, the extravasation is extensive. Hemorrhagic infarcts are thought to result from leakage within damaged vessels following restored blood supply to infarcted areas after lysis or secondary mobilization of a thrombus or em-

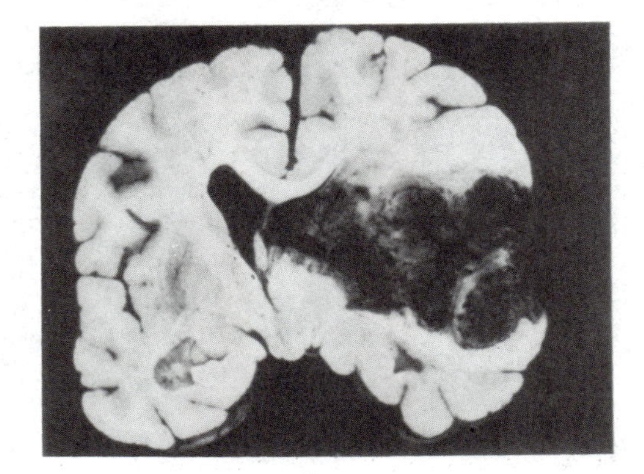

FIGURE 9-7. Hemorrhagic infarct. This type of infarction is particularly found to accompany cerebral emboli. (From Escourolle and Poirier,[20] p. 85, with permission.)

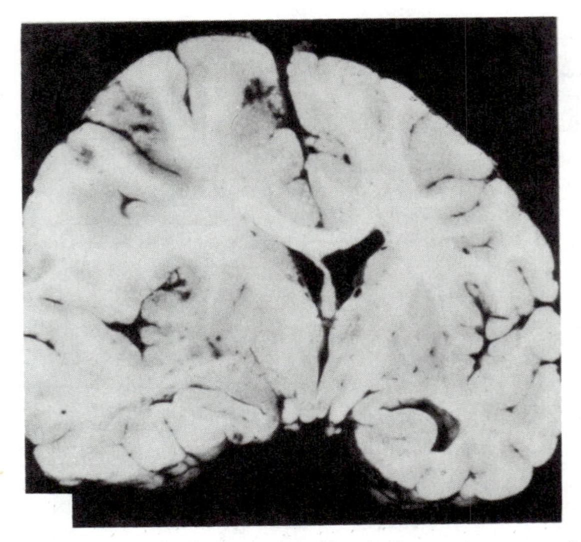

FIGURE 9-8. Recent massive cerebral infarct. Swelling is due to the accumulation of interstitial fluid. (From Escourolle and Poirier,[20] p. 82, with permission.)

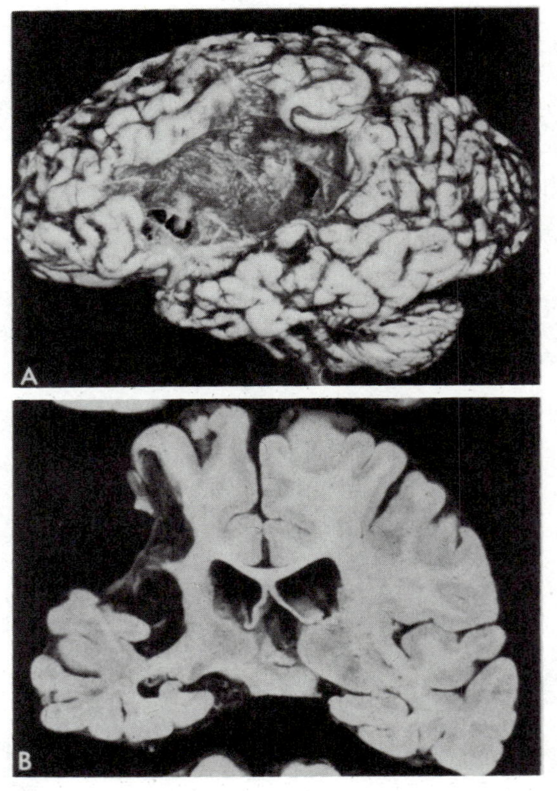

FIGURE 9-9. Old cystic infarct in the territory of the middle cerebral artery. (From Escourolle and Poirier,[20] p. 83, with permission.)

bolus (Fig. 9-7).[16,20] In the acute stage of any cerebral infarct, massive swelling occurs due to the accumulation of the interstitial fluid (Fig. 9-8). Later, this fluid infiltrates the cells. Neurons, glial cells, and small blood vessels all undergo necrosis.[20,24] The size of the infarct may increase for 4 to 5 days.[24] Eventually, the damaged area is removed by the processes of phagocytosis and liquefaction, and a cystic cavity is formed (Fig. 9-9).[20]

Another factor that may influence the amount of brain damage following a stroke is the release by ischemic neurons of vasoactive neurotransmitters into the surrounding tissue.[25,26] (This process is similar to the release of enzymes by dying cardiac cells following a myocardial infarction.) In animals, these released neurotransmitters (specifically, dopamine, norepinephrine, and serotonin) are thought to exacerbate pathophysiologic changes caused by ischemia by constricting local blood vessels and by altering the receptor activity of nearby neurons that do not normally receive monoaminergic inputs.[26] Furthermore, lesions of specific tracts created by the infarction lead to altered neurotransmitter release, and altered receptor binding in distant viable portions of the brain.[25] These alterations result in complex morphologic and functional responses in the distant denervated areas, a process termed neural plasticity. Literature related to neural plasticity has recently been extensively reviewed by Bishop[27] and Craik[28] and will not be discussed here.

PATHOPHYSIOLOGY SPECIFIC TO THE CASE STUDY: CAROTID DISSECTION

The purpose of this section is to provide the reader with a more detailed review of the pathophysiology related to the case under discussion.

Arterial walls are composed of three main layers: the intima, the media, and the adventitia. The innermost layer (intima) consists of three parts, an innermost endothelial lining similar to that found in capillaries, an intermediate layer of delicate connective tissue, and a band of elastic fibers, the internal elastic membrane, that separates the intima and media. The second layer (media) is composed mainly of smooth muscle cells, with variable amounts of elastic and connective tissues interspersed. The third layer (adventitia or externa) consists mainly of connective tissue. The structure and relative thickness of each layer varies according to the size and function of the artery. The layers seen in the internal carotid artery are illustrated in Figure 9-10. The internal carotid is considered a large or elastic artery. The large arteries are specialized for conducting blood. The walls are relatively thin for the size of the vessel, the amount of elastic tissue is greatly increased, and the amount of smooth muscle is greatly decreased as compared with medium-sized vessels. In large arteries, the tissue layers are arranged predominantly in a spiral disposition, in contrast to the circular arrangement seen in smaller vessels.[29]

Carotid dissection refers to a pathologic separation between two of these arterial layers. The most commonly described location for dissection is on a subintimal plane between the internal elastic membrane of the intima and the media,[16,30-34] but it can occur between other layers as well.[31-34] The process of dissection creates a false lumen through which blood can flow (Fig. 9-11). Stenosis, thrombotic occlusion, and secondary emboli with resul-

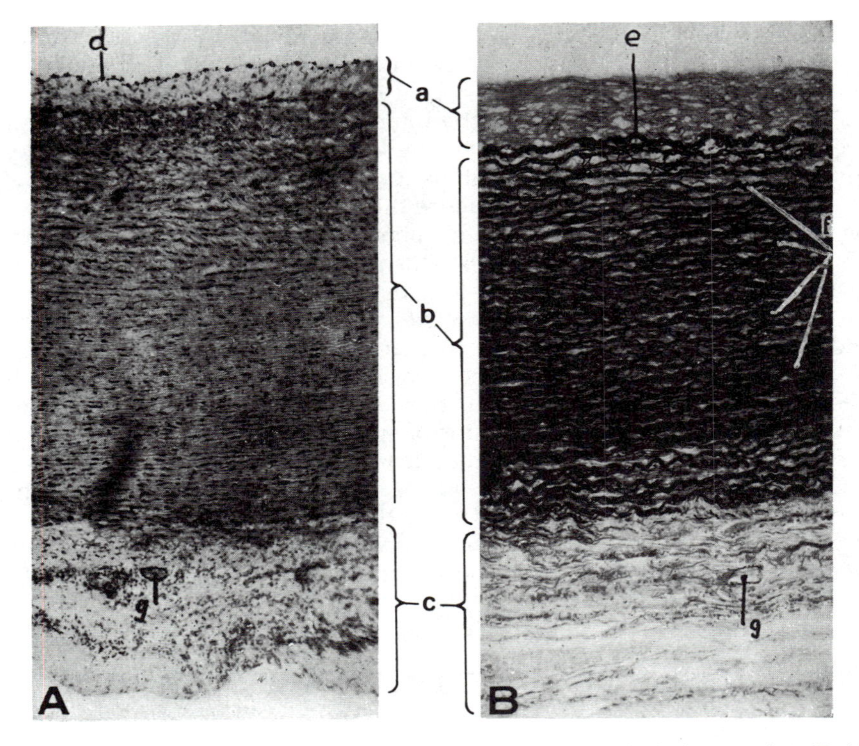

FIGURE 9-10. Cross section through internal carotid artery. Retouched photograph ×85. *(A)* Stained with hematoxylin-eosin; *(B)* stained with resorcin-fuchsin; *a*, intima; *b*, media; *c*, adventitia; *d*, endothelium; *e*, internal elastic membrane; *f*, elastic membranes in media; *g*, vasa vasorum. (From Copenhauer, Bunge, and Bunge,[29] p. 316, with permission.)

tant neurologic deficits may follow.[16,30-35] The lesion produces a characteristic radiographic appearance on angiography, termed the "string sign" (Fig. 9-12). The long, narrow column of contrast material seen following a dissection differs markedly from the typical short, stenotic lesions of atherosclerosis.[35]

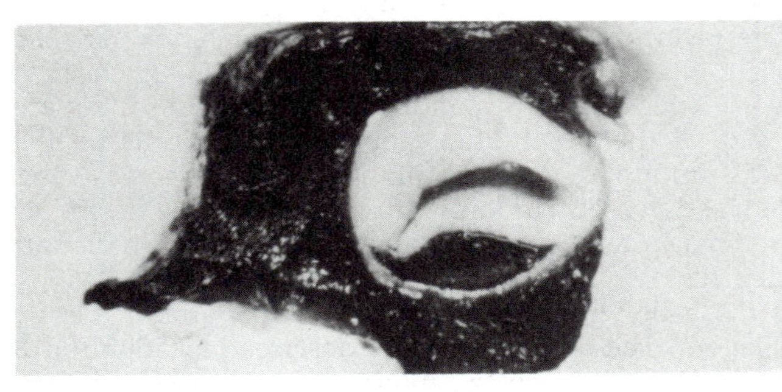

FIGURE 9-11. Dissecting carotid aneurysm from angiography. The lumen is compressed by the crescentic mural hematoma. There is a large hematoma in the carotid sheath. Shown about 3.2 times natural size. (From Hutchinson and Acheson,[24] p. 55, with permission.)

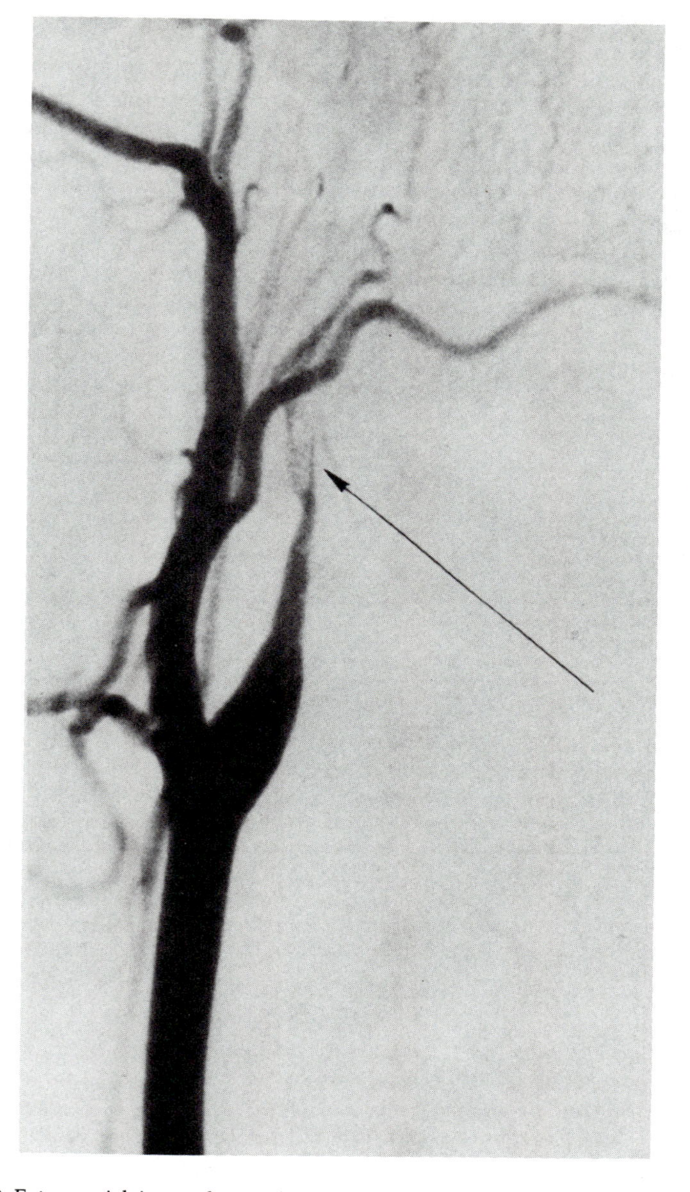

FIGURE 9-12. Extracranial–internal carotid artery dissection manifest by tapered narrowing in the proximal artery. Intraluminal clot and "string sign" *(arrow)* are evident with selective carotid study. (From Zelenock et al,[36] p. 428, with permission.)

Carotid dissection may result from direct trauma to the artery (e.g., head/neck injury, knife or gunshot wounds, or secondary to puncture for angiography) or may be spontaneous in origin. The cause of "spontaneous" carotid dissections is unclear, but it is known that these lesions are *not* associated with hypertension or arteriosclerotic disease. Patients are usually younger than the typical stroke victim and display few, if any, of the common risk factors for stroke.[30-36]

Zelenock and associates[36] reviewed factors postulated by others to contribute to carotid artery dissection. Possible factors include myxoid degeneration, moyamoya arteriopathy, fibrodysplastic disease, medial degeneration, homocystinuria, and developmental and acquired arterial wall defects. Others have postulated mechanical causes, such as heavy coughing that produces tears in the carotid intima,[35] or repeated minor trauma to the neck resulting from cervical rotation and hyperextension, such as occurs in endotrachial intubation and some cervical manipulations.[37,38] Figure 9-13 shows how the movement of neck extension with rotation can cause the transverse processes of the upper cervical vertebrae to impinge on the internal carotid artery causing small tears in the intima. Figure 9-14 illustrates how the internal carotid can be compressed between the angle of the mandible and the

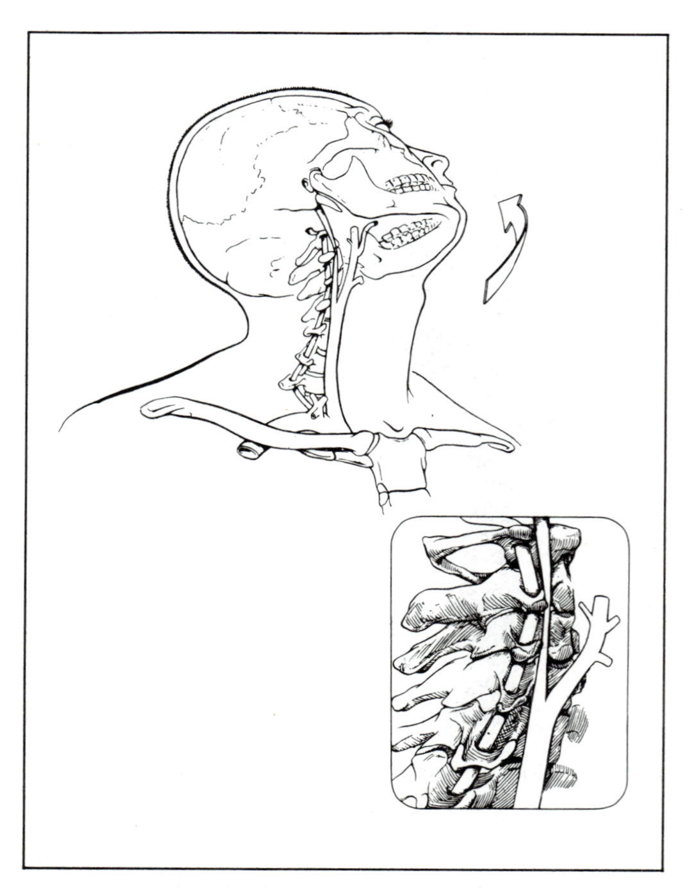

FIGURE 9-13. Stretch-traction-rotation forces applied to the internal carotid artery as it crosses the transverse processes of the second and third cervical vertebrae causing intimal fracture. Mechanical compromise of lumen or thromboembolism may develop as dissection of intramural hematoma progresses or thrombosis occurs on exposed subendothelial tissues. (From Zelenock et al,[36] p. 427, with permission.)

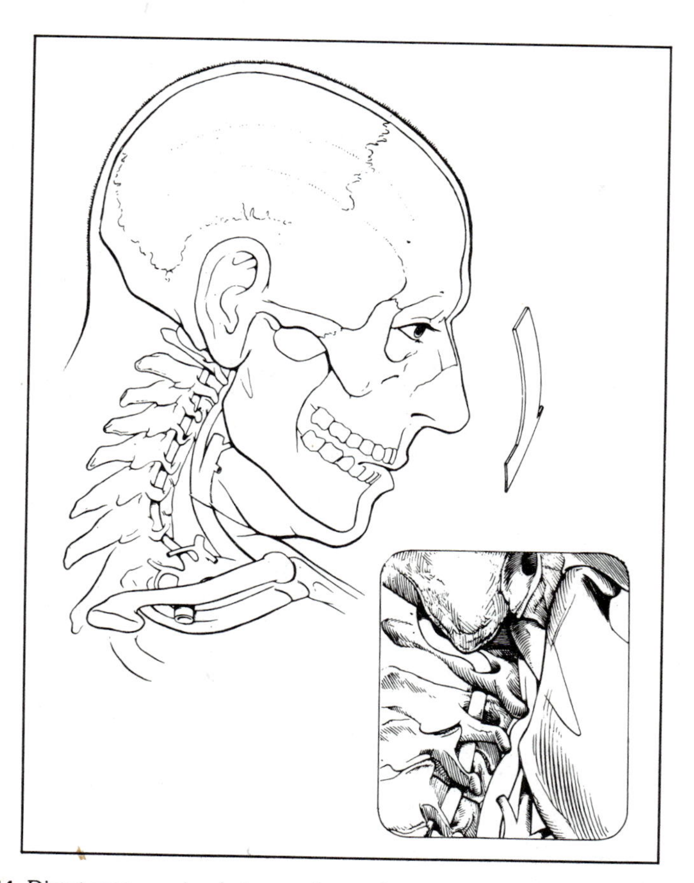

FIGURE 9-14. Direct compression between the angle of the mandible and the upper cervical vertebra may result in mural hematoma or intimal disruption and may initiate dissecting process. (From Zelenock et al,[36] p. 427, with permission.)

upper cervical vertebra during rapid and forceful neck flexion.[30,36] Whether this type of trauma actually leads to a dissection, or only does so if some type of structural defect is already present in the arterial wall, is not known.[36]

The most common clinical presentations are transient ischemic attacks (TIAs), which represent a broader territory of cerebral ischemia than arteriosclerotic stenosis,[33,35,39] and hemifacial or hemicranial pain and Horner's syndrome.[33,35,39] Although many case reports cite hemiplegia,[30,31,36,40] in the two largest series reported, the incidence of hemiplegia was only 7 out of 22[35] and 3 out of 18 cases.[41] Many of those patients with hemiplegia recovered function within a few weeks. In patients with residual deficits, the description of motor and functional abilities at long-term follow-up is scant or nonexistant.[30-42] In children, the process seems to be much more malignant, with 76 percent of reported cases dying as a result of the neurologic sequelae.[32] Several authors suggest that carotid dissection may be a much more common process than previously thought, and that many patients who were actually suffering from an occlusive carotid dissection might have been erroneously diagnosed as having atherosclerotic thrombosis.[35,39,41]

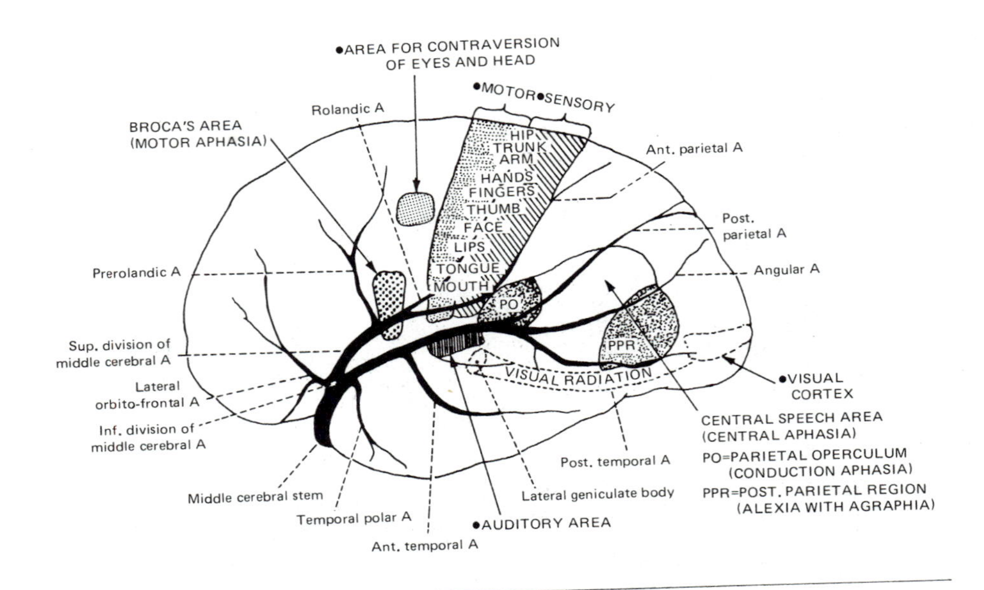

Signs and symptoms	*Structures involved*
Paralysis of the contralateral face, arm, and leg.	Somatic motor area for face and arm and the fibers descending from the leg area to enter the corona radiata
Sensory impairment over the contralateral face, arm, and leg (pinprick, cotton touch, vibration, position, two-point discrimination, stereognosis, tactile localization, barognosis, cutaneographia)	
Motor speech disorder	Broca's area of the dominant hemisphere
"Central" aphasia, word deafness, anomia, jargon speech, alexia, agraphia, acalculia, finger agnosia, right-left confusion (the last four comprise the Gerstmann syndrome)	Central language area and parietooccipital cortex of the dominant hemisphere
Apractagnosia (amorphosynthesis), anosognosia, hemiasomatognosia, unilateral neglect, agnosia for the left half of external space, "dressing apraxia," "constructional apraxia," distortion of visual coordinates, inaccurate localization in the half field, impaired ability to judge distance, upside-down reading, visual illusions	Usually nondominant parietal lobe. Loss of topographic memory is usually due to a nondominant lesion, occasionally to a dominant one.
Homonymous hemianopia (often superior homonymous quadrantanopia)	Optic radiation deep to second temporal convolution
Paralysis of conjugate to the opposite side	Frontal contraversive field or fibers projecting therefrom
Avoidance reaction of opposite limbs	Parietal lobe
Miscellaneous: frontal ataxia	Frontopontine tract (?)
Loss or impairment of optokinetic nystagmus	Supramarginal or angular gyrus
Limb-kinetic apraxia	Premotor or parietal cortical damage
Mirror movements	Precise location of responsible lesions not known
Cheyne-Stokes respiration, contralateral hyperhidrosis, mydriasis (occasionally)	
Capsular (pure motor) hemiplegia	Upper portion of the posterior limb of the internal capsule and the adjacent corona radiata.

FIGURE 9-15. Diagram of cerebral hemisphere, lateral aspect, showing the branches and distribution of the middle cerebral artery and the principal regions of cerebral localization. Also, a list of the clinical manifestations of infarction in the territory of the artery and the corresponding regions of cerebral damage. (From Adams and Victor,[16] p. 536, with permission.)

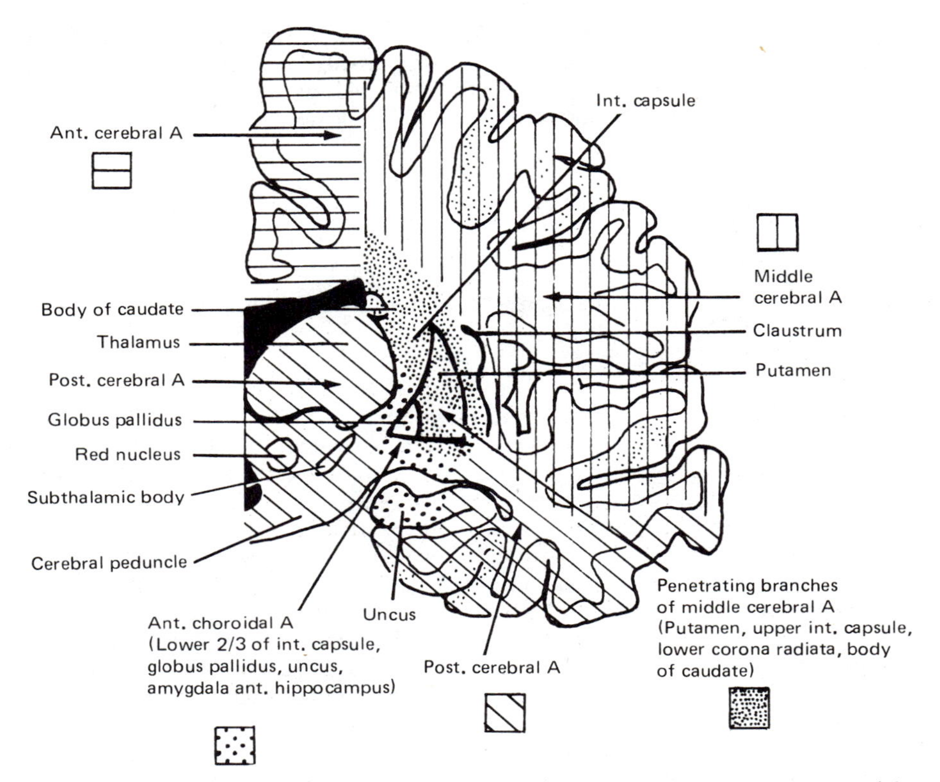

FIGURE 9-16. Diagram of cerebral hemisphere, coronal section, showing the territories of the major cerebral vessels. (From Adams and Victor,[16] p. 538, with permission.)

The proper medical management of these lesions is unknown.[35] Treatments have included surgical repair,[31,36,38,41] or anticoagulant or anti–platelet aggregation therapy.[30,33,40,42]

Although emboli from the thrombus formed at the site of the dissection are not a commonly reported sequelae of carotid dissection,[35,41] this appears to be what happened to the patient in the case about to be discussed. Because of the anatomy of the cerebral arteries (see Fig. 9-5), the most common site for embolic occlusion is in the distribution of the middle cerebral artery (MCA). Figure 9-15 illustrates the cortical branches of the MCA, the principal regions of cerebral localization, and the signs and symptoms associated with occlusion of various portions of the MCA. The penetrating branches of the MCA (Fig. 9-16) supply the putamen, part of the head and body of the caudate nucleus, the outer globus pallidus, the posterior limb of the internal capsule, and the corona radiata.[16]

If the MCA is occluded at the stem (see Fig. 9-15), both the deep penetrating and superficial cortical branches will be blocked, resulting in the classic picture of contralateral hemiplegia, hemianesthesia, and homonymous hemianopia, with aphasia in left-hemisphere lesions and amorphosynthesis in right-sided lesions. Occlusion of the superior division mimics the syndrome of stem occlusion, but with less impairment of alertness. If occlusion is limited to one of the branches of the superior division, further fractionation of the syndrome occurs (see Fig. 9-15). If the inferior division of the MCA is occluded (less common), the usual result (for left-sided lesions) is Wernicke's aphasia. With right- or left-sided lesions, there is usually a homonymous hemianopia, and with right-sided lesions an amorphosynthesis.[16]

CASE HISTORY

This patient was referred for outpatient physical therapy 3 months after her stroke, 1 week following discharge from a local rehabilitation center.

ACUTE HOSPITAL COURSE

This 43-year-old, left-handed woman awoke around 1 AM with a left hemiparesis and an inability to speak. Seven weeks prior to this episode, the patient had an Escherichia coli septicemia, followed by an appendectomy with full and uneventful recovery. For several days prior to the onset of hemiparesis, she had posterior headaches and pain on turning her head. She was admitted to a local hospital, where an emergency CAT scan showed a slight right-hemisphere mass effect. An arteriogram revealed a tapering right internal carotid artery occlusion beginning 1 cm above the carotid bifurcation (positive ''string'' sign).[35] The left internal carotid arteriogram revealed a narrowing over several centimeters that was not hemodynamically significant. There was no evidence of atheromatous disease. There appeared to be embolic occlusion of the superior division of the middle cerebral artery on the right. On examination, the patient was easily aroused and followed simple commands with the right side. There was no understandable speech. There was a left gaze palsy and a left facial palsy. Pupils were equal and reactive to light. The left extremities were flaccid, with absent deep tendon reflexes (DTRs) and no voluntary motion. Babinski's sign was positive on the left.

The following day, the patient was transferred to a larger hospital. Repeat CAT scan revealed a large right frontoparietal low density area with moderate mass effect. Her lumbar puncture was clear. A left carotid bruit was present. Her cranial nerve examination revealed the following results:

I	not tested
II	responds to right-side threat only; disks flat
III, IV, VI	right gaze preferred, but moves left with encouragement; movement of head occurs with attempted left gaze
V	decreased left corneal reflex
VII	central facial paralysis on left
VIII	grossly intact
IX, X	gag present; uvula and palate deviate to right
XI	? present
XII	tongue deviates slightly to left.

Her left extremities were still flaccid, with no voluntary movement, but her DTRs had changed to 3+ throughout on the left. She had a brisk flexor withdrawal reflex to pain in the left lower extremity. She appeared to feel a pinprick on the left but could not localize it with her right hand.

She was arousable from the right side only. Her speech consisted of monosyllables and remained incomprehensible. Her reading and writing were also impaired and incomprehensible, but she made an active attempt at communication. Her ability to copy a block and clock was severely impaired (constructural deficit). She could follow one-step commands but not two-step commands, and she occasionally perseverated her responses. She was able to recognize objects such as a watch, a pen, and tape. There was no left-sided denial; she would use her right hand to move the left upon request. There was evidence of astereognosis on the left; she identified a number drawn in her right palm correctly approximately half of the time, but not at all in the left palm. She recognized coins placed in her right palm, but not in the left.

Her medical history revealed no alcohol abuse, diabetes mellitus, hypertension, or smoking; thus, she had no risk factors for atherosclerotic disease. Her social history revealed a well-educated woman, a former nurse with a master's degree in social work. She was employed as a psychiatric social worker immediately prior to her stroke. She is married with two sons, and family and friends visited daily.

She remained alert throughout her 1 month hospitalization, with some improvement in speech, but almost no return of left-side function. Muscle tone remained flaccid, left upper-extremity strength was 0/5, lower-extremity strength was 2/5 in hip flexors, adductors, extensors (medial hamstrings), and external rotators; the rest of her musculature was 0/5. Passive range of motion (ROM) was normal with the exception of dorsiflexion on the left, which was limited to 5 degrees past neutral.

Functionally, she required verbal cues and minimal assistance of one for bed mobility, and supine-to-sit. She required supervision in sitting and moderate assistance of one for sit-to-stand and transfers. She could stand only with support of a bar and with the knee immobilized in extension, and she was nonambulatory.

The patient was discharged to a rehabilitation hospital after 1 month in the acute hospital. Diagnoses of fibromuscular dysplasia and systemic vasculitis were ruled out. The discharge diagnosis was bilateral carotid dissections with an occlusion of the right internal carotid artery resulting in a lesion in her right (dominant) parietal lobe. She was initially treated with intravenous heparin, fluid restriction, and steroids in an attempt to reduce swelling and decrease further emboli from dissecting vessels. She was taking warfarin (Coumadin) when discharged.

REHABILITATION COURSE

The patient spent 2 months in a rehabilitation facility, receiving intensive daily physical, occupational, and speech therapies. Discharge status was as follows:

ROM: Within normal limits except for left ankle dorsiflexion of only 5 degrees past neutral (with knee extended); left shoulder: 165-

degree flexion, 120-degree abduction, and 65-degree external rotation.

Motor: Muscle tone: mild to moderate resistance to passive movement present in most muscle groups of upper and lower extremities. Active movement: Stage 3 synergy movement[3] at left shoulder and elbow through approximately one-half normal range. Hand function at Stage 4, with wrist and finger extension present but no thumb movement.[3] Lower extremity at Stage 3 recovery, with beginning isolated movements; for example, hip abduction with knee extension through one-half range. Ankle dorsiflexion only with inversion. Trace eversion. Trunk flexion reported as 3/5 and entension as 4/5.

Sensory/Perceptual: Sensation intact with the exception of a minimal decrease to pinprick, temperature, and proprioception in distal left upper and lower extremities. Minimal neglect of left extremities and left environment present.

Pain: Complains of pain in left shoulder, wrist, and foot.

Functional Status: Independent in bed mobility, transfers, and sit-to-stand. Requires supervision for balance in ambulation on level surface and stairs. Uses straight cane, double upright short leg brace with spring dorsiflexion assist, and sling for upper extremity during ambulation. Requires use of railing on stairs. Endurance was 1000 feet, 2 to 3 times.

APPLYING THE DECISION-MAKING MODEL

EVALUATION

The first set of decisions to be made involves which aspects of the patient's performance to evaluate and which tools or methods to use in so doing (see Figs. 9-1 and 9-2). A careful review of the patient's history and verbal report will assist the therapist in selecting key elements to evaluate. The history review will also be used in assessment and goal setting.

Table 9-1 shows a complete list of items to be included in a physical therapy evaluation of a neurologically impaired patient. The decision we face is how to select from this extensive battery those items that are essential to evaluate in depth in the first session for any particular patient. We want to ensure that the patient leaves the first session feeling that something has been done for at least one of her problems; we do not want to spend our time collecting information that is interesting but peripheral to the management of the patient's problems. In reviewing this patient's history, the following problems were noted: (1) pain in the left foot and upper extremity (UE), (2) decreased ROM in the left ankle and UE, (3) disordered active movement control on the left, (4) functional dependence in ambulation, and (5) poor endurance.

At the beginning of the first session, the patient was asked what her chief complaint was and what she hoped to gain from coming to physical therapy. This patient replied that what bothered her most was her difficulty with speech, pain in her left foot, and difficulty walking. This response suggests a need for a special effort to find out from the speech therapist what to

TABLE 9-1. Evaluation Battery for Neurologically Impaired Patients

Demographic Information
Medical History
Psychosocial History
Patient's Chief Complaint
Impact of Disability on Lifestyle
Mental Status
Communication Ability
Mobility
• Range of Motion (ROM)
• Joint Play
• Soft Tissue
–skin condition
–compliance of muscle and connective tissue
–edema
Motor Control
• Muscle Tone
• Strength
• Abnormal Reflexes
• Voluntary Movement Patterns
• Motor Planning Ability
• Coordination
• Balance—static/dynamic
• Developmental Sequence
• Automatic Postural and Equilibrium Reactions
Vital Functions
Autonomic Nervous System
Sensation
Perceptual Evaluation
Pain
Posture
Gait
Functional Abilities
Equipment
Endurance/CardioRespiratory Status

do to assist the patient with her speech. Her response also suggests that in the first session we will want to concentrate the detailed evaluation on her pain, movement patterns in the lower extremity, and gait assessment. Other parts of the evaluation should receive less emphasis or may be deferred to a subsequent session.

How do we choose evaluation tools for these problems? We need tools that will satisfy a dual purpose: (1) provide information about the nature of the problem, and (2) provide an objective measure of progress over time.

Since pain is a priority problem for this patient, we will want to know a great deal of detail about it: location, intensity, duration, and activities that relieve or aggravate the pain. For ROM, we want a tool that tells us degrees of motion in a standardized fashion, but also a qualitative tool that helps us to assess the reasons for the lack of motion (e.g., joint play, joint component movement analysis, and soft tissue analysis). For the disordered active motor control, we want to assess factors that may contribute to the problem independently or in concert. From the list shown in Table 9-1, five factors are selected: (1) muscle tone, (2) strength, (3) movement patterns, (4) balance, and (5) automatic postural and equilibrium reactions.

Muscle Tone

In discussing evaluation of muscle tone, we would like to avoid terms such as "spasticity" and "rigidity," which are subject to so many different interpretations that their usefulness as objective descriptions is close to nil.[43] Instead, we should describe what we do to the patient, or what we ask the patient to do, and the response obtained.

Traditionally, muscle tone has been assessed via deep tendon reflexes (DTRs, or the phasic stretch reflex) and via the response to passive movement at different velocities (tonic stretch reflex).[44] While these measures are useful, we should place more emphasis on assessing the active tonic stretch reflex (muscle response to active movement attempts) because this reflex provides a more direct measure of the ability to recruit agonists and to reciprocally inhibit antagonists.[44,45] The active tonic stretch reflex can be evaluated by measuring the quality and speed of unidirectional and reciprocal movements and can readily be combined with the voluntary movement pattern assessment. More elaborate and qualitative measures of the "active" tonic stretch reflex may be obtained by the step-torque technique or the continuous perturbation technique.[45]

DTRs tell us if the lower motor neuron arc is intact or if the excitability of the spinal motor neuron pool is heightened; but the response to this nonphysiologic stimulus does not necessarily correlate with active movement control or with the tonic stretch reflex (TSR).[44,45] For example, patients with cerebellar disorders have increased DTRs but are typically hypotonic (depressed TSR).[46] Conversely, patients with Parkinson's disease have increased muscle tone but may display normal DTRs.[45]

The responses to passive stretch (resting TSR) and active stretch (action TSR) have been shown to be clearly and quantitatively different in normal people[47] and to vary with the level of contraction in normal people.[48] In patients with movement disorders, the resting and action TSRs also differ from each other and differ from the response pattern seen in normal people.[48,49,50] Andrews, Neilson, and Knowles[51] tested the effect of an alpha-adrenergic blocking agent (phenoxybenzamine) on the TSR and found that the drug had a different effect on the resting TSR than on the action TSR. The resting TSR was reduced, but the action TSR was not. Even though the response to passive stretch was normalized, there was no concomitant improvement in voluntary movement control. Norton and associates[52] have also reported a lack of correlation between "spasticity" (as measured by the response to passive movement) and functional measures of gait performance such as speed of gait.

These data support the idea that the resting and action TSRs may have different neurophysiologic substrates, and that improvement in one (for example, response to passive stretch) may not necessarily correlate with improvement in the other. Since the problem that usually concerns our patients is active movement control, our evaluation of muscle tone should not neglect this aspect of performance (i.e., the action tonic stretch reflex).

Strength

Despite claims to the contrary,[2] clear evidence exists that many patients with central nervous system disorders may, in fact, be weak. They have abnormal recruitment and discharge patterns,[53-55] can show evidence of Type II muscle fiber atrophy,[56,57] and have a decreased ability to generate torque.[58,59] These abnormalities are not always due to inhibition by spastic antagonists,[60-62] although this may be part of the problem in some cases.

Movement Patterns

There are several ways to measure the variety and quality of movements available to the patient in different positions.[2-9] We want to know the dominance of movement synergies, the ability for reciprocal movements, and the influence of movements on other body parts (associated reactions). This will help us to choose the patterns, positions, and level of difficulty appropriate to the patient's abilities.

Balance

We want a measure of both static and dynamic balance because poor balance limits the patient's independence in ambulation, according to the history.

Automatic Postural and Equilibrium Reactions[2,7]

Until these automatic reactions are present, the patient will have little functional carry-over because the degree of concentration required by cortically directed postural and equilibrium responses will require too much effort to be practical.[2] Deficits in these reactions may also play a role in her dependence in ambulation.

For functional assessment, we want to identify the activities for which the patient requires human assistance and to categorize the amount of assistance needed. Gait assessment should include a qualitative measure of gait deviations present so that the nature of the the problem causing the gait deviations can be determined. Time-distance measures can be used to assess gait performance more quantitatively and to measure progress over time.[63] Endurance can be described using time-distance terms.

Sensation is evaluated because it is an important predictor of recovery,[64-66] but the evaluation will focus on distal limbs because the history reveals that sensation was normal everywhere except for these areas. Posture, gait, and functional abilities are evaluated because these are major concerns of the patient. Equipment assessment requires careful evaluation because the type of equipment can influence function and may influence the patient's pain symptoms.

Several items under motor control in Table 9-1 were omitted in this patient's case. Abnormal reflexes were not evaluated in detail. This information would be more useful in the acute state, when the presence or absence of various reflexes could serve as an index of recovery, and when these reflexes could be facilitated or inhibited during work on vital function activities or basic functional patterns such as rolling, supine-to-sit, and sit-to-stand. Now that the patient is at a higher level of function, we can learn more about how to help her by assessing her voluntary movement patterns and automatic postural and equilibrium responses. Motor planning activity did not seem to be a problem. We know that the patient will be seeing an occupational therapist. Coordination was not a primary problem by history, and our evaluation of voluntary motor patterns will reveal if we need to evaluate this in more detail later. Developmental sequence evaluation is deferred because the patient is ambulatory and walking is her primary concern. Vital functions and autonomic nervous system evaluation are deferred because they do not appear to be a problem by history. However, results of the pain evaluation may point out the need to evaluate the autonomic nervous system reactions in more detail later. Perceptual evaluation is deferred to occupational therapy.

Initial Evaluation

Demographic Information:

A 43-year-old woman; diagnosis: carotid dissection with secondary emboli to right middle cerebral artery.

Medical History:

Seven weeks post-appendectomy, with secondary septicemia, resolved. No evidence of atherosclerotic disease, hypertension, or diabetes; no previous medical problems.

Psychosocial History:

Employed full time in counseling profession; married with two sons; supportive family and friends.

Chief Complaint:

Poor speech; pain in her left foot; lack of independence in walking; dislikes present brace.

Impact of Disability on Lifestyle:

Severe; she probably will be unable to resume her former occupation due to speech problems.

Mental Status:

Flat affect; appears depressed, but alert and cooperative.

Communication:

Poor speech with many paraphasic errors and word-finding problems; able to follow all commands during evaluation.

Mobility:

Within normal limits on the right side. Passive ROM on the left side normal except:

UE:	Shoulder flexion	
	Glenohumeral	0–135°
	Combined	0–150°
	Abduction	
	Glenohumeral	0–100°
	Combined	0–110°
	Horizontal adduction	0–20°
	External rotation in 50° abduction	0–45°
	Combined wrist and finger extension	0–45°
LE:	Straight leg raise	0–65°
	Hip abduction	0–35°

Ankle dorsiflexion	
Knee flexed	0–5°
Knee extended	−15° from neutral

At the ankle joint, the calcaneus does not move inferiorly. The talus does not rotate downward and backward to allow dorsiflexion. The foot is hypersensitive to touch (causes pain). Soft tissue in the arch of the foot feels firm and tight; compliance of posterior compartment muscles and musculotendinous junctions is poor. They feel very stiff and hard on both sides, but worse on the left. No edema, skin changes, or vascular or temperature abnormalities are noted.

There is a 1-cm subluxation of the shoulder joint at rest. Lack of mobility in external rotation prevents normal scapulohumeral rhythm and normal mobility in abduction and flexion. No edema or skin changes. Detailed evaluation deferred.

Motor Control:

Muscle Tone: Passive Tonic Stretch Reflex
There is a moderate increase in muscle tone in response to quick passive movement in the following muscles or muscle groups:
Left UE: Pectorals, scapula retractors, biceps, pronators, wrist and finger flexors, thumb flexors, and adductors.
Left LE: Adductors, quadriceps, pelvic retractors, gastrocnemius, soleus, and toe flexors. No clonus.

Strength (0 to 5 scale)	*In Synergy*	*Out of Synergy*
Shoulder	2+	2−
Elbow	2+	2−
Wrist/Hand	3−	3−
Hip	3	2+
Knee	3	2−
Ankle	3−	1

Voluntary Movement Patterns:

Upper extremity:
Stage 3 flexion and extension synergy movements[3] in sitting, with beginning control out of synergy.
Shoulder: Scapular elevation and retraction through half the flexor synergy range; abduction through half the flexor synergy range. External rotation through 15-degree range possible with arm at side. In supine position, patient can maintain 90 degrees of shoulder flexion with elbow extension but no dynamic control.
Elbow: Can flex and extend through full range with gravity eliminated, but not against gravity. Supinates through one-fourth range in elbow flexion.
Wrist: Extends wrist through half the range with elbow flexed or extended.
Hand: Patient has mass grasp and release as well as opposition of thumb to all fingers. However, thumb tends to remain adducted in palm.

Reciprocal movements (tested in sitting) are slow (2 to 3 seconds for one reversal) and often occur only through partial range. Voluntary movements in left upper extremity produce synkinetic movements in right upper extremity and associated reactions of pelvic retraction and 10-degree knee extension in the lower limb.

Trunk: Most difficulty is with rotational movements; tends to "log" roll and keep left trunk, especially pelvic girdle, retracted during supine-to-sit and sit-to-stand activities.

Lower extremity:
Stage 3 synergy[3] movements in supine and sitting.
Able to complete full flexor and extensor synergies with weak ankle dorsiflexion in flexor pattern (anterior tibialis only).
Beginning to isolate movement out of synergy (e.g., hip flexion with knee extension in supine position).
Reciprocal movements at knee and hip are synergy bound and slow (requires 2 to 3 seconds to initiate reversal of movement).
Voluntary effort in lower extremity produces mild associated reactions of pelvic and scapular retraction, shoulder internal rotation, supination, and slight finger flexion, but not elbow flexion.

Balance:
Sitting: Independent; recovers balance upon disturbance.
Standing: Independent; recovers balance only if mild disturbance; otherwise, needs assistance.
Walking: Occasionally falls to left; requires supervision for safety.

Automatic Postural and Equilibrium Reactions:

The patient shows abnormal automatic postural adjustments in trunk during sitting and standing, weight shift, and disturbed balance. The left trunk tends to laterally flex with shoulder and pelvic girdle retraction. Normal protective and equilibrium reactions are absent from the limbs during disturbed balance, but abnormal associated reactions in limbs do not occur; postural tone in limbs remains relatively normal.

Sensation:
Impaired proprioception present in left ankle, toes, hand; sensitivity to pinprick in left foot and hand, as compared to right, is slightly decreased.

Pain:
Left Foot:
Location: Along metatarsal heads and dorsomedial aspect of foot.
Associated Activities: Walking; patient feels brace does not fit properly.
Intensity: Patient describes as very troublesome; prevents her from walking more than a few hundred yards.
Duration: Pain occurs during walking and for several hours afterward.
Left U.E.:
Location: Anterior-superior aspect of shoulder.
Associated Activities: Occur at end of passive shoulder flexion (150 degrees), external rotation (145 degrees), and abduction (110 degrees), or when ambulating without sling.

Intensity: Mild to moderate, depending on day.
Duration: During movement only, or walking without sling.

Posture:

Sitting: Her weight is shifted to the right, trunk and pelvis retracted, with left lateral "C" curve of spine, concave to left. Patient holds her left arm on her lap in shoulder adduction, internal rotation, elbow flexion with wrist slightly flexed. Her lower extremity position is normal.

Standing: Her weight is shifted to the right, left leg forward, knee hyperextended, hip in external rotation, and pelvis retracted. Prefers arm in sling to avoid shoulder pain.

Gait:

She ambulates with cane and short leg brace on level surface. When stair climbing, she uses the rail and supervision of one person for balance. Gait deviations include:

	Stance Phase	*Swing Phase*
Hip	Retracted pelvis; no hyperextension	Retracted pelvis; apparent hip external rotation
Knee	Hyperextension or wobbles in flexion	Decreased flexion
Ankle	Foot flat at initial contact; no push off	No dorsiflexion

Ambulation:

Shortened stance phase on left.
Shortened step length on right.
Decreased weight shift to left.
Velocity is 0.24 m/sec.

Functional Abilities:

Independent in all activities except walking and stairs, which require supervision of one for balance.

Equipment:

Straight cane, double upright short leg brace with Klensak ankle and spring dorsiflexion assist. Sling for left arm. Adaptive bathroom equipment.

Endurance:

She does not walk outside the house except to get into a car. Ambulation is limited to a few hundred yards within the house; she sits most of the day.

ASSESSMENT

In assessing the evaluative findings, the therapist makes two decisions: (1) which of the clinical problems displayed by the patient should be treated by physical therapy, and (2) the most likely cause of each problem to be treated. Decisions about the cause of the problems will lead logically to prioritization of goals and choice of treatment methods.

In the case just presented, we would identify the major problems to be treated by physical therapy. They are listed in Table 9-2. The reader will probably note that there are several problems displayed by the patient that are not on this list. We chose only those problems for which we plan to set measurable goals and actively treat. Information about other problems will be used to make decisions about the cause of the primary problem or to make treatment choices. For example, the patient's aphasia is a major problem, but it does not appear on our problem list because its treatment is not our major focus; nor are we adequately trained to treat aphasia. However, we will use our knowledge about this problem in planning treatment. We can use suggestions from the speech therapist for shortening verbal directions to the patient or for facilitating speech by the patient during treatment sessions. Improvement of speech is *not* an outcome goal of this treatment, but knowledge about this problem is necessary for treatment planning. In a similar vein, the patient's flat affect and possible depression are not problems we will address directly, but they will influence our choice of treatment and the types of communications we pursue with other health professionals involved in this patient's care management.

The problems of abnormal muscle tone and impaired sensation help to explain the cause of the patient's abnormal motor control and will influence our choice of treatment; but these problems are not the primary focus of our treatment, because they are not what the patient complains about. The patient complains about pain and being unable to walk, not about increased resistance to passive movement. Thus, these are the problems for which we should develop goals and outcome measures. Treatment of abnormal tone is a means to an end, not an end in itself. If we change the patient's muscle tone, but not her motor control or functional ability, the treatment has not been a success because we have not addressed the problems of concern to the patient.

Analyzing the probable cause of the problems to be treated will lead to decisions about appropriate goals, goal priorities, and treatment methods. In this case, there are several factors that could be contributory to the patient's pain in the left foot and shoulder. Examination of her brace revealed that the toe plate did not extend to the ball of the foot. This allowed much flexibility in the brace, especially motion about the tarsometatarsal joint. Because she lacks mobility in dorsiflexion, particularly downward and backward rotation of the talus about the talocrural joint, the dorsiflexion motion must be transferred forward to the transverse tarsal and tarsometatarsal joint, hypermobilizing these joints and possibly explaining the pain. The spring assist in the Klensak ankle brace provides a quick stretch to her triceps surae during swing, which could inhibit her anterior tibialis and facilitate the plantar flexors—exactly opposite to the normal movement pattern. However, her "spasticity" is not severe (no clonus, only moderate resistance to passive movement, no evidence of associated reactions in ankle). So the role of this quick stretch in producing an abnormal movement pattern and ankle pain may not be that significant. In the shoulder, her lack of proximal muscle control about the scapula and lack of humeral external rotation prevent the normal scapulohumeral rhythm,[67] and thus cause impingement of the greater tuberosity on the acromion in positions of extreme abduction and flexion, producing pain.[2,3,68]

TABLE 9-2. List of Problems, Goals, and Outcomes

PROBLEM	GOAL: 3 MONTHS	OUTCOME: 3 MONTHS
1. Pain: Left Foot	Reduce intensity of pain to minor.	Intensity of pain reduced, but not yet "minor."
	Reduce associated activities of pain to only following ambulation of >15 minutes duration.	No pain when ambulating in house, but pain after longer walks, e.g., excursions to shopping mall.
	Reduce duration of pain to $<\frac{1}{2}$ hour after walking a long distance ($\frac{1}{2}$ mile or $>$).	Duration varies from a few minutes after ambulation to several hours. Sometimes feels pain the next day more than immediately after the activity.
	No hypersensitivity to touch left foot and leg.	Hypersensitivity greatly reduced. Now restricted to a small area on dorso medial aspect of foot over transverse tarsal and tarsometatarsal joints.
Left Shoulder	No pain during ambulation without sling for $<\frac{1}{2}$ hour.	Able to go without sling during ambulation for 15 minutes or less about house with no pain. Still needs sling out of house and for longer excursions.
	No pain during passive shoulder movement to end of available range.	No pain on *passive* shoulder ROM. Pain on *active* shoulder flexion or abduction beyond 40°.
2. Abnormal Mobility: Left Ankle	0–10° dorsiflexion in knee flexion; neutral dorsiflexion in knee extension. (Since the patient has had limited dorsiflexion for 3 months, and right side is also limited, goal was not set higher.)	0–5° dorsiflexion in knee flexion; -10° from neutral in knee extension.
	Increase compliance of posterior compartment muscles, and soft tissues in ankle and foot.	Compliance of gastrocnemius almost equal to right; soleus still quite stiff and immobile. Soft tissues in arch of foot feel nearly like right side.
	Normal calcaneal and talar motion during dorsiflexion to neutral in knee extension.	Talus moves posteriorly during available dorsiflexion in normal pattern when knee is flexed, but cannot complete its normal pattern when knee is extended. Feels limited by leg muscle tightness (gastrocnemius-soleus) rather than by ligamentous tightness or lack of joint play.

TABLE 9-2—*continued*

PROBLEM	GOAL: 3 MONTHS	OUTCOME: 3 MONTHS
Left Shoulder	0–150° glenohumeral flexion. 0–165° combined flexion. 0–120° glenohumeral abduction. 0–140° combined abduction. 0–60° external rotation. No subluxation at rest.	0–160° glenohumeral flexion. 0–170° combined flexion. 0–140° glenohumeral abduction. 0–160° combined abduction. 0–60° external rotation. 1/4 inch subluxation at rest.
3. Abnormal Motor Control a. Decrease in variety of movement combinations on left	Stage 4 synergy control left UE.	Still in Stage 3,[3] left upper extremity but can pronate and supinate forearm with elbow at side in 90° flexion (a Stage 4 activity). Stage 3 movements are now 3/4 range, and patient can bring left hand to mouth and touch top of head while sitting.
	Moves shoulder in small circle in supine with 90° shoulder flexion and elbow extension.	Moves shoulder in 6-inch-diameter circle in supine with 90° shoulder flexion and full elbow extension.
	Ability to segmentally roll.	Can segmentally roll when asked to do so, but automatic pattern is still to "log" roll.
	Pelvic protraction in supine-to-sit and sit-to-stand activities.	Pelvis still retracts in supine-to-sit activities, but movement is near normal in sit-to-stand activities.
	Stage 4 synergy control in left LE.	Stage 4 synergy control left LE.
	Active eversion with non-weight bearing knee extension.	Active eversion through available range in supine with knee extension and in sitting.
	Active dorsiflexion with knee extension in standing.	Can activate all dorsiflexors in standing with knee extension, but movement does not occur due to tight plantar flexors.
b. Slowness of reciprocal movements	Reciprocal movements through full active range with no associated reactions in trunk or extremities with 1-second lag or less for reversal.	Left UE: Reciprocal movements still slow and poorly performed with scapula and shoulder, but have improved at elbow and hand, where reciprocal movements are performed through 3/4 range with 1-second lag between reversals. Active movement of left UE still produces mild synkinetic movements in right hand, but no longer causes associated reactions in left trunk or left LE.

TABLE 9-2—*continued*

PROBLEM	GOAL: 3 MONTHS	OUTCOME: 3 MONTHS
		Left LE: Reciprocal movements are better proximally, and in total patterns. Can perform hip/knee/ankle flexion and extension in supine out of synergy, with 2-second lag between reversals. Isolated reciprocal movement at knee or ankle still has 2-3 second lag and occurs through 1/2 ROM or less. Associated reactions in left UE during reciprocal LE movements have decreased to forearm pronation and finger flexion through partial range.
c. Weakness Left Lower Extremity	Out of synergy Hip 3+	Out of synergy Hip 3+ (extensors weaker than flexors)
	Knee 3 Ankle 2	Knee 3− Ankle 3−
Left Upper Extremity	Shoulder 3− Elbow 3− Wrist/hand 3+	Shoulder 2 Elbow 3− Wrist/hand 3+
d. Abnormal sitting and standing postures	Sitting: Symmetrical weight. Spine straight. No pelvic retraction.	Sitting: Weight is symmetrical. Spine straight. No pelvic retraction. Places left hand to side, palm on mat.
	Standing: Feet even, weight borne symmetrically. No knee hyperextension. Only mild pelvic retraction. No arm sling.	Standing: Weight kept on right leg. If feet even, knee must hyperextend to accommodate lack of dorsiflexion. Pelvic retraction improved, but still present. Able to go without sling for short periods (<15 minutes).
e. Lack of normal automatic postural and equilibrium responses on left side	Normal postural adjustments of trunk in sitting during weight shift and disturbed balance.	Sitting: Shows normal postural adjustments in trunk and extremities in active weight shift. On disturbed balance, shows normal pattern of equilibrium responses in leg, with slight lag in timing, and shows partial protective extension pattern in left UE. The UE reaction is too slow to be functional, but pattern is normal. Distal components (e.g., finger extension) much better than proximal.

In the upper extremity, the patient's lack of mobility in her shoulder seems clearly linked to her abnormal motor control, which is worse proximally. In the lower extremity, the situation is not as clear. Her soft tissues have decreased compliance to a degree inconsistent with the "spasticity" she displays (i.e., no clonus, not much resistance to rapid passive stretch, and although she has no equilibrium reactions in the foot, neither does she display abnormal associated reactions in the ankle with disturbed balance or effort). It is possible that true weakness of the dorsiflexors, more than inhibition by spastic antagonists, accounts for her lack of mobility in the gastrocnemius-soleus group. If weakness is truly the problem, she may do better with a brace that provides a plantar flexion stop (to prevent toe drag) but that allows active movement into dorsiflexion without a spring assist. At this time, the patient has some ability to actively dorsiflex, but she may not be using it because the brace does all the work for her. Thus, the muscle does not get a chance to hypertrophy. Another troublesome symptom is her hypersensitivity to touch in the foot. She does not exhibit other signs of heightened flexor reflexes or autonomic dysfunction (skin, vascular, or sweating changes) or reflex sympathetic dystrophy. What is at the root of this hypersensitivity is unclear. It may be an early sign of impending reflex sympathetic dystrophy. If the pain on weight bearing does not improve, she could be a candidate to develop a full-blown reflex sympathetic dystrophy[69] in the foot with associated vascular and skin changes.

Her motor control problems seem more dominated by an inability to recruit muscles rapidly than by abnormal muscle tone and associated reactions. Another dominant feature of her motor control problems is abnormal postural responses of the trunk in both static and dynamic activities. Her functional dependence in gait and poor endurance are probably due to a combination of the pain, abnormal motor control, and deconditioning resulting from markedly reduced activity levels over the previous 3 months.

SETTING GOALS

The next decision to be made is the setting and prioritization of treatment goals. For goals to be useful in evaluating the effectiveness of treatment, they must be defined in measurable terms and be time limited. How much progress do we expect to make toward a certain goal and within what time frame?

To make decisions about goals, we must review the patient's history for factors that give an indication of how rapidly we can expect recovery or progress toward goals and long-term recovery potential. This information is then integrated within our assessment of the patient's problems. Several factors indicating a favorable prognosis for motor and functional recovery are noted in this patient's history:

1. No loss of consciousness.
2. Minimal involvement of vital functions, brain stem structures, and tracts innervating brain stem structures, as indicated by the cranial nerve examination (thus decreased problems with respiration and risk of pneumonia).

3. Early (2 days post-onset) signs of recovery in eye movements to the left, indicating recovery of function in corticobulbar and other brain stem tracts.
4. Early (2 days) improvement in sensory function (i.e., flexor reflex in response to pinprick indicates recovery of segmental reflexes and possibly long loop reflexes involving brain stem centers such as the reticular formation).[44,45] Early recovery of flexor-withdrawal reflex has also been associated with better cognitive recovery in traumatic brain injured adults.[70] Awareness of pinprick on the left indicates recovery of sensory function to a level of at least the thalamus; but inability to localize, along with evidence of astereognosis, indicates continued impaired function of the cortex, especially the parietal lobes and sensory integrative functions.[16] Recovery of sensation is one of the best indicators of a favorable prognosis for motor and functional recovery.[64–66]
5. Early (2 day) change in deep tendon reflexes from zero to 3+ indicates recovery of segmental reflexes and motor neuron pool excitability. This may indicate recovery of areas of reticular formation that provide excitatory drive to alpha motor neuron pools via segmental interneuronal pools, and thus it may be a favorable sign for long-term motor recovery.[44]
6. Supportive, interested family and friends.
7. Young age, and absence of risk factors for additional vascular pathology (i.e., no hypertension, atherosclerosis, diabetes, or tobacco or alcohol consumption).
8. Significant improvement in motor and functional ability from the time of acute discharge to the time of the discharge from the rehabilitation facility. This indicates that the patient has shown both neurologic recovery and the ability to learn compensatory patterns for her present residual deficits.
9. Little evidence of perceptual problems or apraxia.
10. Recovery of speech function may be a favorable sign for parallel recovery of sensory integrative function needed for more highly skilled motor recovery.

Signs that are not favorable to recovery are as follows: (1) more than 24 days elapsed before transfer to a rehabilitation facility;[65] (2) muscle tone was still flaccid and severe weakness was present 1 month after onset;[64] and (3) decreased range of motion in left ankle has not improved and may continue to interfere with functional compensation.

In reviewing all these factors, we seem to have an individual who has excellent potential for continued recovery and who has the general health status and family support to help her make use of this potential.

Having reviewed this information, we are now ready to set and prioritize goals. The goals we expect to achieve following 3 months of treatment are listed in Table 9-2. The goals relate directly to the problems and are expressed in measurable terms. They are listed in order of priority, which was determined from the assessment of the problem. Pain is what is bothering the patient most. In turn, we have assessed the pain as being caused primarily by lack of mobility, but also by lack of motor control. Her functional dependence in gait is probably due to a combination of pain and lack of mobility and motor control, especially abnormal postural and equilibrium reactions. This leads to a natural sequence for treatment. Endurance is listed last because it will be difficult for the patient to work on endurance effectively until she has less pain and is able to do more without help from another person. While all of the patient's problems receive attention in treatment, early sessions focus on the key underlying problems (pain, lack of mobility), and later sessions can focus more on motor control and gait if progress is made toward alleviating the pain and impaired mobility. While the reason for the pain and impaired mobility may be the lack of motor control, at this point if we began to work on motor control, it would be difficult for the patient to respond because her responses would be dominated by the symptoms of pain and impaired mobility.

FREQUENCY AND METHOD OF TREATMENT

Very little hard evidence is available upon which to base decisions about the appropriate frequency of treatment for hemiplegic patients who have passed the acute rehabilitative phase. While good evidence exists to support the superiority of specialized rehabilitation hospital care (where, presumably, treatment is more frequent) over general hospital or home care in the acute phase of stroke,[71-73] very few studies examine the response to rehabilitation in patients in the chronic disability phase. One study that did examine this question of treatment frequency in stroke rehabilitation was done in England by Smith and associates.[74] Three different intensities of treatment were compared. The "intense" therapy group received outpatient therapy for half of a day, 5 days per week; the "moderate" group received therapy for half a day, 3 days per week. The "control" group received a home program and weekly visits by a home health worker not trained in physical therapy. The control group lost ground in functional status, while the groups receiving therapy maintained or gained in functional status. The "moderate" intensity used in this study would be unheard of in the United States. In our geographic area, a frequency of 1 hour, three times per week would be considered "intense" and appropriate for a patient, fairly soon after rehabilitation discharge, who displays good potential for recovery by history, as does this patient. In this case, we wanted to choose the highest frequency possible for the patient, within the constraints of her home situation and our department. Getting the patient to and from the hospital more than three times per week seemed too great a burden to place on her family—and on the patient herself, considering her poor endurance. Also, after so much time in the hospital, time at home, with the opportunity to visit with friends and family, was considered important for her mental health. Because improved mobility was a goal, the frequency of three times per week was thought necessary to maintain carryover of gains made in each session and to monitor the effects of treatment. These decisions are based on clinical experience with previous patients and could easily be biased; but since little information from the literature is available on this point, clinical experience (of oneself and colleagues) is the only evidence available for use in this decision.

Decisions about the method of treatment depend, to a great extent, on assessment of the cause of the problem. In this case, the pain and abnormal mobility about the ankle were treated by a variety of means. First, the patient received an orthotics consultation. A new plastic solid ankle foot orthosis was recommended and ordered. This would prevent hypermobilization of the transverse tarsal and tarsometatarsal joints, support the subtalar joint and prevent excessive pronation, remove dynamic stretch to the triceps surae, and allow active dorsiflexion. As an interim measure, a heel lift was placed on the left shoe to decrease the extreme stretch input to the calf during gait that occurred with the Klensak brace, and the spring in the brace was replaced with a solid rod. In treatment, the patient received ice chip packs to the calf and sole of the foot for 15 minutes to inhibit the gastrocnemius muscle and decrease the hypersensitivity of the cutaneous receptors. The decreased sensitivity allowed the patient to tolerate a deep friction massage to her calf, which focused on the intermuscular fascia and musculotendinous junctions. The purpose of the massage was to increase tissue compliance. Although heat would have been better for improving tissue compliance, ice was chosen for its inhibitory effects on the cutaneous receptors and muscle. Following massage, the patient received gentle traction to the calcaneus and gentle passive mobilization of the talus during passive dorsiflexion in her pain-free range. This was followed by active exercises to facilitate dorsiflexion first in long sitting, then with weight bearing in sitting and standing.[2-5] The patient was taught a home program of stretching, in sitting, with knee flex to 90 degrees, foot flat using pressure over the knee and weight shift to left (rocking forward over knee).

After several weeks, the skin's hypersensitivity to touch had decreased, and functional electrical stimulation (FES) to the ankle dorsiflexion was attempted. However, the patient could not tolerate a high enough intensity to produce a contraction, even in the noninvolved side. After trying repeatedly, for several sessions in a row, a decision was made to wait until a later date and try the FES again. The patient had a very negative psychological reaction to the FES and was already very depressed, so it was best not to push her to accept this modality at this time. However, it would be an ideal tool to facilitate the newly active evertors and to inhibit the overactive gastrocnemius-soleus.

The problems of pain and abnormal mobility in the left shoulder were approached by working on improved motor control of the proximal stability muscles in the shoulder and scapula, and by stopping movements and activities that produced pain. Only pain-free movements were used. The normal scapular movements were performed by the therapist during attempts at active movements by the patient, so that upper-extremity motion always recurred with relatively normal scapulohumeral rhythm. Holding and short-arc movements were used in side-lying, supine, and weight-bearing postures of sitting, all fours, and standing with assistance proximally to support the shoulder in a normal position. Work on the motor control of the upper extremity was closely coordinated with occupational therapy. Both occupational and physical therapy worked on proximal stability and scapular control. Work with more distal control in physical therapy focused on weight bearing and postural activities and equilibrium responses; in occupational therapy, work on distal control focused on more purposeful, goal-directed movements, such as two-handed functional activities or using the left upper extremity to assist in dressing activities.

Motor control activities in the lower extremity focused on improving pelvic protraction in rolling, in supine-to-sitting, and in sit-to-stand movements. Pelvic control was assessed as a key to her posture control, balance, and abnormal movement pattern in the lower extremity. Lack of reciprocal movements focused on the ability to alternate knee flexion with knee extension because knee control was a key factor in her abnormal gait. At this time, she practiced in supine and sitting positions because standing was too advanced a position for this activity (i.e., it required postural control beyond the patient's ability). However, the foot was kept on the mat or floor, so that the patient learned to perform reciprocal knee movement even in the presence of cutaneous input from the sole of the foot. Later, weight bearing on the sole of the foot would make reciprocal movements even more difficult. (But this function is necessary for gait.) The other two motor patterns that received focus through a variety of exercise techniques were hip flexion with knee extension, and dorsiflexion (balanced eversion/inversion) with knee extension. Progression was from combining these movements in non–weight bearing to semi-upright to standing positions. To improve sitting and standing positions, work focused on the trunk, especially the ability to rotate and laterally flex and shift weight symmetrically first in sitting, later in standing. Many of the exercises used for proximal control in the upper and lower extremities (i.e., for scapula and pelvis) could readily be combined with work on trunk patterns needed for posture control in sitting and standing.[2,3,7] Automatic postural and equilibrium reactions were facilitated in sitting and standing by first working on proximal stability control in side-lying and supine positions, then on normal alignment in sitting. Slow weight shifting with assistance into the normal postural pattern of the trunk and proximal joints was used in the first few weeks. As the patient improved with this control, movements could become more rapid, and assistive movements could focus on distal components of the normal postural responses.

Early sessions focused more on control in sitting; later sessions used kneeling, half kneeling, and standing. Although Nashner[75–77] has found that many normal postural responses in the lower extremity occur distal to proximal, he has not examined the trunk in detail; we must remember that these distal-to-proximal responses were seen in normal people with a normal and stable trunk. In hemiplegic patients with poor trunk stability, these postural patterns are often out of phase or poorly organized and variable.[78] Sessions during the first few weeks of treatment included practice time with walking, both on level surface and stairs, to help achieve functional independence. Even though the gait pattern was not ideal, and some bad habits were necessary to achieve independence, the psychological benefits of independent ambulation were considered to be more important for this patient at this point in time. Once the patient achieved independence in ambulation, endurance training was approached by encouraging the patient to walk longer distances, and more frequently at home, but being careful to progress only within the limits of her left-foot pain. At this point in her treatment, the goal was not to reinforce poor quality movement patterns through emphasis on endurance activities, but to focus on better motor control, leaving true endurance work until later, when her motor control would hopefully be improved and her gait pattern more normal.

MEASUREMENT OF OUTCOMES

Outcomes were measured as progress toward the goals stated in Table 9-2. The outcomes after 3 months can be seen in Table 9-2.

REASSESSMENT

The process of reassessment involves examination of the progress toward the defined goals. The therapist makes judgments about the reasons for the progress, and based on these judgments, sets new goals and makes treatment changes, if indicated. The reasons for progress fall into three basic categories: (1) physical interventions (in this case, physical therapy treatment, since the patient is not on medication or other treatments aimed at these goals), (2) psychosocial factors, and (3) natural recovery/regression factors. In most situations, all three of these categories of factors will interact to produce the observed effect. Trying to ascertain the nature of these interactions may seem an impossible task. However, all of us do make these judgments, whether we realize it or not. Often the judgments are based on an unconscious store of experience regarding how these factors can interact to produce the responses seen in a particular patient. If we believe a lack of progress is most influenced by the patient's psychological state, we may make it a priority to get the patient referred to a social worker or psychologist for more extensive care. If we feel our treatment has not been correct, we may change it. Sometimes we will do both.

In assessing this patient's progress after 3 months of treatment (see Table 9-2), we see that she has reached and surpassed some goals and fallen short in reaching others. Examining exactly what has happened will help us to formulate our "plan of attack" for the next 3 months of treatment.

A good deal of progress has been made in reducing her foot pain, but the pain has not been eradicated. The pain seems to be clearly related to the abnormal movement mechanics about the ankle in weight bearing and walking, and it coincides with her slow progress in increasing ankle range of motion and muscle compliance of the plantar flexors. Much of her pain reduction is due to the stability provided the forefoot by the new brace (which prevents hypermobilization of the transverse tarsal and tarsometatarsal joints) and improved mobility of the calcaneus and, secondly, the talus, during dorsiflexion movements. The problem with ankle stiffness is particularly vexing in this case in light of the unusually advanced motor recovery about the ankle displayed by this patient. The patient can activate all of the ankle muscles out of synergy in a variety of positions (but not in weight-bearing positions). The ankle muscles even contract in a normal pattern in equilibrium reactions that are non–weight bearing (see Goal 3e), a response that often lags well behind voluntary movement control. If we could help her gain the ability to get her foot flat on the floor, without pain, it seems likely that all these muscles would function in that position as well. The problem at the ankle is also the key to many of her standing posture and gait deviations. Until she can get her foot flat, she cannot hope to get rid of the knee hyperextension and pelvic retraction, which are compensatory postural adjustments that allow the patient to move her torso over an ankle that will not dorsiflex.

Thus, while work would continue on pelvic, hip, and knee control, the major focus of treatment during the next 3 months would be normalizing ankle movement, especially in a weight-bearing posture. Surface electromyographic monitoring might be helpful at this point to record activity of the plantar flexors and dorsiflexors during reciprocal non–weight-bearing and weight-bearing activities. Recording the muscle activity would help to determine if the lack of mobility into dorsiflexion was due more to active or to passive resistance factors in the plantar flexors, and thus help to direct the treatment approach.

From palpation, the problem seems to be due more to passive resistance, and thus the massage to her soft tissues would continue; but massage would now be preceded by heat applications. The patient now has little problem with hypersensitivity (thus, ice is omitted), and heat will be more effective in increasing compliance in the soft tissues.

In working on the ankle motion, the patient is ready to progress from passive mobilization to more work in standing, with the therapist providing the normal movement pattern about the ankle and knee (similar to what was done to facilitate shoulder control by moving the scapula in a normal pattern for the patient). Providing the normal joint alignment during weight bearing should help facilitate the contraction of the ankle muscles (which we know are present) in a normal postural pattern. Work in kneeling is ideal at this stage to refine hip control and to facilitate the pattern of knee flexion with hip extension. Kneeling avoids the problem of abnormal ankle mobility, which interferes with normal pelvic and hip alignment in upright posture. Because the patient still has pain and mobility problems about the ankle, walking endurance for longer distances will not be stressed or encouraged. Walking longer distances may irritate the ankle joint. While walking in the house without her brace is detrimental to her ankle joint, the activity is of such great psychological benefit to this patient that she should be encouraged to continue doing this, but with frequent rests and careful monitoring of foot pain, stopping when pain occurs. Endurance training could now be approached by having the patient work on the stationary bicycle, since she has control out of synergy at hip and knee and since she will also practice partial weight bearing on her left upper extremity, facilitating shoulder stability muscles in a nonpainful position during this activity. Some type of endurance training will be particularly motivating to this patient because she used to run 4 to 5 miles a day prior to her stroke.

Excellent progress has been made with her pain and mobility in the left shoulder, where the patient has surpassed some of the set goals. Although she has made good progress in motor control of the upper extremity in many respects, she clearly has had more improvement in her distal control (at elbow and hand); her progress in proximal control, though present, has lagged behind. This amount of distal recovery is unusual in a stroke patient[3,66] and may be due more to natural recovery than to the treatment intervention. Work would proceed with distal motor patterns but would also focus much more heavily on proximal control, because this is where her natural recovery is lagging and where she needs the most facilitation and assistance. She is a prime candidate to develop a painful shoulder, especially as her motor recovery continues, unless she learns to move with a more normal scapulohumeral rhythm during flexion and abduction. Since she has such good motor return distally, she will be highly motivated to use the hand functionally, and frequently may do so with an abnormal movement pattern at the shoulder. Because her shoulder control is such a key problem, several sessions will be scheduled with occupational therapy, where joint treatments can occur. Thus, each specialist can observe the other's techniques, and the treatment programs can be coordinated to reinforce the goals of treatment.

The patient has made good progress with her trunk control, especially in sitting. Her slower progress in standing and in gait is due mainly to her problems about the ankle, as discussed earlier.

In short, after 3 months of treatment experience with this patient, and observing the progress she has made thus far, her key problems now appear to be lack of mobility and abnormal motor control about the left ankle joint and left scapula. Treatment techniques should focus on these problems. As progress is made toward alleviation of these problems, concentrated treatment could progress to more work on reciprocal movement control, particularly about the knee and in the hand, correction of gait deviations, and more attention to long-distance endurance in walking, rather than biking.

DISCHARGE PLANNING

Since the patient has made significant progress toward most goals, discharge was not considered at this time. After another 3 months, the patient's progress will again be reassessed. It is expected that progress will be slower and gains less dramatic. At that time, the patient may have enough improvement to allow her to do more on her own in a home program. If so, the frequency of her physical therapy visits can be reduced. Even when "formal treatment" stops for this patient (determined by when she no longer progresses toward set goals), she should continue to come to physical therapy for 6-month or 1-year follow-up visits.

If she begins to loose some of her functional ability, she may need to return for a short-term course of intensive treatment, followed by a revised home program. A patient such as this, with a permanent chronic disability, will most likely continue to have a flexible course in her functional abilities that will require periodic intervention by the various rehabilitation therapies to maintain her at her optimal functional level.

SUMMARY

This chapter introduced a model for analyzing the process of clinical decision making in physical therapy and illustrated the application of that analysis model to the case of a 43-year-old stroke victim. Since I believe that clinical decisions should proceed from a knowledge base of the anatomy and pathophysiology involved with the disorder being treated, this chapter included a basic review of the general anatomy and pathophysiology of stroke, along with a more detailed review of the specific disorder under discussion, that is, carotid dissection with secondary embolus to the right middle cerebral artery. Following the presentation of the patient's case history, six major decision-making steps were reviewed, and the factors that contribute to the decisions that were made at each step were analyzed. The discussion covered decisions made during evaluation, assessment, goal setting, treatment planning, reassessment, and discharge planning. The need to understand the influence and interaction of physical, cognitive, and psychosocial factors in this decision-making process was stressed.

REFERENCES

1. Office of Scientific Health Reports, NINCDS, NIH: *The National Survey of Stroke.* Stroke 12(2), Suppl 1, Mar/Apr 1981.
2. Bobath, B: *Adult Hemiplegia: Evaluation and Treatment*, ed 2. William Heinemann, London, 1970.
3. Brunnstrom, S: *Movement Therapy in Hemiplegia.* Harper & Row, New York, 1970.
4. Knott, M and Voss, D: *Proprioceptive Neuromuscular Facilitation: Patterns and Techniques*, ed 2. Harper & Row, New York, 1968.
5. Stockmeyer, S: *An interpretation of the approach of Rood to the treatment of neuromuscular dysfunction.* Am J Phys Med 46:900–956, 1967.
6. Johnstone, M: *Restoration of Motor Function in the Stroke Patient.* Churchill-Livingstone, 1978.
7. Carr, J and Shepard, R: *Physiotherapy in Disorders of the Brain.* William Heinemann, London, 1980.
8. Sullivan, P, Markos, P, and Minor, M: *An Integrated Approach to Therapeutic Exercise: Theory and Clinical Application.* Reston Publishing, Reston, Va, 1982.
9. Farber, C: *Neurorehabilitation.* WB Saunders, Philadelphia, 1982.
10. Basmajian, JV (ed): *Therapeutic Exercise*, ed 3. William & Wilkins, Baltimore, 1978.
11. Wolf, S, et al: *EMG feedback in stroke: Effect of patient characteristics.* Arch Phys Med Rehabil 60:96–102, 1979.
12. Baker, L, et al: *Electrical stimulation of wrist and fingers for hemiplegic patients.* Phys Ther 59:1495–1499, 1979.
13. Baker, M, et al: *Developing strategies for biofeedback: Applications in the neurologically handicapped patient.* Phys Ther 57:402–408, 1977.
14. DeJong, G and Branch, L: *Predicting the stroke patient's ability to live independently.* Stroke 13(5):648–655, 1982.
15. Lobitz, C and Shepard, K: *Effect of compatibility on goal achievement in patient-therapist dyads.* Phys Ther 63:319–324, 1983.
16. Adams, RD and Victor, M: *Cerebrovascular diseases.* In *Principles of Neurology*, ed 2. McGraw-Hill, New York, 1981, pp 529–593.
17. O'Brien, M: *Total Care of the Stroke Patient.* Little, Brown & Co, Boston, 1978.
18. Mohr, JP, et al: *The Harvard Cooperative Stroke Registry: A prospective registry of patients hospitalized with stroke.* Neurology 28:754, 1978.
19. Wylie, E and Ehrenfeld, W: *Extracranial Occlusive CVD: Diagnoses and Management.* WB Saunders, Philadelphia, 1970.
20. Escourolle, R and Poirier, J: *Manual of Basic Neuropathology*, ed 2. WB Saunders, Philadelphia, 1978.
21. Marshall, J: *Management of Cerebrovascular Disease*, ed 3. Blackwell Scientific Publications, Oxford, 1976.
22. Brice, JG, Dawsett, DJ, and Lowe, RP: *Hemodynamic effects of carotid artery stenosis.* Br Med J 2:1363, 1964.
23. Chiang, J, et al: *Cerebral ischemia: Vascular changes.* Am J Pathol 52:455–465, 1968.
24. McCall, AS, Fletcher, PJ, and Hutchinson, E: *Pathology.* In Hutchinson, EC and Acheson, EJ: *Strokes: Natural History, Pathology and Surgical Treatment.* WB Saunders, Philadelphia, 1975, pp 36–105.
25. Davis, J, Miller, R, and Lefkowitz, R: *A possible role for neurotransmitter receptors in stroke.* In Scheinberg, P (ed): *Cerebrovascular Diseases: Tenth Princeton Conference.* Raven Press, New York, 1976, pp 149–152.
26. Moskowitz, M and Wurtman, R: *Acute stroke and brain monoamines.* In Scheinberg, P (ed): *Cerebrovascular Diseases: Tenth Princeton Conference.* Raven Press, New York, 1976, pp 133–166.
27. Bishop, B: *Neural plasticity. I–IV.* Phys Ther 62:1122–1131, 1132–1143, 1275–1283, 1442–1451, 1982.
28. Craik, R: *Clinical correlates of neural plasticity.* Phys Ther 62:1452–1462, 1982.
29. Copenhauer, W, Bunge, R, and Bunge, M: *Baily's Textbook of Histology*, ed 16. Williams & Wilkins, Baltimore, 1971, pp 305–366.
30. Stringer, W and Kelly, D: *Traumatic dissection of the extracranial internal carotid artery.* Neurosurgery 6:123–130, 1980.
31. Ojemann, RG, Fisher, CM, and Rich, JC: *Spontaneous dissecting aneurysms of the internal carotid artery.* Stroke 3:434, 1972.

32. Manz, H, Vester, J, and Lavenstein, B: *Dissecting aneurysm of cerebral arteries in childhood and adolescence.* Virchows Arch a Path Anat Histol 384:325–335, 1979.
33. Pollati, E, Gaist, G, and Poppi, M: *Resolution of occlusion in spontaneously dissected carotid arteries.* J Neurosurg 56:857–860, 1982.
34. Rhoton, A and Friedman, W: Discussion of article by Chapleau and Robertson: *Spontaneous cervical carotid artery dissection: Outpatient treatment and continuous heparin infusion using a totally implantable infusion device.* Neurosurgery 8:83–87, 1981.
35. Fisher, CM, Ojemann, RG, and Roberson, GH: *Spontaneous dissection of the cervico-cerebral arteries.* Can J Neurol Sci 5:9–19, 1978.
36. Zelenock, G, et al: *Extracranial internal carotid artery dissection.* Arch Surg 117:425–432, 1982.
37. Beatty, RA: *Dissecting hematoma of the internal carotid artery following chiropractic cervical manipulation.* J Trauma 17:248–249, 1977.
38. Countece, K, Vijayonathan, T, and Barrese, C: *Cervical carotid aneurysm presenting as recurrent cerebral ischemia with head turning.* Stroke 10:144–147, 1979.
39. Mokr, B, Sundt, T, and Houser, W: *Spontaneous internal carotid dissection, hemicrania and Horner's Syndrome.* Arch Neurol 36:677–680, 1979.
40. Chapleau, C and Robertson, J: *Spontaneous cervical carotid artery dissection: Outpatient treatment with continuous heparin infusion using a totally implantable influsion device.* Neurosurgery 8:83–87, 1981.
41. Ehrenfeld, WK and Wylie, EJ: *Spontaneous dissection of the internal carotid artery.* Arch Surg 111:1244–1301, 1976.
42. McNut, D, Dreisbach, J, and Marsden, R: *Spontaneous dissection of the internal carotid artery.* Arch Neurol 37:54–55, 1980.
43. Landau, WM: *Spasticity: The fable of a neurological demon and the emperor's new therapy.* Arch Neurol 31:217–219, 1974.
44. Lance, JW and McLeod, JG: *A Physiological Approach to Clinical Neurology,* ed 3. Butterworth & Co, Boston, 1981, pp 43–153.
45. Neilson, PD and Lance, JW: *Reflex transmission characteristics during voluntary activity in normal man and patients with movement disorders.* In Desmidt, JD (ed): *Cerebral Motor Control in Man: Long Loop Mechanisms. Clinical Neurophysiology,* Vol 4. Karger-Basel, 1978, pp 263–299.
46. Holmes, G: *The cerebellum of man.* Brain 62:1–30, 1939.
47. Neilson, PD: *Frequency-response characteristics of the tonic stretch reflexes of biceps brachii muscle in intact man.* Medical and Biological Engineering 10:460–472, 1972.
48. Neilson, PD: *Interaction between voluntary contraction and tonic stretch reflex transmission in normal and spastic patients.* J Neurol Neurosurg Psychiatry 35:853–860, 1972.
49. Neilson, PD: *Voluntary and reflex control of the biceps brachii muscle in spastic-athetotic patients.* J Neurol Neurosurg Psychiatry 35:589–598, 1972.
50. Neilson, PD and Andrews, CJ: *Comparison of the tonic stretch reflex in athetotic patients during rest and voluntary activity.* J Neurol Neurosurg Psychiatry 36:547–554, 1973.
51. Andrews, CJ, Neilson, PD and Knowles, L: *Electromyographic study of the rigidospacity of athetosis.* J Neurol Neurosurg Psychiatry 36:94–103, 1973.
52. Norton, B, et al: *Correlation of gait speed and spasticity of the knee.* Phys Ther 55:355–364, 1975.
53. Grimby, L, Hannerz, J, and Ranlund, T: *Disturbances in the voluntary recruitment order of anterior tibial motor units in spastic paraparesis.* J Neurol Neurosurg Psychiatry 37:40–46, 1974.
54. Young, RR, and Shahani, BT: *A clinical neurophysiological analysis of single motor unit discharge patterns in spasticity.* In Feldman, RG, Young, RR, and Koella, WP (eds): *Spasticity: Disordered Motor Control.* Symposia Specialists, Miami, 1980, pp 219–231.
55. Rosenfalch, A and Andreassen, S: *Impaired regulation of force and firing pattern of single motor units in patients with spasticity.* J Neurol Neurosurg Psychiatry 43:907–916, 1980.
56. Brooke, MH and Engel, WK: *The histographic analysis of human muscle biopsies with regard to fiber types. 2. Disease of the upper and lower motor neuron.* Neurology 19:378–393, 1969.
57. Chokroverty, S, Reyes, MG, Rubino, F. Barronk: *Hemiplegic atrophy.* Arch Neurol 33:104–110, 1976.
58. Knuttson, E and Murtensson, A: *Dynamic motor capacity in spastic paresis and its relation to prime mover dysfunction, spastic reflexes and antagonistic co-activation.* Scand J Rehabil Med 12:93–100, 1980.
59. Watkins, MP, Harris, BA, and Kozlowski, BA: *Isokinetic testing in patients with hemiparesis: A pilot study.* Phys Ther 64:184–189, 1984.

60. SAHRMANN, SA AND NORTON, B: *The relationship of voluntary movement to spasticity in the upper motor neuron syndrome.* Ann Neurol 2:460–465, 1977.
61. KNUTTSON, E AND RICHARDS, C: *Different types of disturbed motor control in gait of hemiparetic patients.* Brain 102:405–430, 1979.
62. DEITZ, V, QUINTERN, J, AND BERGER, W: *Electrophysiological studies of gait in spasticity and rigidity.* Brain 104:431–449, 1981.
63. HOLDEN, M, ET AL: *Clinical gait assessment in the neurologically impaired: Reliability and meaningfulness.* Phys Ther 64:35–40, 1984.
64. PRESCOTT, RJ, GARRAWAY, WM, AND AKHTAR, AJ: *Predicting functional outcome following acute stroke using a standard clinical examination.* Stroke 13:641–647, 1982.
65. STERN, P, ET AL: *Factors influencing stroke rehabilitation.* Stroke 2:213–218, 1971.
66. MOSKOWITZ, E, LIGHTBODY, F, AND FREITAG, N: *Long term follow-up of the post stroke patient.* Arch Phys Med Rehabil 53:167–172, 1972.
67. PERRY, J: *Normal upper extremity kinesiology.* Phys Ther 58:265–278, 1978.
68. BOBATH, K: Letter to the Editor. Phys Ther 52:44–45, 1972.
69. SUBBARAO, J AND STILLIVELL, GK: *Reflex sympathetic dystrophy syndrome of the upper extremity: Analysis of total outcome of management of 125 cases.* Arch Phys Med Rehabil 62:549–554, 1981.
70. BOOKSTEIN, NA: *Early Flexer Withdrawal as a Prognotic Indicator in Severe Head Injury.* Thesis, Medical College Virginia/Virginia Commonwealth University, Richmond Va, 1978.
71. ANDERSON, TP, ET AL: *Stroke rehabilitation, evaluation of its quality by assessing patient outcomes.* Arch Phys Med Rehabil 59:170–175, 1978.
72. ANDERSON, TP, BALDRIDGE, M, AND ETTINGER, M: *Quality of care for completed stroke without rehabilitation: Evaluation by assessing patient outcomes.* Arch Phys Med Rehabil 60:103–107, 1979.
73. REIGENSON, J: *Stroke rehabilitation: Outcome studies and guidelines for alternative levels of care.* Stroke 12:372–375, 1981.
74. SMITH, DS, ET AL: *Remedial therapy after stroke: A randomized controlled trial.* Br Med J 282:517–520, 1981.
75. NASHNER, LM: *Organization and programming of motor activity during posture control.* Prog Brain Res 50:177–184, 1979.
76. NASHNER, LM: *Adapting reflexes controlling the human posture.* Exp Brain Res 26:59–72, 1976.
77. NASHNER, LM, WOOLLACOTT, M, AND TUMA, G: *Organization of rapid responses to postural and locomotor-like perturbations of standing man.* Exp Brain Res 36:163–76, 1979.
78. BADKE, M AND DUNCAN, P: *Patterns of rapid motor responses during postural adjustments when standing in healthy subjects and hemiplegic patients.* Phys Ther 63:13–20, 1983.

Chapter 10

CLINICAL DECISION MAKING: ORTHOPAEDIC PHYSICAL THERAPY

STANLEY V. PARIS, N.Z.S.P., M.C.S.P., P.T.

Orthopaedic physical therapy embraces perhaps the broadest field within our profession and may be the most basic science of all our practice. Whatever we do as clinical physical therapists, we will be seeking to enhance the functioning of the musculoskeletal system. This improvement is true not just for neck and hip pains, but for chest conditions, pediatrics, sports, neurology, and so forth. It is therefore necessary for all therapists to have a basic knowledge of orthopaedic physical therapy so that they may practice their particular specialties as effectively as possible. Since the spectrum of physical therapy is so broad, it is necessary that I limit my presentation to that which is practiced under the specialty area of orthopaedics and further limit it to the area that I shall be presenting, a simple neck condition. To present this information in a meaningful fashion, I have divided the contents into two categories: (1) orthopaedic principles and practice, and (2) evaluation and treatment of the simple neck condition.

ORTHOPAEDIC PRINCIPLES AND PRACTICE

BASIC SCIENCE GAP

There are two components for determining clinical decisions. The first consists of the scientific knowledge base, known as the basic sciences, which includes factors proven by clinical trial and controlled studies; the second is the empirical or intuitive approach derived from our clinical experiences.

The basic sciences supporting orthopaedic physical therapy, particularly that of the spine, are, at best, very meager. This lack of a knowledge base is not the case, for instance, in a joint such as the knee, where the anatomy, mechanics, and pathology appear to be well understood by most of the "authorities." There are, of course, some differences and preferences regarding how the knee might be treated, but these preferences are based on interpretation of the known data and, in fact, are quite similar in method and purpose.

The human spine is a highly developed, extremely complex structure. Unlike the knee, efforts to understand the spine have only just begun. Only in recent years has its neurophysiology been explored and its neuroanatomy investigated.[1-3] Furthermore, only in the last decade have societies been formed with a specific goal of developing knowledge in these areas (Cervical Spine Research Society, International Society for the Study of the Lumbar Spine, and Scoliosis Society). Much remains to be done. The small pool of what is known permits practitioners to do and justify almost whatever they wish. Some clinicians attempt to relate their practice to basic science, while others disregard it entirely, explaining their practice by simply stating "it works." Still others develop their own theories that are totally unsupported by what is known or even by sound logic. Much of what we do is based on intuition. Intuition is a process in clinical practice common to the more experienced clinician. Ask such persons why they performed a certain procedure or made a particular choice, and they may not at first have an answer. On further inquiry, however, it is quite likely that they will be able to recall a similar case in which they found that the choice they just made was quite effective. Hopefully, they will not reply as technicians that they always do it in that way, or worse still, it is done that way because they were taught so.

A PHILOSOPHY ON DYSFUNCTION

It is philosophy that decides our approach or, if you wish, bias. Philosophy is necessary for practice, but it must not become so rigid that it inhibits not only our own professional growth but those of us whom we influence. My personal philosophy of practice may be summarized in seven general principles related to dysfunction:

1. *Joint injuries,* including such conditions referred to as osteoarthritis, instability, and the after effects of sprains and strains, are not diseases but dysfunctions.
2. Dysfunctions are manifest as either increases or decreases of motion from the expected normal or by the presence of aberrant movements. Thus, dysfunctions are represented by *abnormal movement.*
3. Where the dysfunction is detected as limited motion, the treatment of choice is *mobilization* (manipulation) of joint structures, stretching of muscles and fascia, and the promotion of activities that encourage a full range of movement.
4. When the dysfunction is manifest as increased movement, laxity, or instability, the treatment is not mobilization of the joint in question, but *stabilization* by instruction about correct posture, stabilization exercises, and correction of any limitations of movement in neighboring joints that may contribute compensation.
5. Degenerated cartilage resulting in a loss of joint space can be made to *regenerate* by altering alignment and stresses and by promoting

frequent use at low loads. Therefore, it is reasonable to assume that in physical therapy, by stretching restricted capsules and myofascia, correcting postural alignment, and utilizing means to alter alignment, it should also be possible not only to halt but to reverse the degeneration or aging process.

6. The physical therapist's *primary role* is in the evaluation and treatment of dysfunction, whereas that of the physician is the diagnosis and treatment of disease.
7. In this age where, in some medical schools, the study of the anatomy of the extremities is an elective, and where spinal dissection is rarely required, we in physical therapy have the added responsibility of developing our knowledge of the structure and function of the neuro-muscular-skeletal system so that we may safely assume the leadership in the conservative treatment and management of this system.

The last principle is a challenge to our profession and not just to orthopaedic physical therapists. It is a challenge that we are not sufficiently prepared to accept, but it is one that we must rise to meet. If we do not, then another profession will fill the gap. The history of physical therapy is full of lost opportunities and inroads made by other professional groups, such as chiropractors, physician assistants, licensed practical nurses, correction therapists, nurse practitioners, and others. The professions that were developed to fill the gaps that we have not filled are already quite numerous and include athletic trainers, chest physical therapists, and movement therapists.

One can argue against such a philosophy, but support can also be gathered. The approach that we, as orthopaedic physical therapists, should have to our patients and the medical profession is as outlined above. It is not unrealistic, and it is wholly practical. Note that the philosophy avoids our being associated with the term diagnosis. Nothing could do us more harm in our progress as a profession than the word "diagnosis." Regardless of its exact definition, and regardless of those physicians and health educators who say that we physical therapists can use the term, it is in my view somewhat presumptuous of us, if not dishonest; above all, it is threatening to our medical colleagues.

Professionally, we are not sufficiently trained in biochemistry and laboratory and diagnostic procedures to make a meaningful diagnosis. Furthermore, if we were to undertake such training, we would, like the medical profession, be ignoring what it is we are meant to concentrate on most—dysfunction. We need to work with physicians in a cooperative vein and not in a threatening one. We treat dysfunction, and we do it best when working with the physician who treats the disease.

CHANGING PRACTICE

The changing practice laws that permit evaluation and treatment without practitioner referral must elicit mixed emotions in all physical therapists. On the positive side, however, such laws permit the opportunity to see our patients over an extended period and to follow up on our treatments. This opportunity will be invaluable in the development of a data base for our profession.

All too often, we have received prescriptions ordering us to see a patient for perhaps three times a week for 3 weeks and then to refer back to the physician. Thereafter, we did not see the patient again. Whatever happened to the patient's problems 3 months or a year later was usually lost to our records. Only the physicians might know the answers to the questions that we would have asked, and it is unlikely that they would have asked such questions. As a result, there has been very little opportunity for us to follow a patient long term, and rarely, therefore, do we know the effects of our ministrations.

Now all that is changing, for we shall be able to follow our patients for prolonged periods. This will mean that when we have a patient with osteoarthrosis of the hip, with joint-space narrowing as seen on the radiograph and a tight capsule as detected by clinical evaluation, we shall be able to treat and follow this patient. Our treatments must be effective to be justifiable. In the case of the hip, we may, for instance, treat the patient three times a week for 2 months and then 1 week every 3 months. Over a period of 5 to 10 years, we might be able to establish that by restoring normal capsular extensibility and by modifying the patient's activity, the joint space has indeed regenerated, thus halting the degenerative or aging process of that cartilage. This improvement has been done surgically by Pauwels[4] and Maquet,[5] among others. We should believe that physical therapists, by maintaining function and encouraging light but frequent and correct use of a joint, could achieve the same end.

ORTHOPAEDIC PHILOSOPHY

Since the gap between basic science and clinical practice is admittedly great, there will remain, at least for the present, a divergence of practice. Set forth in Figure 10-1 is a very simple and concise classification of the major emphases by various individuals or professions prominent in the conservative management of spinal conditions. Of course, justice is not done to any of these groups by such a concise presentation, and it is offered merely as a guide.

To advance beyond being technicians, clinicians must independently evaluate and decide on treatment programs. Then they must take professional responsibility for their courses of action. Should there be a conflict in the physician's "orders," then they must initiate and negotiate a compromise. When such is not possible, they cannot treat the patient other than as technicians. Even then they do not escape legal responsibilities.

To justify full responsibility, we must know what it is we are doing—or at least know as well as can be expected of us. The knowledge gained through textbooks, classes, and practical experiences gives us the confidence to make meaningful and effective decisions. We need to ask, "What is that knowledge base?"

The knowledge base we must demonstrate to treat orthopaedic cases effectively includes: (1) functional anatomy, (2) biomechanics, (3) clinical syndromes, (4) a complete system of evaluation, (5) skills in manual techniques, and (6) awareness of supportive services and professionals.

The scope of this presentation does not permit a detailed discussion of these six components. However, the next section will deal with the common

School of Thought — Summary
(principal theory and technique)

1. Based on Relieving Nerve Root Pressure
   Chiropractic - moves vertebra - specific
   Cyriax - moves disk - nonspecific
   McKenzie - moves disk - nonspecific

2. Based on Relieving Pain
   Maitland - oscillates to eliminate reproducible signs
   Maigne - mobilizes osteopathically "no pain & contrary motion"

3. Based on Restoring Function
   Osteopathy - joint and body systems - specific
   Mennell - joint play - specific
   Kaltenborn - arthrokinematics (convex-concave) - specific
   Paris - dysfunction, mechanistic, - specific

FIGURE 10-1. Summary of schools of thought.

clinical syndromes of the spine, as well as with a system of evaluation suitable for the detection of the appropriate dysfunctions.

COMMON SPINAL SYNDROMES

It is possible to examine a patient without having any knowledge of the common spinal syndromes and to collect just the objective data. A knowledge of the possible syndromes, however, will lead clinicians along paths of inquiry that may give further elucidation and may sharpen the eventual focus on the patient's condition. Hence, syndromes should be considered before proceeding to the evaluation.

PHILOSOPHY AGAIN

This progression brings us back to philosophy; for whenever we examine a patient, we do so with our inherent biases. These biases may be helpful, but they usually obstruct objective assessment. We must remember the words of Hollinshead,[6] who stated that if an examiner looks hard enough for something he thinks he sees, he will usually find it. This bespeaks of a trap into which novices often fall.

Most clinicians who examine the spine, regardless of their professional degrees, do so with an inadequate knowledge of anatomy and biomechanics, and most important of all, with an all-too-narrow perspective on clinical

TABLE 10-1. List of Principal Spinal Syndromes

1. Myofascial Restrictions
2. Ligamentous Strains and Sprains
3. Acute Facet Strain and Synovitis
4. Facet Restrictions
5. Sacroiliac Subluxations
6. Sacroiliac Displacement
7. Disk Degeneration
8. Stenosis—Lumbar Spine
9. Spondylosis—Cervical Spine
10. Spondylolisthesis
11. Kissing Vertebrae
12. Dysfunction (Lesion) Complex

possibilities. In this manner, some clinicians see only disk diseases, while others see weak abdominal muscles or loss of back extension or vertebral subluxations. Not until recently have orthopaedic specialists looked beyond the intervertebral disk as the culprit of low back and cervical pain.[7-10] The numbers of such individuals are small. But due to their influence and their acceptance of an ever-broadening range of diagnostic possibilities, they have had a significant influence on medical education and practice in the care of the spine and, in particular, of the lumbar spine. Of course, there is no agreement among them, and none should be expected. Healthy differences of opinions stimulate discussion and debate and lead to research. Fortunately, such activities are finally taking place at an increasing level in open forums and in the professional journals and societies. Perhaps during the next decade, most professional journals will forsake their present biases and move to a more common base on the broader classifications such as those in Table 10-1.

Each of the spinal syndromes depicted in Table 10-1 cannot be presented in any detail, but the salient points about each can.

This list has been compiled over the years, and it continues to undergo revision. One recent addition was spinal stenosis, which, although referred to first by Verbiest,[11] did not really come to our consciousness until Kirkaldy-Willis and Hill[8] began a series of studies that were later reinforced by computerized tomography, which enhances our visualization of this condition.

On the other hand, facet restrictions and subluxations have finally gained the recognition they deserve. In the literature, the facet syndrome was first described by Ghormley[12] in 1933. Unfortunately, in the next year, Mixter and Barr[13] were to make the preoperative diagnosis of a herniated disk, and thus the surgeons directed their attention to disk prolapse and not to the more posterior facet. The facet has not been forgotten over these past 50 years by persons such as the Mennells,[14,15] Stoddard,[16] and Paris,[17,18] who have suggested that the facet was perhaps the most prominent cause of low back pain. It finally received the recognition it deserved when Rees[19] and, later, Mooney and Robertson[7] and Carrera and associates[20] noted the importance of facet pathology to low back pain and sciatica. Change arising from the facet may alter reflexes and straight leg raising and may give not only central low back pain, but also pain down either leg. Our investigations of spinal facet anatomy and neuroanatomy have enabled us to find what we believe is the first interarticular facet adhesion and to identify that seven nerves innervate this joint.[3,21]

Conditions involving the sacroiliac joint and the myofascia await further clinical attention. Myofascial restrictions are recognized around most joints of the body, notably the hip, shoulder, knee, and ankle. Restrictions of the spine, however, do not receive the recognition they deserve. Fortunately, the sacroiliac is beginning to receive much-needed attention from persons such as Kirkaldy-Willis and Hill[8] and Park.[22] Movement of the joint is still being debated, but the evidence for it is overwhelming.

Given the complexities of spinal anatomy and function, and the difficulties in determining exact diagnoses, it is not surprising that our limited knowledge would lead us to wish for a single pathologic entity such as "prolapsed disk." Alternatively, we could recognize that we really do not understand the pathology.

The principal feature of each syndrome will be presented in the form of a table, and the more subtle points will be discussed in the text. Such tables and discussions can only serve to highlight the distinguishing features of these syndromes.

MYOFASCIAL RESTRICTIONS

Myofascial restrictions (Table 10-2) may occur by themselves due to overuse or overstrain and will invariably accompany any other injury in the low back. The patient complains of "tight" muscles and may show limitation of active movements, most noticeably, forward bending. These restrictions obviously limit function and may lead to adverse changes in other structures, such as the facet and disk.

Treatment should be directed at relieving the cause of the muscle stress wherever possible. If this resulted from simple overuse, then the cause is in the muscle, and we will attempt to stretch those muscles. If the cause, however, resides in an injury to the facet joint and the muscle pain is secondary to guard against further injury, then we will need to treat both facets and

TABLE 10-2. Myofascial Restrictions

FACTS
- Perhaps the most common dysfunction
- Subtle subthreshold changes
- Pain widespread in the back

CAUSES
- Poor posture (lordosis)
- Unaccustomed activity
- Overuse (rarely, if ever, a tear)
- Secondary to other dysfunctions

SIGNS AND SYMPTOMS
- Restriction of forward bending
- Free sidebending (in neck, may need to support arms)
- Altered tone to touch—less elasticity

TREATMENT
- Correct posture and advise on use
- Correct other dysfunctions
- Contract-relax-stretch (see Fig. 10-2A)
- Sustained stretch (see Fig. 10-2B)

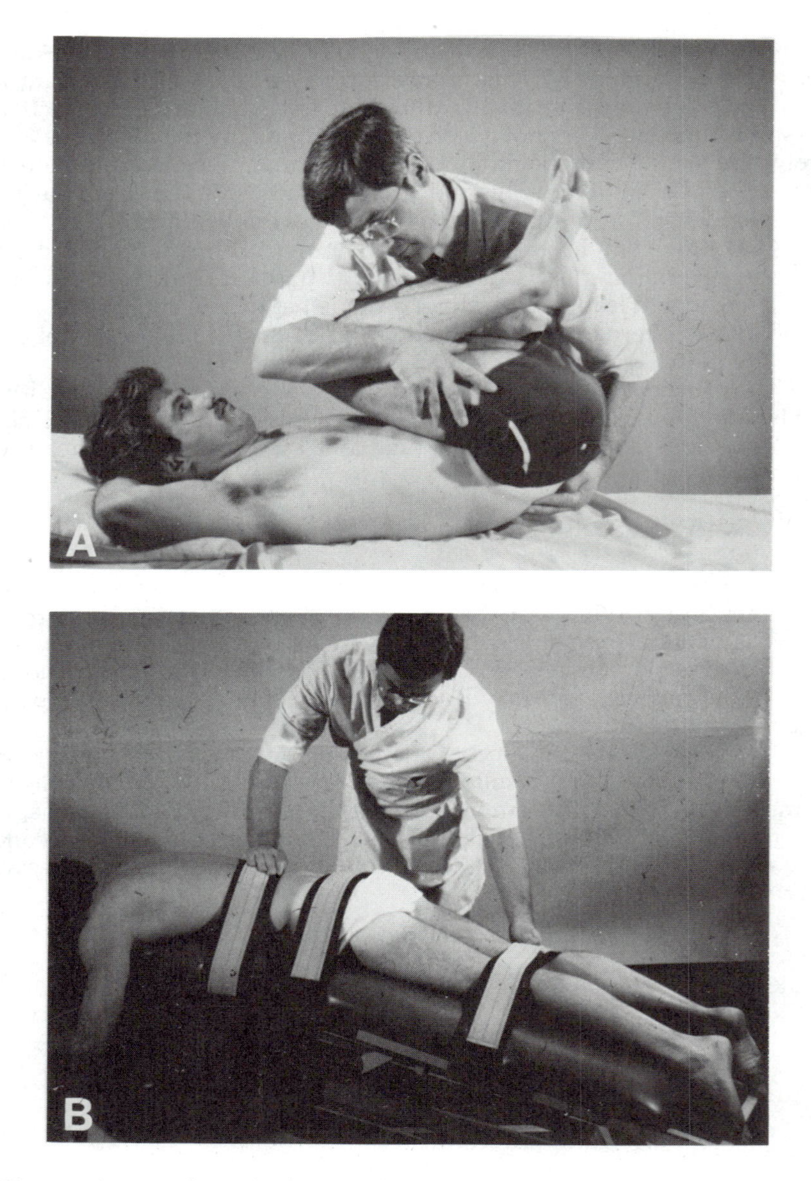

FIGURE 10-2. *A,* Manual stretch of the myofascia. Here, a contract-relax-stretch technique is used. *B,* Mechanical stretch of the myofascia.

muscles. For the muscles, the techniques of neuromuscular facilitation, which consist of contract, relax, and stretch, are quite useful. Figure 10-2A illustrates a method of a sustained stretch performed manually. When the patient is either too large for the therapist or when the muscle contracture has been present for some time, a mechanical assist, as illustrated in Figure 10-2B, can be quite useful. The methods of contract-relax are well known in reducing the muscle's tendency to resist stretch. When using a

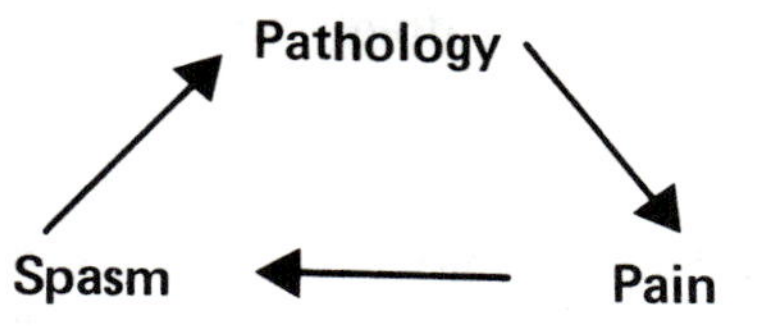

FIGURE 10-3. Incorrect triad.

mechanical stretch, the muscle will resist; therefore, the mechanical stretch will be applied for at least 15 minutes. A duration of 20 minutes seems to be more effective, and the possible reason is that the stretch reflex of muscles has been fatigued.

Muscle Guarding

A clinical note needs to be made concerning the term *muscle spasm,* which is apparently often used in clinical practice to describe several muscle states, with little attempt to differentiate between them. *Dorland's Illustrated Medical Dictionary* defines spasm as "an uncontrolled, involuntary jerk." But we do not see this behavior in a patient who displays "tight" musculature when sitting, standing, or lying prone. The simple triad set forth in Figure 10-3 is quite incorrect.

In this triad, pathology leads to pain, pain to spasm, and spasm to the pathology once again. This is, of course, an oversimplification. Pathology, or as I prefer to call it, dysfunction, may lead to nociception (noxious stimuli) that, if not at a conscious level, will lead to a state of involuntary muscle holding rather than to an appreciation of pain. This holding will limit or alter joint function and, thus, aggravate the dysfunction. Therefore, the basic triad shown in Figure 10-4 is suggested.

Dysfunction leads to nociception and involuntary muscle holding. This triad presents a much better framework within which to begin our understanding of muscle dysfunction as either a primary lesion following, for instance, overuse after digging in a garden, or a secondary lesion to, for instance, a facet joint problem or after ligamentous injury.

The complaint of pain brings the patients to us. They do not come because their back has lost a few degrees of movement or because one shoulder does not elevate as high as the other. They come because they hurt, and they come to seek relief from discomfort. For us to imagine that, in non-traumatic cases such as osteoarthrosis of the hip and degenerative conditions

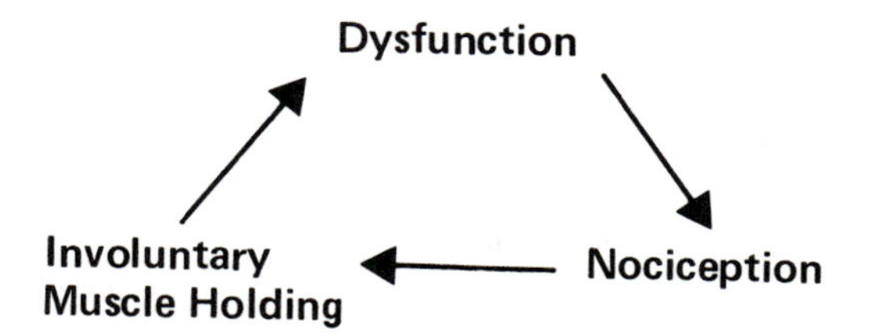

FIGURE 10-4. Correct basic triad.

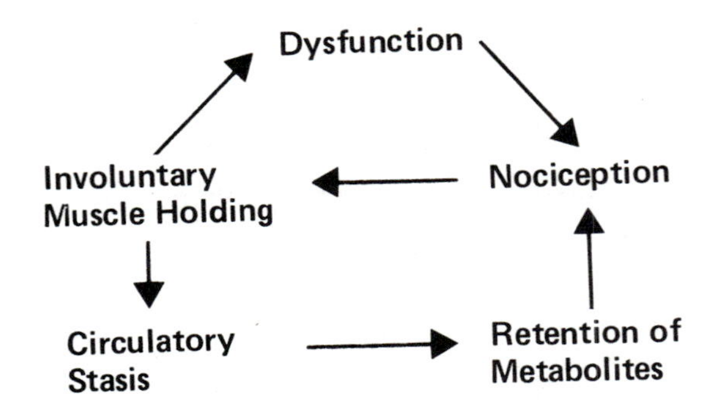

FIGURE 10-5. Expanded diagram.

of the spine, there was nothing wrong before the patients began to complain of pain is to totally misunderstand the degenerative process. Degeneration begins, progresses, and causes minor nociception long before it reaches the conscious level.

Should the condition causing the involuntary muscle holding not resolve itself, the result will be increased circulatory stasis. The stasis will lead to retention of metabolites such as lactic acid, which will further increase nociception. Thus, we can now expand on the diagram, as shown in Figure 10-5. Please note that although we have further nociception, we still do not have any description of pain.

The next stage, shown in Figure 10-6, is the addition of what I call, for lack of histologic evidence, "chemical muscle holding." This phenomenon is the second type of muscle holding. The first is involuntary.

Chemical muscle holding is believed to be present when, for example, the patient lies face down and, after being made comfortable, continues to display a unilateral or bilateral increase in back muscle tone. This tone has a firm and somewhat inelastic response to touch. These muscles may have lost much of their extensibility, perhaps due to retention of metabolites. Therefore, these muscles may offer restriction to both active and passive motions. This chemical muscle holding state responds well to heat and massage but returns rapidly when activities are resumed, unless the underlying dysfunction is adequately corrected. At about this stage, the patient may become aware of pain.

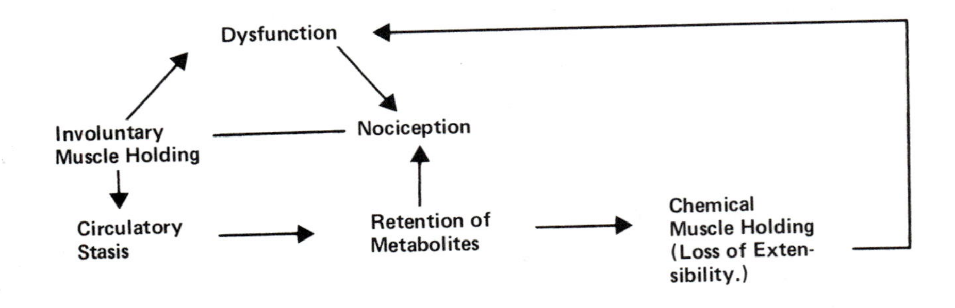

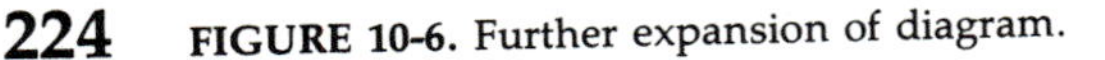

FIGURE 10-6. Further expansion of diagram.

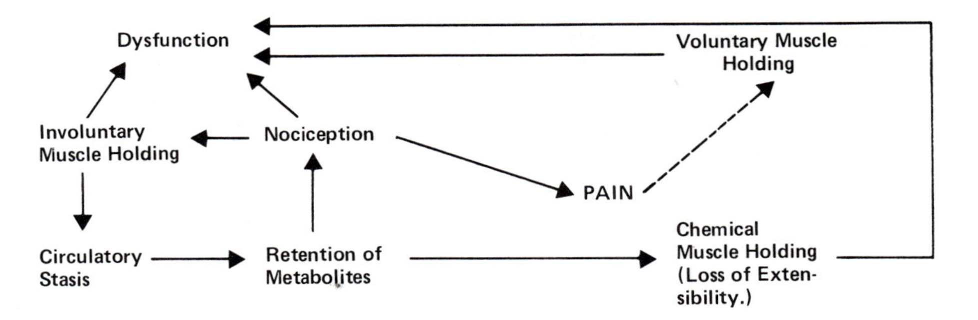

FIGURE 10-7. Final diagram, with inclusion of pain.

The key to our managing joint conditions is our understanding of the role played by pain. If, for instance, a patient is referred with a painful shoulder with abduction limited to 90 degrees, and after 2 weeks of therapy, abduction is increased to 120 degrees and the patient reports relief of pain, would we discharge that patient? We would be in agreement that discharge at this point would be a disservice since much function remains to be regained. The complaint of pain would probably return again because the joint is not satisfactorily rehabilitated and is liable to further injury.

But what of the spine? All too often, the clinician lacks the knowledge of the techniques to adequately assess the spine. Hence, when the patient ceases to complain of pain, a discharge is usually arranged. It should not be surprising, therefore, that with the continuing existence of uncorrected dysfunctions, back pain continues to recur; and at each recurrence, the degenerative process is most likely increased, and progress toward a serious condition may be underway.

Figure 10-7 presents the last diagram in this series and the missing word. *Pain* in this diagram has been shown to be the latent response to dysfunction. The relief of pain does not mean the relief of dysfunction. What finally brings on pain? It could be a combination of any one of a number of factors, including: (1) advancing of the dysfunction, (2) further injury, (3) premenstrual or other forms of stress, and (4) depression.

LIGAMENTOUS INJURIES

Basically, there are two causes of ligamentous injuries. The first is one of gradual onset usually caused by the stresses of poor posture (Table 10-3). The patient compensates for the loss of movement at an adjacent segment. If a surgeon, for instance, has fused the lumbosacral segment, then the segment immediately above that, between the fourth and fifth lumbar vertebrae, will need to compensate for this loss of movement. Other common compensatory relationships include the sacroiliac joint in response to a tight hip and the midcervical region in response to upper-thoracic restrictions common in post-menopausal women.

Ligamentous conditions are difficult to envision but, no doubt, are represented by a weakening, frank separation or disruption of the ligamentous fibers. Once such a weakening has occurred, the ligament will easily extend whenever a stress is placed upon it, and input from nociceptive axons will

TABLE 10-3. Ligamentous Strains and Sprains

CAUSES
- Obesity, poor posture
- Secondary to neighboring restrictions (e.g., upper-thoracic kyphosis, hip restrictions)
- Trauma (e.g., motor vehicle accidents)

SIGNS AND SYMPTOMS
- Dull ache on assuming a fixed posture
- Constant need to change posture
- Associated involuntary muscle holding
- Aggravated by menstrual cycle

TREATMENT
- Postural reeducation and weight loss
- Temporary support—corset or brace
- Exercises to support ligaments
- Heat and massage to associated muscle states

soon be triggered. Since we understand that ligamentous pain arises from a weakened ligament that, whenever stretched, will reproduce pain and perhaps trigger muscle guarding, it makes good sense to reduce the stress on these ligaments. Correct posture or neutral postures, particularly where they are supported by adequate muscle action or appropriate sitting and resting positions, will reduce this stress. In time, the ligaments will recover. We believe that recovery does take place because the patient not only complains of less discomfort, but on examination, less movement is present, thus indicating that ligaments have regained some of their integrity.

FACET STRAIN

Facet strains occur and result most probably in synovitis whenever an individual experiences a sudden twinge of pain or a sudden blocking against moving in a certain direction (Table 10-4). Of course, some authorities consider that this may be due to a disk prolapse; but disk prolapses are soft and unlikely to restrict motion. Furthermore, these sudden catches or blockings of movement are not uncommon in the thoracic region, where it is generally recognized that disk prolapses are rare. It could be a muscle strain, but isometric contraction does not reproduce the pain. Nipping of a nerve has been suggested, but healthy nerves do not hurt when pressed upon and only reproduce pain once they have become ischemic. It looks like the sensitive facet capsule has been nipped and is responsible for these kinds of signs and symptoms.

Once injured, the joint may just be stiff; if the capsule is caught, a situation that exists when movement of side bending toward the painful side is acutely limited by pain, movement will not be possible. The more common situation of just restriction will be that demonstrating a *capsular pattern*. This means that movements involving the injured facet will be those that are most restricted (Table 10-5). For low cervical facets on the left side, the capsular pattern is most likely to restrict side bending and rotation to the right, but all other movements are less restricted. Once muscle guarding is established, all movements may be limited to varying degrees. This is something that

TABLE 10-4. Acute Facet Strain and Synovitis

FACTS
- With or without painful blocking
- Will demonstrate capsular pattern
- Pain unilateral, posterior thigh to the knee

CAUSES
- Sustained stretch or overstretch
- Unaccustomed overuse
- Awkward movement "catch"

SIGNS AND SYMPTOMS
- Pain demonstrating capsular pattern
- If painful blocking—associated muscle guarding (picture capsular impingement)
- Considerable muscle guarding

TREATMENT
- If painful blocking—manipulate to release impinged structure
- Rest from activity but not function
- Maintain neutral postures
- Gate with neurophysiologic techniques
- Manipulate restrictions 10 days after initial injury

most individuals soon recognize after they have injured their facets and begun to treat themselves by stretching and twisting the tightened muscles. Failure to do this by an apprehensive or previously injured patient may only result in increasing the stiffness.

If blocking is present, the therapist will need to manipulate the patient to relieve the trapped capsule. One common technique involves traction in the following manner. The head and neck are given traction along the long axis of the spine and then strongly rotated toward the side of the discomfort. The neck is then brought back to the long axis position and released gently. If, at any time, this procedure brings on the patient's pain, it should be abandoned.

Movements should be maintained following a facet injury. Oscillations may assist mobility by helping to block the pain and by relieving muscle guarding.[23] Any restrictions that remain could be manipulated after 10 days,

TABLE 10-5. Facet Restrictions

FACTS
- Follows uncorrected acute facet synovitis
- Most are asymptomatic

CAUSES
- Acute facet strain with resultant adhesions
- Repeated minor abuse leading to osteoarthrosis
- Poor posture—restricted use

SIGNS AND SYMPTOMS
- Capsular pattern of restriction
- Minimal discomfort

TREATMENT
- Manipulation

because the joint will then have a good tolerance and seems to respond better at that time.

FACET RESTRICTIONS

Facet restrictions result from uncorrected synovitis or disuse that occurs after formation of adhesions (Fig. 10-8). Restrictions may happen after loss of extensibility of an immobile facet joint capsule. Usually, these conditions do not hurt; but like any stiff joint, its tolerance to insult is decreased and might therefore be subjected more frequently to sprains.

We frequently find facet restrictions adjacent to painful segments and therefore attempt to remove the stiffness to reduce the stress on the painful segment. This approach works quite effectively.

Figure 10-8 illustrates intra-articular facet adhesions, and Figure 10-9 shows a method of stretching these by manipulation.

Sacroiliac conditions have not received a great deal of attention in the medical literature, although a recent article[8] and book[16] have attempted to place the joint in perspective. Dissection studies have shown that the innervation of the joint is such that surgical approaches to the lumbar spine, including rhizotomy, laminectomy, and spinal fusion, may well result in the relief of pain from the sacroiliac joint because the nerve to this joint will have been severed.[3] As a result, failure to recognize the role of this joint in the

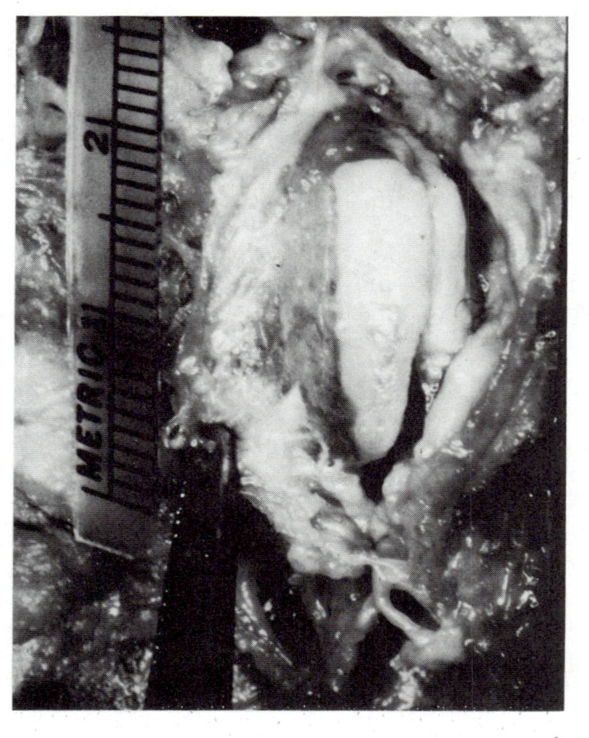

FIGURE 10-8. An intra-articular facet adhesion. Note the adhesion just to the right of the center, which serves to bind down the capsule to the bone end.

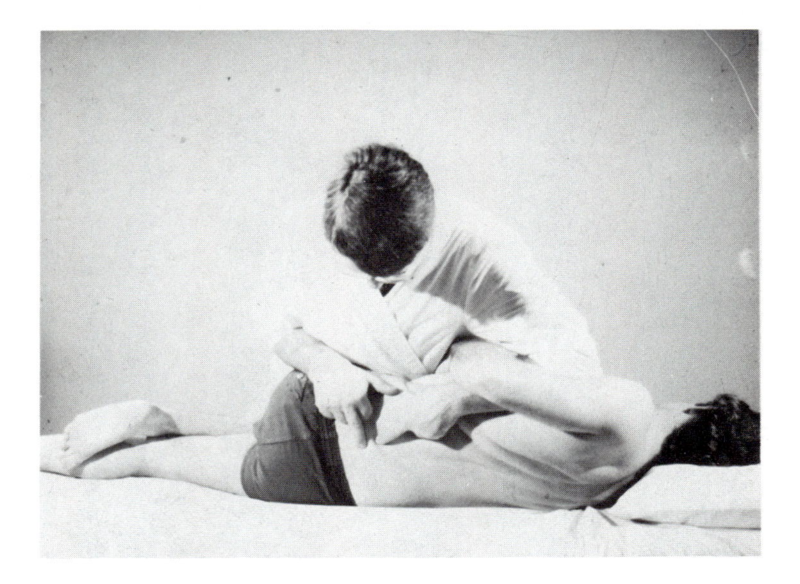

FIGURE 10-9. Manipulation to stretch adhesion. This technique, localized as much as possible to the limited segment, would serve to distract the facet joint and thus place a stretch on the adhesion.

reduction of low back pain may cause surgeons to misinterpret the methods by which their procedures have produced pain relief.

SACROILIAC SUBLUXATIONS

Subluxations are more common in younger women. However, they are not unknown in athletic men up to their mid-fifties, as illustrated in Figures 10-10 and 10-11 resulting from trauma while riding a mechanical bull.

The most common condition involving the sacroiliac joint is subluxation that will result whenever the ligaments to the joint have become lax (Table 10-6). Women are affected more often than men, possibly because the joint is smaller and is located further from the hip, which increases the leverage upon the sacroiliac joint. Furthermore, a woman during childbearing years may experience hormonal changes concomitant with pregnancy that help soften the ligaments of the pelvis and thus lead, still further, to the tendency toward subluxation. Other causes, again principally in women, include the tendency to stand on one leg with the pelvis dropped, and repeated minor trauma from slips and falls.

The treatment is postural correction and support using corsets or sacroiliac belts. The purpose of this approach is to reduce the stress on the joint and to allow the ligaments time to regain their normal strength. Several months may need to elapse before the patient is free of symptoms. It might also be helpful to correct any restrictions of motion in neighboring joints, such as the hip or within the low back, to relieve the strain on the sacroiliac joint.

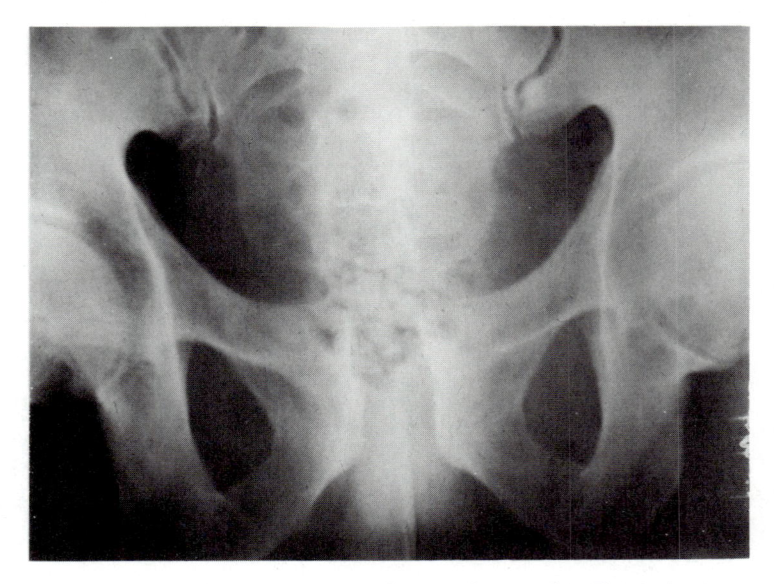

FIGURE 10-10. Note the rather large space at the symphysis pubis. This is due to a traumatic separation.

SACROILIAC DISPLACEMENT

Sacroiliac displacements (Table 10-7) are uncommon in men because the joint is somewhat larger and thus more stable. Displacements are most likely to occur following hypermobility, when an additional force is sufficient to

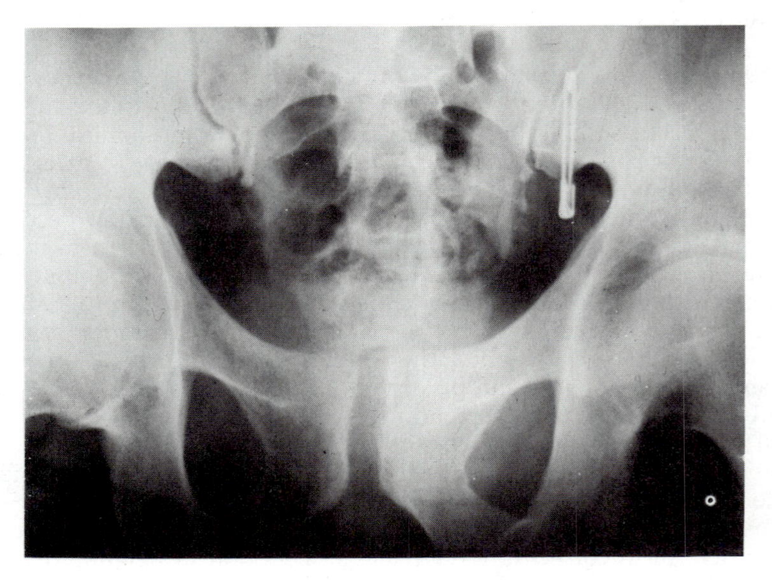

FIGURE 10-11. The same patient as in Figure 10-10, but now the symphysis pubis has been reduced by the application of a sacroiliac binder.

TABLE 10-6. Sacroiliac Subluxations

FACT
More frequent in women during childbearing years
CAUSES
Persistent one-leg standing
Repeated minor trauma
Childbirth and intercourse strains
SIGNS AND SYMPTOMS
Low pelvis on affected side
Hypermobility to passive motion tests
Posterior sacroiliac ligaments tender to palpation
TREATMENT
Support and posture
Injection
Correction of any neighboring restrictions

take the articular surfaces beyond their normal limits, causing a hitch on some articular incongruity. This state can be detected by passive motion testing, whereupon it will be seen that the joint is barely moving compared with the good side, or by observing structural defects in the pelvis, illustrating a rotary lesion. These structural defects are difficult to describe without viewing a patient who actually has the problem. The treatment of choice is manipulation to restore the joint to its normal alignment, after which it may be found to be hypermobile.

DISK DEGENERATION

For several decades, ever since Mixter and Barr[13] delivered their paper on disk herniations, the disk has been thought to be the principal cause of all low back pain and pain referred from the back. However, while the disk may cause most of the serious low back problems, it is rarely, if ever, the initial cause of low back pain (Table 10-8). All patients who have a proven disk

TABLE 10-7. Sacroiliac Displacement

FACTS
Uncommon in men
May follow hypermobility
CAUSES
Sudden violent trauma (e.g., fall on ischial tuberosity)
Golf swing in presence of limited hip extension
SIGNS AND SYMPTOMS
Low or high ilium on affected side
Lying-to-sitting leg length change
Restriction of sacrum on forward bending
TREATMENT
Manipulation

TABLE 10-8. Disk Degeneration

FACTS
- Rarely, if ever, a primary condition
- Preceded by a history of minor attacks of increasing frequency and severity

CAUSES
- Postural misuse and abuse
- Uncorrected myofascial dysfunction
- Repeated vibratory and/or rotary stresses
- Often trivial final insult

SIGNS AND SYMPTOMS
- Objective neurologic signs (i.e., objective numbness to pin prick and weakness in same segment myotome)
- Myelogram and/or CT scan must agree with clinical neurologic findings

TREATMENT
- Attention to other dysfunctions
- Reduce work and postural stress
- For neurologic signs, consider positional distraction

herniation with the classic neurologic signs of loss of skin sensation and muscle weakness when both are segmentally related and where the myelogram confirms these findings, will already have a history of backaches. The typical history of low back pain reveals increasing frequency and severity. These previous bouts are typical of myofascial, ligamentous, and facet dysfunctions. If these dysfunctions had been treated in a timely manner, the development of the disk herniation might have been prevented.

Since other pathologies, such as myofascial and facet restrictions or ligamentous strains, predispose toward disk conditions, the patient will be evaluated to detect if any of these are present. These pathologies will be treated in addition to the signs from the disk herniation.

The disk herniation, if symptomatic, will usually result in neurologic signs due to either pressure or irritation of the nerve root. For this, our role is to attempt to reduce that pressure or irritation of the nerve root, and the most useful method is positional distraction, illustrated in Figure 10-2B.

STENOSIS—LUMBAR SPINE

Stenosis of the lumbar spine is a condition that gained very little attention prior to 1972.[8,11] It is generally described as a narrowing of the spinal canal and intervertebral foramen caused by degeneration of the disk and other segmental elements, such as vertebral body and facet joints (Table 10-9). This narrowing irritates or compresses the spinal cord and nerve roots and produces signs and symptoms of neurogenic claudication. This claudication is to be distinguished from intermittent claudication of vascular origin. Claudication of vascular origin comes on with exercise and disappears soon with rest. Neurogenic claudication, on the other hand, although triggered by exercise, does not ease very readily with rest and may continue for several hours or even days following the onset.

The physical therapy for patients diagnosed as having spinal stenosis is geared toward improving the patients' health and general posture. In terms

TABLE 10-9. Stenosis—Lumbar Spine

FACTS
- In population older than 55 years of age
- Associated ill health

CAUSES
- Poor posture
- Obesity, diabetes
- Degenerative disk, facet, ligaments

SIGNS AND SYMPTOMS
- Bilateral low-extremity symptoms
- Bizarre signs and symptoms
- Effort neurogenic claudication relieved by forward bending

TREATMENT
- Posture, weight loss, negative heel
- Corset
- Surgery

of improving general health, emphasis will be placed on diet and exercise. For posture, we may need to stretch out tight lumbar myofascia and strengthen the abdominal muscles to reduce lordosis. Excessive lordosis, or indeed any lordosis, will decrease the size of the intervertebral foramen through which the lumbar nerves must exit. Our effectiveness in treating stenosis has not been proven, and most such cases will require surgery for decompression of neural structures, which is usually followed by spinal fusion.

SPONDYLOSIS—CERVICAL SPINE

Spondylosis is a degenerative condition characterized by the formation of osteophytes between the lateral interbody articulations of the cervical spine (Table 10-10). These changes may result in either irritation or compression of

TABLE 10-10. Spondylosis—Cervical Spine

FACTS
- Degeneration of cervical segments
- In population older than 45 years of age
- Associated upper-thoracic kyphosis

CAUSES
- Poor posture—forward head
- Restricted upper-thoracic motion
- Compensatory hypermobility in mid-cervical spine

SIGNS AND SYMPTOMS
- Hypermobility—at least initially
- Ligamentous and nerve root pains
- Kypho-lordosis of thoracic-cervical spine

TREATMENT
- Posture correction
- Manipulation of upper thoracic spine

the cervical nerve root, leading to pain, weakness, and numbness in the upper extremity. It is more common in women and appears to be related to a pronounced kyphosis of the upper thoracic spine that causes the mid-cervical spine to increase its range of motion. This increased range of motion leads to instability and a bony attempt at stabilization by the production of osteophytes. The osteophytes, in turn, irritate and compress nerve roots and give rise to the signs and symptoms of that condition.

Treatment consists of posture correction, mobilization to the upper-thoracic area to decrease the strain on the neck, and traction to assist in relieving the immediate symptoms of nerve root irritation and compression.

SPONDYLOLISTHESIS

Spondylolisthesis is a forward slip of a vertebrae, usually the fifth lumbar on the sacrum, and is due most commonly to a stress fracture of the pars interarticularis of the neural arch (Table 10-11). The vertebra then slips forward and is restrained by the intervertebral disk and the longitudinal ligaments of the spine. Such a restraint may not be sufficiently firm, and as a result, instability may arise.

On examination, the patient's lumbar spine will demonstrate a step that can be palpated between the spinous processes. During active movements, any instability may show as a shaking motion. If during either prone or supine lying, the step in the low back disappears, it can then be assumed that the slipped vertebra is quite mobile and a situation of instability is present. If the instability does not result in any neurologic signs, then the method of approach is conservative and surgery is not generally required to create a fusion. The conservative approach is advisable. The patient should reduce stressful activities, such as twisting, lifting, and carrying objects, and a program for strengthening the abdominal muscles and relieving any tight lumbar myofascia should be implemented. With this approach, the condition should not progress to a point at which surgical fusion would be required.

TABLE 10-11. Spondylolisthesis

FACT
- Unilateral or bilateral slip

CAUSES
- Stress, fracture

SIGNS AND SYMPTOMS
- Visible step on standing
- Muscle hypertrophy is unstable
- Shaking on initial forward bending step disappears on lying if hypermobile

TREATMENT
- Exercises for stability
- Correct any myofascial imbalances in the pelvic area

TABLE 10-12. Kissing Vertebrae

FACT
Bony impingement between either lumbar spinous processes or cervical laminae

CAUSES
Body type—short stocky
Loss of disk height
Poor posture—hyper lordosis

SIGNS AND SYMPTOMS
Central pain relieved by forward bending
Associated muscle guarding and restricted range of forward bending

TREATMENT
Posture correction
Myofascial stretches
Injection or surgery

KISSING VERTEBRAE

The term kissing vertebrae was first coined by Baastrup.[24] It is described as a bony impingement between the spinous processes of the lumbar vertebrae (Table 10-12). This condition may develop due to narrowing of the intervertebral disk and is aggravated still further by an increased lumbar lordosis. Dissections have shown a similar condition to exist between the cervical laminae.

One of the most common signs of patients suffering from this condition is the tendency to gain relief by bending forward or by pulling the knees to the chest. This is a helpful maneuver for any patient with tight myofascia, but it produces almost immediate relief, however temporary, for those patients with kissing vertebrae.

The treatment is to reduce the pressure, and the best method for this is to lessen the lordosis by stretching any tight myofascia and by giving strengthening exercises for the abdominal musculature.

DYSFUNCTION (LESION) COMPLEX

In cases of chronic spinal pain, that is, pain continuing for 3 or more months without improvement, the patient usually presents with more than one syndrome. No longer is the condition a simple facet synovitis, stiffness, or myofascial restriction. Indeed, the facet, muscles, ligaments, and the disk will now all be involved (Table 10-13). All elements of this lesion complex must be treated to help the patient. Most patients who present with a chronic disk herniation requiring surgery will not receive the relief of symptoms expected following surgery if the syndromes of the lesion complex have not been treated.

A vast number of patients fall into this category. Depending on the specialists they see, only one element of a condition may be treated. The approach to these problems should be multidisciplinary and will involve not just the treatment of syndromes by a physical therapist, but the management of diet, medication, lifestyle, and stress. Only a total approach will assist these patients with the most difficult of spinal problems.

TABLE 10-13. Dysfunction (Lesion) Complex

FACT
- Multiple signs and symptoms of a chronic nature

CAUSES
- Uncorrected dysfunction
- Failure or denial of conservative therapy
- Excessive trauma, such as a motor vehicle accident

SIGNS AND SYMPTOMS
- Multiple; principally those of ligaments, myofascia, and facet
- Muscle holding states abound
- Behavioral changes are prominent

TREATMENT
- Behavior modification
- Stress control and management
- Soft tissue techniques
- Posture correction and moderate exercise instruction
- Pain management

There is no excuse for the health care community to allow a simple dysfunction to develop into a dysfunctional (lesion) complex. All too often, the patient is a healthy person who is suffering from a disability that produces moderate pain. The pain is treated by the medical practitioner or by the physical therapist, and perhaps the underlying dysfunction is ignored. The pain is relieved, but the dysfunction continues to develop. Each time it recurs, the pain may not be any more severe, but the dysfunction certainly is. Eventually, the first of several surgeries may be performed. The patient becomes increasingly dependent on the surgeon and the medical team, who increasingly fail to assist the patient. The end result is a mental and physical cripple. It is not the patient but the system that has been at fault. Our goal must be to prevent this chain of events from taking place wherever possible.

EVALUATION

Now that we have the syndrome(s) before us, we can begin to examine the patient to try to find the syndrome(s) that match the patient's complaint.

The goal of the evaluation is not, however, to determine the syndrome(s) or the magnitude of the pain—for we will not be treating these components. Indeed, the goal is to determine the objective signs that, when treated, will relieve the syndrome(s) and remove the pain. This point is most important in patient care and follows along my previous comments on pain.

It is important to develop a consistent routine for both questions and procedures when examining the spine. To be inconsistent is to run the risk of missing key questions or tests, or at the very least, of collecting data in a less-meaningful manner. Clinical decision making is, to a large degree, determined by experience and, therefore, intuitive thinking. The information that makes up our experience, collected in a consistent manner, will permit our personal computer (brain) to readily draw upon these data and give us the correct answer. In computer language, they state "garbage in equals garbage out." Therefore, what we feed into our personal computer must not be garbage.

Now a word of caution. As we proceed through the evaluation process, there will emerge a finding or findings that will point very strongly to the presence of a particular syndrome or dysfunction. The clinician who is overly anxious to reach an understanding of the condition may prematurely latch onto an early finding and quite inadvertently exclude the significance of further data. It is important that when we examine a patient, we first collect all the data before drawing any conclusions about the patient's problems and the best treatment. Unlike physicians, physical therapists tend to make assumptions too quickly. A physician is accustomed to examining the patient and then delaying a decision until the results of laboratory and other tests are available. Physical therapists, by contrast, feel that they must know exactly what is wrong and exactly how they should proceed at the end of their evaluations. This notion leads to premature judgment and incorrect decisions. All that needs to be done at the end of the initial evaluation is to inform the patient of the findings to date, give basic instructions in posture and management, and explain that treatment will commence at the next visit. There are exceptions to this format, for example, when the condition is minor and quite simple. But as a rule, a patient should not be treated on the first visit other than by explanation and instructions in posture and activities.

THE USE OF AN EVALUATION BOOKLET

When examining a patient who has a back problem, an evaluation booklet can be used. The booklet has both advantages and disadvantages. The advantages include: neatness, consistency, and the assurance that on its completion, all of the necessary questions will have been asked and the appropriate tests will have been conducted. A further advantage is that with a form, the data can be completed in far greater detail than by longhand, simply by checking off information. Speed is important. If we have to stop to write every finding, we not only add to the cost of service, but we interrupt the flow of the procedure. Evaluation booklets are of particular value in communicating with other health professionals. Rather than having to pour through handwritten notes, they can see features of particular interest to them and can seek clarification on anything that is not recorded. In this manner, the physical therapist, physician, and psychologist can all work together productively and more cohesively.

A major disadvantage of a booklet is that it may limit inquiry or impede the ability to listen to the patient. The clinician may become intent on completing the form and not on following leads or directions of inquiry, because the form does not have space at that particular juncture. The habit of adding extra notes must be developed if the form is to fulfill its purpose.

THE 15-STEP EVALUATION

The components within the evaluative process include:

1. interview by patient coordinator/receptionist
2. pain assessment

3. initial observation
4. history and interview
5. structural observation
6. active movements
7. upper and/or lower quarter evaluation
8. neurologic assessment
9. palpation for condition
10. palpation for position
11. palpation for mobility
12. radiographic and other reports
13. summary of objective findings
14. plan of treatment for objective findings
15. prognosis.

Remember that each of the steps will be pursued in the order outlined, and within each step a routine will be followed. There are exceptions, of course. One such exception to adhering to this order is in the case of an acute trauma for which consulting the roentgenogram and roentgenogram report prior to evaluating the patient is certainly indicated. Otherwise, the roentgenogram and other reports are consulted rather late in the evaluation because they tend to bias the judgment of the examiner. Notice that each step represents a different topic. The experienced clinician may, while still completing the evaluation booklet, opt to combine certain steps according to the patient's posture. For instance, when the patient is standing, the clinician may not only conduct the structural and active movement evaluation, but may also do some of the neurologic assessment to lessen the amount of movement required of the patient. For our purposes, we will proceed in a mandatory step-by-step manner and not according to the patient's position. The patient will not be permitted to direct the evaluation, and the presence of others in the evaluation room should be discouraged.

CASE STUDY

A NECK PROBLEM

What follows is a typical neck condition with some minimal radiating pains. Each step is discussed, and then the particular findings on our patient, whom we shall call Mrs. Simple Neck, are outlined.

Step 1—Interview

The evaluation of the patients begins the moment they walk into the clinic's reception area. Here, the environment is established to collect the data that will be part of the eventual outcome. The first person to have contact with the patients may be the receptionist or, depending on the size of the clinic, a patient care coordinator. Either way, certain data are collected to begin the process. Data will include:

1. patient's name and personal information
2. insurance coverage and a discussion of treatment costs

EVALUATION SHEET
Biomechanical and Neurophysiological

Mr. / (Mrs.) / Miss Simple Neck Home Ph. ______ Bus. Ph. ______

Address ______ State ______ Zip ______

Birth Date 45+ Present Occupation Bookeeper, H/W Presently at Work Yes ✓ No—Since ______

Sedentary — Light ✓ Heavy—Very Heavy—Activities ______ Weight M Mar. Status M+3

PATIENT'S COMPLAINT Pain in the upper right neck, radiating to right shoulder and up over head to behind the right eye.

HOW SUSTAINED Not sure. Was first noticed after a long car drive following a vacation in which she slept on a uncomfortable pillow.

FIGURE 10-12. Form for recording the interview by the patient care coordinator/receptionist.

3. statement about patient's complaint
4. statement about the cause of the patient's complaint.

These data are recorded on the top of the face page of our evaluation booklet. These tasks may be performed by patient care coordinators. These people are knowledgeable about the clinic and about the patients' immediate needs. They set the tone of the clinic by showing interest, warmth, and empathy. They explain that a detailed evaluation will soon take place and, by discussing fees and insurance coverage, answer any uncertainties in the patients' minds.

At our clinic, we see evaluation as a two-way street. We evaluate the patient, and the patient evaluates our environment, warmth, competence, and procedures.

Figure 10-12 shows the information collected by the patient care coordinator. This information forms the beginning of the patient booklet. In summary, our patient is 45 years old, a bookkeeper and a housewife, married with three children. Her complaint is of pain at the base of the neck radiating up to the base of the skull and over the head to almost behind the right eye. There is further radiation into the right shoulder. The patient recalls that these symptoms occurred following a long car drive and after one or more nights spent sleeping on a rubber pillow.

Step 2—Pain Assessment

The patient care coordinator then directs the patient to complete the pain assessment page in the evaluation booklet. This assessment is based on the work by Melzack and consists of the McGill Pain Questionnaire, a free-body diagram, and some additional questions (Fig. 10-13). These questions should be part of the patient's record for *all* orthopaedic conditions and are beneficial in evaluating a patient's pain.

The questionnaire tests three classes of pain (somatic, affective, and evaluative) that are used to describe subjective pain experience. Although

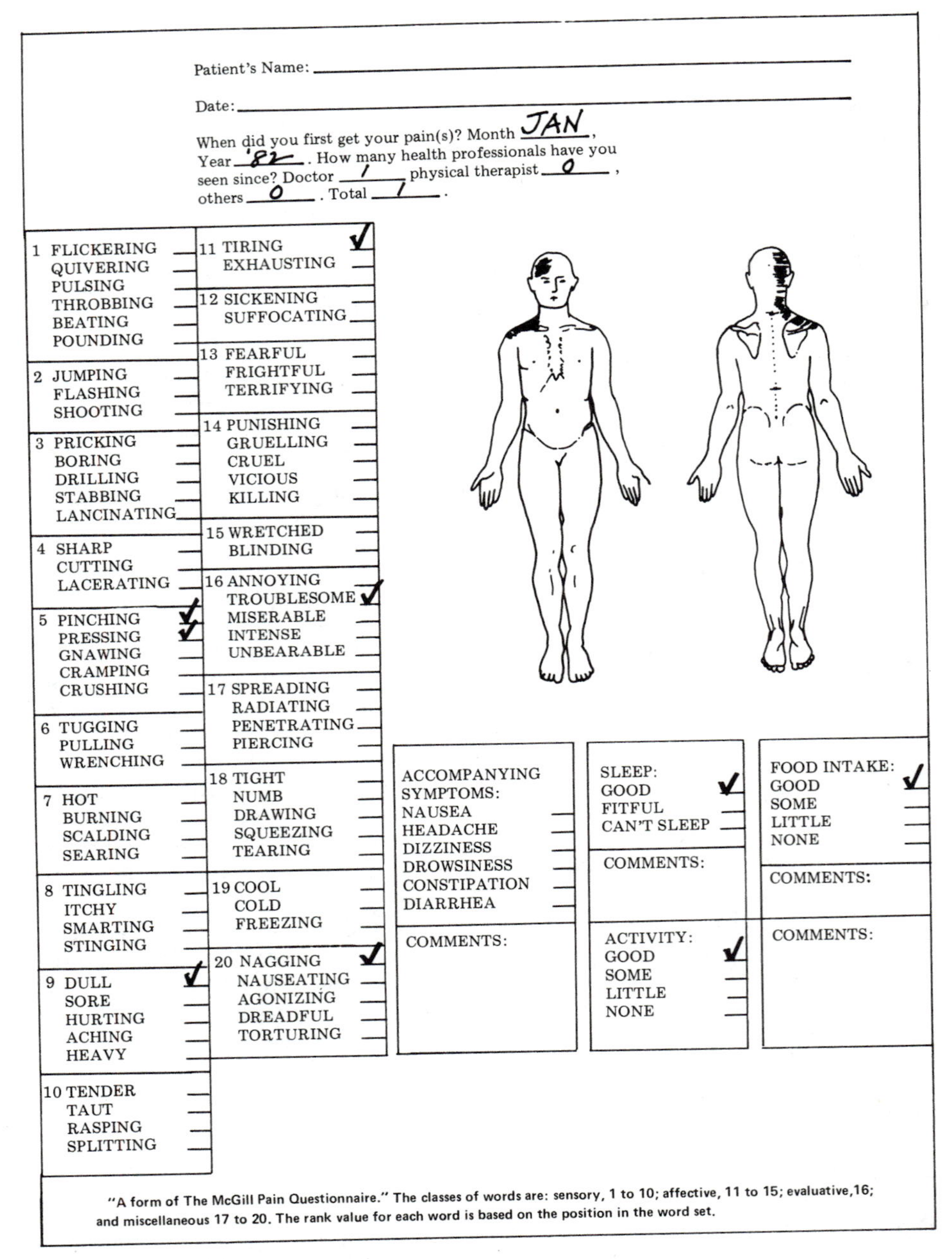

Patient's Name: ______

Date: ______

When did you first get your pain(s)? Month JAN, Year '82. How many health professionals have you seen since? Doctor 1 physical therapist 0, others 0. Total 1.

1 FLICKERING, QUIVERING, PULSING, THROBBING, BEATING, POUNDING

2 JUMPING, FLASHING, SHOOTING

3 PRICKING, BORING, DRILLING, STABBING, LANCINATING

4 SHARP, CUTTING, LACERATING

5 PINCHING ✓, PRESSING ✓, GNAWING, CRAMPING, CRUSHING

6 TUGGING, PULLING, WRENCHING

7 HOT, BURNING, SCALDING, SEARING

8 TINGLING, ITCHY, SMARTING, STINGING

9 DULL ✓, SORE, HURTING, ACHING, HEAVY

10 TENDER, TAUT, RASPING, SPLITTING

11 TIRING ✓, EXHAUSTING

12 SICKENING, SUFFOCATING

13 FEARFUL, FRIGHTFUL, TERRIFYING

14 PUNISHING, GRUELLING, CRUEL, VICIOUS, KILLING

15 WRETCHED, BLINDING

16 ANNOYING, TROUBLESOME ✓, MISERABLE, INTENSE, UNBEARABLE

17 SPREADING, RADIATING, PENETRATING, PIERCING

18 TIGHT, NUMB, DRAWING, SQUEEZING, TEARING

19 COOL, COLD, FREEZING

20 NAGGING ✓, NAUSEATING, AGONIZING, DREADFUL, TORTURING

ACCOMPANYING SYMPTOMS: NAUSEA, HEADACHE, DIZZINESS, DROWSINESS, CONSTIPATION, DIARRHEA

COMMENTS:

SLEEP: GOOD ✓, FITFUL, CAN'T SLEEP

COMMENTS:

ACTIVITY: GOOD ✓, SOME, LITTLE, NONE

FOOD INTAKE: GOOD ✓, SOME, LITTLE, NONE

COMMENTS:

COMMENTS:

"A form of The McGill Pain Questionnaire." The classes of words are: sensory, 1 to 10; affective, 11 to 15; evaluative, 16; and miscellaneous 17 to 20. The rank value for each word is based on the position in the word set.

FIGURE 10-13. Pain assessment form.

this form can be scored, it more importantly provides the patients with the words to more accurately describe their pain than perhaps they could have brought to mind from their own vocabulary. Use of the questionnaire also: (1) allows the physical therapist to save time; (2) shows the patients that we are concerned about their pain; (3) allows us to look for key and significant pain words; and (4) allows us to make a fairly accurate determination about the degree of emotional involvement experienced by the patient and the need, therefore, for psychological counseling.

On the questionnaire, words are divided into separate categories. The exact interpretation of these words is not significant, but it does provide information about possible pathology. Category 1 suggests a vascular disorder; categories 2 to 8, neurogenic; and categories 10 to 20, emotional liability.

The rest of the form gives the patients additional opportunities to express their conditions and to provide the clinician with a statement about their general health. Only experience will determine the value of these questions.

As a rule, most patients will mark from four to eight categories to describe pain. Persons who mark 6 or more categories may be getting a "little into their pain," and certainly those who mark 10 or more have reached this stage and may initially be helped more by clinical psychology than by physical therapy. Patients who have marked 16 categories or more are unlikely to respond to therapy procedures. In fact, such patients should be confronted with this information. The evaluation is first completed. Then the patients are offered an explanation about the clinician's findings and prognosis as if the information on the pain questionnaire were quite normal. Then the pain assessment is discussed. The patients are gently but firmly told that physical therapy will be unable to assist people who have marked 16 or more categories. Therefore, it is suggested that additional help be provided by the clinical psychologist concerning how the pain is being handled by these patients. The patients are told that this approach will help both them and the physical therapist.

Occasionally, patients may run their pencil around the entire page or either check off every category or shade in the entire body. It is obvious in such cases that a physical therapist will be unable to help patients with such emotional problems. Although other aspects of their behavior may be normal, this one certainly is not and will require intervention by another professional, quite possibly a psychiatrist.

Our patient, Mrs. Simple Neck, draws her pain and checks off words that are quite typical in cervical problems and therefore will not require additional assistance.

Step 3—Initial Observation

By the time the patients have completed the pain questionnaire, some 15 to 20 minutes may have elapsed since they first arrived at the clinic and met with the patient care coordinator. Now at last, they are ready for the clinician to begin evaluation.

The clinical evaluation may take from 20 to 45 minutes, depending on the complexity of the condition and the experience of the clinician. Acute conditions for which patients have great difficulty in standing and walking do not warrant a complete evaluation because the active movements would be unnecessarily aggravating to those conditions. All that needs to be done with such patients is to assess the presence of those factors that we may be able to help. On the other hand, complex conditions may take several visits to fully evaluate. This reality does not mean, however, that we could not have begun some treatments at each of these visits.

In our case, Mrs. Simple Neck will receive a full evaluation by the physical therapist. The patient care coordinator now passes the evaluation booklet to the therapist. The therapist needs only a few seconds while walking to the reception area to observe the patient's name, condition, and cause, as well as to glance at the patient's pain chart and note the words marked. This aspect is simple, fast, and effective, and has not involved the costly time of the physical therapist. On arriving at the reception area, the therapist greets the patient by name, as follows: "Good morning Mrs. Simple Neck. I'm Good Hands, your physical therapist." At that point, a handshake is initiated by the therapist, and the patient is asked to walk to the designated room.

Several significant factors have just occurred in patient management, and several more are about to take place. Those that have just occurred included the respect paid to the patient by the manner of greeting, including the offering of a handshake. But just as important, the therapist did not greet the patient by making the mistake of saying, "Good afternoon. How are you? I'm . . ." and so forth. Patients should not be greeted by a question about their condition. Turning their attention from a subjective perception of pain to an objective measurement of their function is paramount. Of course, during the evaluation and each visit, the question, "How do you feel?" will be asked, but this will be done after the evaluation or reassessment and not before it. It is important that patients be assessed objectively at each opportunity and not be misled or directed by their pain through a subjective description of pain.

When patients recognize a greeting and rise to shake hands, observations about posture, movement, and pain expression both before and after they initiate their motion are already underway. Concern is unlikely to show on a clinician's face since it should be your intention to project only warmth and confidence. The relationship between therapist and patient has begun.

At all times, the clinician should be aware of the placebo factor existing in all patient care relationships. If a placebo pill is 30 percent effective, then probably physical therapy administration that includes an in-depth inquiry accompanied by touch and passive movement may rate as high as a 50 percent placebo. As much as we would like to think that our results are more scientific than a placebo, we must nonetheless admit to a placebo factor and manipulate this factor to the advantage of the patient.

As we enter the treatment room, which will be private, quiet, well lit, and tastefully decorated, the patients are asked to rest. Having observed their gait, their selection of either a high stool or a treatment table is now observed. Note that they are asked only to rest and not to sit down. The latter is an order from someone in a white coat. The former is more likely to show natural behavior expressing the patient's condition. In low back pain of discogenic origin, we know that pressure is greatest during sitting and less during standing or lying. As a result, patients with a disk condition may choose to remain standing or request to lie on the treatment table. On the other hand, patients with an acute facet strain may wish to avoid sitting in the low chair and opt instead to rest against the end of the treatment table or high stool and then gradually place weight fully on the back. Various other syndromes present different behaviors. Those patients with ligamentous conditions (which may include the early stage of disk disease) will sit down quite easily at first but will not be able to sit still for any period of time

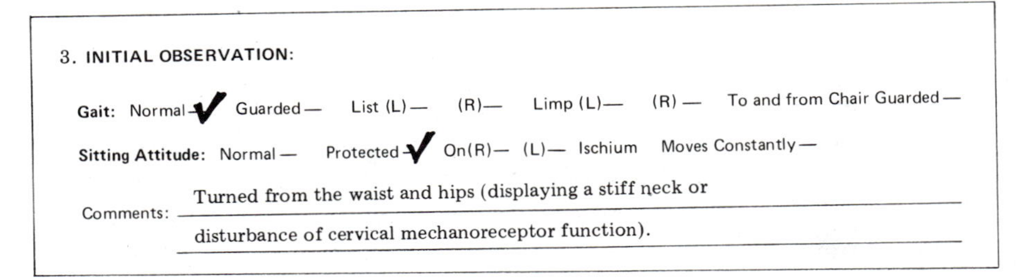
3. INITIAL OBSERVATION:

Gait: Normal ✓ Guarded— List (L)— (R)— Limp (L)— (R)— To and from Chair Guarded—

Sitting Attitude: Normal— Protected ✓ On(R)— (L)— Ischium Moves Constantly—

Comments: Turned from the waist and hips (displaying a stiff neck or disturbance of cervical mechanoreceptor function).

FIGURE 10-14. Initial observation section of the form.

without constantly adjusting position. Those patients with myofascial conditions will sit down without any problem and will often remain quite still.

In our cervical case, Mrs. Simple Neck moved easily from the waiting room and sat down in the chair without any effort. Then she turned her entire body, rather than just her head, to better face the examiner. In this manner, she displayed some loss of cervical motion and alteration in postural mechanoreceptor activity (Fig. 10-14).

Step 4—History and Interview

Now begins the history taking by the clinician and a type of interview where two people begin to make a decision about whether the relationship will continue. This aspect of treatment is often ignored but is significant nonetheless.

The questions that can be used are set forth in Figure 10-15. But before beginning to ask them, the patients are told that you wish to ask them some questions concerning their conditions. When completed, you would be grateful if they could then tell you if there was anything that they would like to add. In this manner, you hope to prevent the patients from giving a rambling account for each question. Answers should be brief and to the point. The information will be collected as efficiently as possible. We certainly must remember to provide the patients with the opportunity at the end to add anything further. Usually, however, at the completion of the questions, patients will simply report in response to a request for additional information, "No, I think you have my history."

A major concern is the reliability of a patient's history. Memory can be deceptive. Patients may forget previous incidents, including even hospitalizations and surgery. Such forgetfulness may permit the examiner to feel that a simple condition prevails whereas, in fact, it could be much more serious. We know from experience, for instance, that a patient who has had an insidious onset of pain over a period of many weeks and without a history of injury may, in fact, have a serious disease process. As clinicians, we must be aware of this possibility and do everything possible to safeguard the patient from this oversight.

It is virtually impossible to be sure that patients covered by workmen's compensation are giving a reliable history. If a clinician were to ask a group of people assembled at a conference or a meeting how many of them have never had low back pain, not more than 5 percent will have a pain-free history. By contrast, when you examine patients covered by workmen's

4. **HISTORY AND INTERVIEW:**

A. Present Status: (use body chart)

1. Precisely where did the pain commence? high right neck
2. Where did the pain spread to? see diagram
3. Where is the pain now (past 48 hours)? Diagram
4. Do you have any pins and needles, etc.? Yes—
5. Does it throb — twinge — burn — other — ?
6. What in particular makes your pain worse? reading in bed, rubber pillows, long drives.
7. What if anything eases your pain? rest, aspirin, heat and massage

9. Can you get comfortable at night? Yes ✓ No —
10. How does your back feel on rising in the morning? Stiff ✓ Sore ✓ Fine —
11. Once you start moving about, does it worsen — ease ✓ ?
12. What is it like at the end of the day? Worse — Easier ✓
13. What is the effect of coughing? — ve
14. Do you have any problem with your bladder? Yes —
15. Do you have any sensation in the S4 region? Yes —

B. Previous History (leave blank if inappropriate)

1. Have you ever had anything similar before? Yes — No ✓
2. How often? ______
3. Are they increasing in frequency? Yes — No —
4. Are they increasing in severity? Yes — No —
5. Are they changing in character? Yes — No — If yes, describe ______
6. Usual cause? ______
7. Hospitalization? Yes — No ✓ Surgery? Yes — No ✓ Report available? — Summarize ______

C. Miscellaneous

1. Just prior to this onset were you completely free of symptoms? Yes ✓ No —
2. What if any treatments have you had for this current problem? none
3. Did they help? Yes — No — ______
4. Are you presently taking any medications? Yes ✓ What? aspirin On steroids? Yes —
5. Do you have Respiratory Tract Infection? Yes — Rheumatoid Arthritis? Yes —
6. At the present time are you getting better — worse — stable ✓ ?
7. Now is there anything else that you think I should know? no

FIGURE 10-15. History questionnaire.

compensation, you will find that at least 90 percent will deny ever having had low back pain before.[1]

Obviously, they are choosing to give less than the complete story. They fear that to give a history of back pain, particularly if it originated in a former employment situation, may complicate the whole process of reimbursement and coverage. They wish only to have their pain treated. They therefore run the risk of unknowingly covering up a possibly serious situation. It is our responsibility to recognize this and to protect the patients against an understandable dishonesty.

Step 5—Structural Observation

Now this patient's neck and trunk can be examined in detail. This examination is begun by asking the patient to suitably disrobe. She is asked to step behind the screen and to undress to the waist, leaving on only her bra and skirt.

There can be no exceptions to having the patients adequately disrobe. Prudery or embarrassment has no place in the health professions. If there is a problem with a male therapist asking a female patient to disrobe, then a female assistant needs to be present. Using a gown is simply not permissible because it prevents a full structural assessment and, later, a meaningful observation of active movements.

The patients now stand with their back to the clinician. Their general appearance is noted and will include their weight, spinal curves, and the presence of surgical scars that will require explanation. The next step is to assess the patients' sacral base. Sacral base means the tilt of the sacrum. If, for instance, it is tilted anteriorly, an excessive lordosis would be present. If the sacrum is tilted laterally, scoliosis, which may be due to either a short leg, a rotated pelvis, or a pelvic anomaly, would be present.

In Mrs. Simple Neck's condition, she displayed a sacrum tilted to the right with a long "C" curve convexity to the right (Fig. 10-16). On exploring the reasons for this, we see that her right iliac crest was low, as was her posterior inferior iliac spine and right greater trochanter. However, her knees

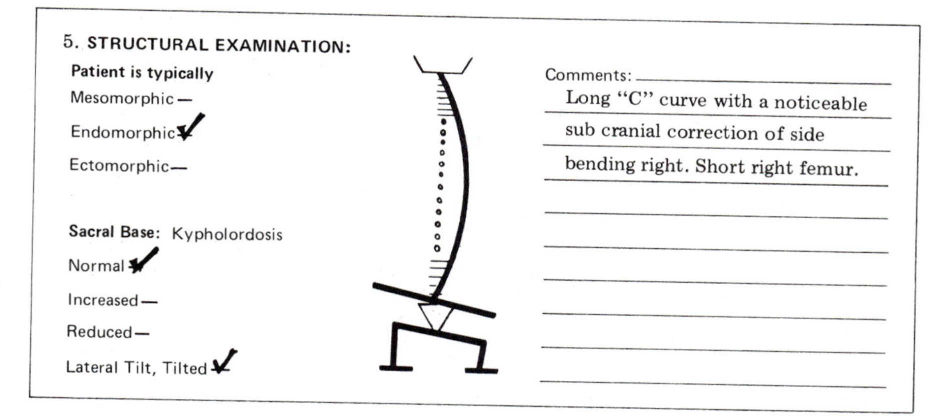
5. STRUCTURAL EXAMINATION:

Patient is typically

Mesomorphic—

Endomorphic ✓

Ectomorphic—

Sacral Base: Kypholordosis

Normal ✓

Increased—

Reduced—

Lateral Tilt, Tilted ✓

Comments:

Long "C" curve with a noticeable sub cranial correction of side bending right. Short right femur.

FIGURE 10-16. Structural observation section of the form.

were level. These findings point to a difference in the length of the femoral shaft and are indicative of a short right femur.

The right convexity carried all the way to her cervical spine, and since her eyes were level, it can be assumed that there may well be a structural side bending of the head to the right. This might be easier to understand by looking at the drawing placed on the patient's structural outline in Figure 10-16.

Step 6—Active Movements

To the novice, testing the active movements of the cervical spine would appear to be a very simple task; but it is not. Movements of the head and neck will involve at least three functionally different regions. The first of these is the subcranial region, the second is the mid-cervical spine, and the third is the upper-thoracic spine.

The first step, therefore, is to test the subcranial area. This test is carried out by having the patient gently restrict forward bending and side bending to the subcranial region. The therapist assists the patient in this procedure by placing light fingertip pressure under the chin and just under the occiput. This proprioceptive localization assists the patient in the motions of nodding. Next, the fingers are placed on either side of the occiput, and side bending is instructed. Rotation is difficult to assess actively in this region and therefore is omitted.

In the subcranial region, Mrs. Simple Neck demonstrated on backward nodding a tendency for the head and nose to deviate to the right side. Biomechanically, this finding can be interpreted as the subcranial area moving freely on the left and being limited on the right. She also demonstrated a limitation of side bending to the right, but this finding is understandable since the cervical spine has a convexity to the right (see her structural examination). The head is already in right side bending to keep the eyes level, and thus, the remaining available range will appear limited. Because her right side bending is limited actively, we will need to assess whether or not the end feel, that is, the resistance felt at the end of passive range, is normal or abnormal for this region during passive movement testing.

Figure 10-17 represents our findings on active movement. Note the simple movement diagram and the key at the side. These movement diagrams can be freely drawn anywhere in the patient's record to note progress. Next, we test the mid-cervical region by having the patient perform the same movements again but now over a wider arc. Knowing what movement alterations were present in the subcranial area will permit us to better assess

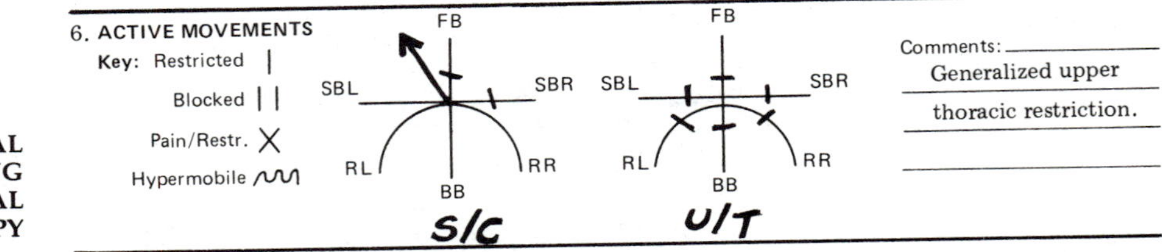

FIGURE 10-17. Active movements section of the form.

7. **UPPER QUARTER** – Screen

Shoulder

(L) Limited –	Painful –	Capsular –	Non-Capsular –
(R) Limited –	Painful –	Capsular –	Non-Capsular –

(R) (L)

Crepitus right sd.

Thoracic Outlet ______

Other ______

LOWER QUARTER

Hip

(L) Limited –	Painful –	Capsular –	Non-Capsular –	FABER ______ inches
(R) Limited –	Painful –	Capsular –	Non-Capsular –	FABER ______ inches

Sacroiliac Normal – ASIS gap – ve ASIS compression – ve

Positional fault – ve; describe ______

Provocation	(L)	(R)		(L)	(R)
Fwd. Torsion	–	–	Hyper		
Bkwd. Torsion	–	–	Hypo		

FIGURE 10-18. Upper- and lower-quarter evaluation section of the form.

any alterations in the mid-cervical region. Mrs. Simple Neck showed no restrictions in this region, so we moved on to test the upper-thoracic area.

Mrs. Simple Neck had begun to develop an upper-thoracic kyphosis as a result of this increased curve. This finding is not unexpected in women over the age of 40. We find all of her movements to be generally limited in this area, thus placing a greater need for motion on the mid-cervical spine.

Step 7—Upper and/or Lower Quarter Evaluation

For our patient, we need only evaluate what may be referred to as the upper quarter: the shoulder, the arm, and the cranio-mandibular joint. Given her description of pain as originating in the right subcranial area and radiating down no further than the shoulder and up over the right side of the head, only minimal attention will be paid to the arm. The shoulder was checked out as having normal movement. On the other hand, since the cranio-mandibular joint can refer pain to the upper neck and cranium, this joint was checked in more detail.

The evaluation was performed with the patient in a standing position for the arm and in a sitting position for the cranio-mandibular joint. Her evaluation was virtually normal except for some crepitus in the right cranio-mandibular joint. This finding was briefly noted in the evaluation booklet (Fig. 10-18).

Step 8—Neurologic Assessment

Again Mrs. Simple Neck's evaluation was normal. Since there were no findings, a large "OK" was placed in the appropriate area (Fig. 10-19).

8. NEUROLOGICAL:

Lower Quarter Examination:

	Left	Right
L1, 2 Psoas.		
L3 Quads.		
L4 Tib. Ant.		
L5 E.H.L.		
S1 F.H.L.		
S2 Hams.		

Reflexes:

	Left	Right
Abds T1-12		
Knee Jk. L4		
Ankl. Jk. S1		
Plantar. UMN		

L. R.

SLR ________° ________°

or ________cm ________cm

Laseque — —

Kernig — —

Dural stretch — range ________

Compression — Distraction —

Quadrant Test: (L) — (R) —

Keys

Muscle Strength

0 – No contraction
1 – Trace
2 – Poor
3 – Fair
4 – Good
5 – Normal

Reflexes

0 – Absent
1+ – Diminished
2+ – Normal
3+ – Increased
4+ – Clonus

Vertebral Artery:

L – ve R – ve

Range Full – Restricted –

E.M.G.: Performed –

Comments (sensation) ________

Upper Quarter Examination: O.K.

	Left	Right
C1-2 apr tk chin in		
C1-2 ppr psh chin up		
C3 press hd nk lat		
C4 diaphragm		
C4 shoulder shrug		
C5 biceps		
C6 wrist extensors		
C7 triceps		
C8 thumb extensors		
T1 hand intrinsics		

Reflexes:

	Left	Right
Biceps C5, 6		
Triceps C7		
Brac. Rad. C5, 6		

Compression – Distraction —

Quadrant Test: (L) – (R) –

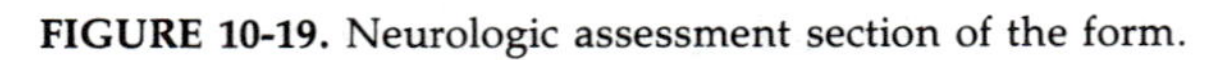

FIGURE 10-19. Neurologic assessment section of the form.

PALPATION:

9. Condition:

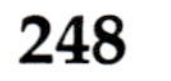

10. Position:

Transverse process of atlas prominent on the right.

Key:

X Tender
⊗ Center Pain
//// Guarding
↕ Reflex Contr.

Key:

0 – Ankylosed
1 – Considerable Restriction
2 – Slight Restriction
3 – Normal
4 – Slight Increase
5 – Considerable Increase
6 – Unstable

11. Mobility:

Segment	FB	SBL	SBR	RL	RR	BB
O/A	2	1	1	0	0	2
A/A						
C2/3						
U/T	2	2	2	2	2	2
T2/3	2	2	2	1	1	--

FIGURE 10-20. Palpation, condition, position, and mobility section of the form.

Step 9—Palpation for Condition

To this point, we have concentrated on collecting as much "non-tactile" information as is reasonable. Now we use our hands to learn what changes in tissue tension are present. To perform this examination, the patient lies supine with the neck supported on a soft pillow. The therapist then palpates the skin, subcutaneous areas, muscles, ligaments, and finally, the facet joints of the cervical spine, as well as the muscles of the cranium and face. The cranio-mandibular joint is palpated further.

Mrs. Simple Neck displayed tenderness over the facet joints of C1-2 and C2-3, with some associated muscle guarding in that area (Fig. 10-20).

Step 10—Palpation for Position

It was not surprising to find an apparent shift of the atlas to the right, thus bringing the transverse process of the atlas more prominent between the mastoid process and the mandible. This shift to the right was due to a relative side bending of the head to the right (remember that because of her scoliosis, Mrs. Simple Neck has to side bend her head to the right to keep her head level). This observation was noted on her chart (see Fig. 10-20).

Step 11—Palpation for Mobility

Our awareness of active movements that we attempted to localize to the subcranial, mid-cervical, and upper-thoracic regions is now made more accurate and more localized by passive movement testing. A variety of techniques are available, and those noted below are representative.

To test the subcranial area, the examiner may choose to place the palpating fingers on the transverse process of the atlas and then to gently nod, side bend, and rotate the head, feeling the relative movement between the occiput and the atlas. During these tests, it is noted that all movements are restricted, in particular, side bendings left and right of the occiput on the atlas. These findings are recorded in Figure 10-19, a key to which accompanies the figure. It will be noted that the occiput/atlas was restricted in forward bending and in side bending. No rotation is recorded, but this is due to the biomechanics of the joint and not to its pathology. The movements of both the atlas and axis and the C2-3 joints are normal, and therefore, to avoid cluttering the grid diagram, no results are recorded. The mid-cervical spine is examined and found to be normal, and thus no results are recorded. The upper-thoracic area is also examined and found to be generally restricted. Hence, the numeral "2" is placed on the grid for this area. T2-3, however, required special mention because it was particularly limited in its rotations.

Step 12—Radiographic and Other Reports

Mrs. Simple Neck had no roentgenograms or other reports other than the physician's referral. That part of the evaluation booklet where this information would be recorded is shown in Figure 10-21.

12. RADIOLOGICAL Key: ✓If done ✗If report with this record

Impression ______

Standard Views Taken: Yes— Regions ______ Viewed: Yes —

Special Studies: Myelogram—Discogram—Venogram—Tomography—
Results ______

Functional Radiology: Request area SC— C—T— L— S/I—

Standard — Special—Emphasize ______

Result ______

FIGURE 10-21. Radiographic and other reports section of the form.

Step 13—Summary of Objective Findings

Having completed the evaluation, the clinician now needs to review the data and make a listing of those findings that are amenable to physical therapy procedures. This list could be quite long, but practically speaking, the list of "significant" findings will rarely exceed seven items. The basis, therefore, for deciding on the significant findings is to set out those from the evaluation that we feel can be improved with physical therapy intervention. These conditions have been set out in Figure 10-22.

Step 14—Treatment Plan for Objective Findings

Figure 10-22 shows a list of treatments opposite the summary of significant findings. Each of these shall now be presented and discussed.

1. Short Right Femur

A short right femur may seem irrelevant to a pain in the right upper neck radiating over the head and into the right arm. In our patient's case, however, structural evaluation revealed that she had a long "C" curve continuing all the way to the subcranial region. This meant that her head, in order to have the eyes level and facing the front, would need to side bend to the right, thus creating a considerable postural strain in this region. Correcting her leg lengths through the use of a heel lift and thus leveling her pelvis should assist in reducing, if not correcting, the long "C" curve. As a result, the head would sit more level on the neck, and there would be less compressive forces on the side of her discomfort.

2. Long "C" Curve, Convex Right

We have already referred to having the heel lift and the effects it may have on the curve. The patient also needs to increase her awareness of this condition because it was noticed during an evaluation that she tended to stand on her left leg, dropping her pelvis to the right and, therefore, increasing the

AREAS EXAMINED: U/C ✓ M/C ✓ U/T ✓ T — L — S/I — Upper Quarter ✓ Lower Quarter —

---

13. SUMMARY OF SIGNIFICANT FINDINGS | **14. TREATMENTS PLANNED**

	13. Summary of Significant Findings	14. Treatments Planned
1.	short right femur	¼" insole heel lift
2.	long "C" curve, convex right	lift plus awareness, alter leg stance
3.	tenderness A/A and A/O joints	— — — — — —
4.	restr. U/T, Noticeably T2/3	manipulation
5.	restr. A/O on the right	manipulation
6.	atlas prominent on the right	possibly manipulation
7.	forward head posture	posture and awareness

PAIN TYPE: Facet ✓ Muscular ✓ Ligamentous — Neurogenic — Dural — Discogenic —

IMPRESSION: Facet Str. ✓ Facet Blk. ✓ Instability — Soft Tissue — Postural ✓ Discogenic — Lesion Complex —

PRESENT STAGE: Immediate — Acute — Sub Acute — Settled ✓ Chronic — DEGREE: Min. — Mod. ✓ Severe —

---

15. PROGNOSIS: 10≠3 PAIN QUESTIONNAIRE COMPLETED: Yes ✓

Month	Yr.	1	2	3	4	5	6	7	8	9	10	11	12	13	14	15	16	17	18	19	20	21	22	23	24	25	26	27	28	29	30	31
			✓																													

FIGURE 10-22. Summary of significant findings, plan of treatment, and prognosis, as well as attendance chart.

"C" curve. By correcting this posture and, in fact, encouraging one-leg standing on the right side, we may further help reduce the tendency toward the "C" curve with convexity to the right. Any reduction in this curve should improve the function of the spine and decrease the stress in the subcranial region.

3. Tenderness Atlantoaxial (A/A) and Atlanto-Occipital (A/O) Joints

There is no treatment planned for this tenderness. Although it represents a significant finding, we feel that it is not tenderness we treat, but the cause of the tenderness, which so far as we have identified is due to a long "C" curve and, as we shall soon see, to other restrictions as well.

4. Restriction Upper Thoracic (U/T), Noticeably Between the Second and Third Thoracic Vertebrae (T2-3)

These restrictions shall be manipulated. Our reason for manipulating is that by improving the movement here, we will reduce the need for compensation and, hence, improve strains at the subcranial regions where some of the pain appears to be arising.

5. Restriction Atlanto-Occipital (A/O) on the Right

This restriction is no doubt secondary to the long "C" curve resulting in the head being side bent right on the curve. As a result, the atlas has moved to the right (the atlas always moves in the direction of the head motion), and in our patient, it has apparently become stiffened with time.

Manipulation to the atlanto-occipital joint on the right side should reduce this restriction. There are a number of techniques from which the appropriate maneuver may be selected.

6. Atlas Prominent on the Right

This prominence is no doubt due to the subluxation of the atlas as a result of the head being constantly side bent to the right and thus having forced the atlas to that side. Once the heel lift corrects the curve and manipulation is applied to the restricted atlanto-occipital level, the atlas should return to its normal position by itself. If this is not the case, the atlas will then be manipulated by a technique combining distraction and slow but steady overpressure to the vertebrae in the direction of its intended correction.

We have now used manipulation in three instances on this patient. Manipulation is primarily directed at restoring motion. This restoration should have a number of beneficial effects for our patient, including improving range of motion, reducing stress at other levels, and increasing the firing of mechanoreceptive mechanisms to assist in the blocking of pain and the reduction of muscle guarding. We also need to recognize the psychological and/or placebo effects of manipulation, since it combines the technique of placing the hands on the patient as well as some very definitive maneuvers. These psychological effects are not to be discouraged, for patients in pain need all the help they can get.

7. Forward Head Posture.

A forward head posture will result in relative backward bending of the head on the neck and, as a consequence, increased compression and resulting restrictions in that region. A patient's headache could, therefore, be increased by this compression. By teaching more correct positions, primarily one in which the head is drawn back, the head will produce a relative forward bending to the upper-cervical spine, thus relieving the compression in the suboccipital region.

These are the principal findings and treatments and a synopsis of the basis for these treatments. Much more could be said about each. Unfortunately, many of the treatment decisions are based purely on clinical experience. Very little proof exists for their effectiveness compared with other treatment modalities, and therefore, as professionals, we need to recognize that clinical trials must be conducted to determine the effectiveness of these modalities.

As a general rule, the significant findings of the evaluation and the treatment plan should now be reviewed with the patient (Steps 13 and 14).

Then the patient is told that about 10 treatments could lead to improvement, but a few more may be necessary depending on her degree of participation in the treatment. The tasks expected of her are outlined, and she is told that she will be reassessed at each visit to gain a better idea of her progress. There are many forms of this communication. The experienced therapist usually has little problem in satisfying the patient's need for an answer.

SUMMARY

In this evaluation of a patient with neck pain, I have attempted to show how, rather than treating pain with heat, massage, and traction, an orthopaedic physical therapist will use a complete differential evaluation to detect the problem. The more I am aware of possibilities, the more I shall find, and the greater will then be the likelihood of my being able to help the patient.

There has to be a limit to the amount of time allocated for and the details sought in the evaluation. Realistic limits placed on us are dictated by time and, therefore, economics. On occasion, a stiff hip or a flat foot may be a key factor in the production of pain in the head and neck; but these events are rare, and one should first treat the obvious and only resort to other possibilities when the patient's condition has failed to respond in the expected manner. The evaluation did produce sufficient data to account for the patient's pain reference and disability. From experience, it would seem that the proposed treatment should help relieve the pain and minimize dysfunction in a reasonable period of time. If the relief of symptoms and return of function did not proceed as expected, then we would need to reevaluate the patient to learn where the initial evaluation went wrong.

CONCLUSION

Orthopaedic physical therapy covers a number of areas in health care. I have centered this presentation on the cervical spine to give a little depth to that part of the profession that is of particular interest to me. It is a lifelong study. I get from it only what I put into it. As each year passes, I am increasingly encouraged that we will eventually have a much better understanding of spinal pain and its cause and treatment. Further, I am being increasingly convinced that spinal pain and spinal dysfunction can benefit by specialized orthopaedic physical therapy to a degree far greater than can be offered by any other health disciplines. These are, therefore, exciting times for the professional clinician committed to moving toward excellence.

REFERENCES

1. Wyke, BD: *American Academy of Orthopaedic Surgeons Symposium on Idiopathic Low Back Pain.* CV Mosby, St. Louis, 1982.
2. Bogduk, N: *The anatomy of the lumbar intervertebral disc syndrome.* Med J Aust 1:878–881, 1979.
3. Paris, SV: *Anatomy as Related to Function and Pain: Lumbar Spine Symposium.* In *Clinical Orthopaedics and Related Research, Symposium on Evaluation and Care of Lumbar Spine Problems.* Orthopaedic Clinics of North America, 14:3, July, 1983.
4. Pauwels, F: *Biomechanics of the Normal and Diseased Hip.* Springer-Verlag, Berlin, 1976.
5. Maquet, P.GH.J.: *Biomechanics of the Knee.* Springer-Verlag, Berlin, 1976.

6. HOLLINSHEAD, WH: *Anatomy for Surgeons, Vol 3, The Back and Limbs,* ed 2. Harper & Row, New York, 1969.
7. MOONEY, V AND Robertson, J: *The facet syndrome.* Clin Orthop 115:149–156, 1976.
8. KIRKALDY-WILLIS, WH AND HILL, RJ: *A more precise diagnosis for low-back pain.* Spine 4:102–109, 1979.
9. FARFAN, HS: *Mechanical Disorder of the Low Back.* Lea & Febiger, Philadelphia, 1973.
10. FINNESON, BE: *Low Back Pain,* ed 2. JB Lippincott, Philadelphia, 1980.
11. VERBIEST, H: *Neorogenic intermittent claudication in cases with absolute and relative stenosis of the lumbar vertebral canal, etc.* Clin Neurosurg 20:204–214, 1972.
12. GHORMLEY, RK: *Low back pain with special reference to the articular facets.* JAMA 19:1773–1777, 1933.
13. MIXTER, WJ AND BARR, JS: *Rupture of the intervertebral disc with involvement of the spinal canal.* N Engl J Med 210–215, 1934.
14. MENNELL, JB: *Physical Treatment by Movement, Manipulation and Massage.* J & A Churchill, London, 1934.
15. MENNELL, JM: *Back Pain.* Little, Brown & Co, Boston, 1960.
16. STODDARD, A: *Manual of Osteopathic Technique,* ed 3. Hutchinson, London, 1980.
17. PARIS, SV: *The theory and technique of specific spinal manipulation.* NZ Med J 62:320–321, 1963.
18. PARIS, SV: *The Spinal Lesion.* Pegasus Press, New Zealand, 1965.
19. REES, WES: *Multiple bilateral subcutaneous rhizolysis of segmental nerves in the treatment of the intervertebral disc syndrome.* Annals of General Practice 26:126, 1971.
20. CARRERA, GF, ET AL: *Computed tomography of the lumbar facet joints.* Radiology 134:145–148, 1980.
21. SELBY, DK AND PARIS, SV: *Anatomy of facet joints and its clinical correlation with low back pain.* Contemporary Orthopaedics 3(12):1097–1103, 1981.
22. PARK, W: Personal communication.
23. CODMAN, EA: *The Shoulder.* Thomas Todd, Boston, 1934.
24. BAASTRUP, C: *On the spinous process of the lumbar vertebrae and the soft tissues between them, and on pathological changes in that region.* Acta Radiol 14:52, 1933.

Chapter 11

CLINICAL DECISION MAKING IN ORTHOPAEDIC PHYSICAL THERAPY: THE LOW BACK

RICHARD NYBERG, P.T.

The case study to be presented demonstrates the complexities confronting the orthopaedic physical therapist working with a patient who has significant low back pathology. The objective is to identify the decision-making process an orthopaedic physical therapist undergoes when evaluating and managing the difficult low back case. However, decision making and good judgment are dependent upon a sound knowledge base. Therefore, the information necessary for an orthopaedic physical therapist to exercise proper judgment is also presented. The rationale for management choices is provided within the case study. The intention is to assist physical therapists interested in treating patients with vertebral-structural-mechanical pathology by identifying important subject matter and the bases for selecting certain methods of management. The case study concerns a patient with multiple physical findings of a long-standing nature. The problem is a chronic one by orthopaedic standards because the symptoms have persisted for over a few months and the patient had clinical signs of discouragement, despair, increased irritability, and depression.[1] The methods of clinical evaluation and test interpretation are reviewed first. The significant clinical evaluation and radiologic and electrodiagnostic findings are then identified. A written description of the verbal report by the therapist to the patient about his condition is included.

The therapeutic approach decided upon, the goals expected, and the overall prognosis are explained from a treatment standpoint. The techniques used are discussed in terms of intention, effect, and result. The selection of each specific therapy given is analyzed. Patient instruction and education are outlined in order to demonstrate the contribution of the home program in the overall management of the patient. A final analysis is provided to indicate the present stage of the condition and to summarize the specific objectives based upon data from the evaluation.

EVALUATION

HISTORY AND INTERVIEW

The patient, Bad Back (BB), is a self-referred, 37-year-old man who was initially seen on March 16, 1981, at the Atlanta Back Clinic by an orthopaedic physical therapist (OPT). The initial interview revealed that the patient was employed as an epidemiologist in Atlanta, Georgia. BB had evidently experienced recurrent but nondebilitating lower back discomfort since his college days. The present episode of pain occurred while lowering a heavy object from an overhead shelf approximately 2 months before being evaluated. The exact mechanism of the injury and the specific movements during the lift could not be recalled by the patient. Therefore, the examiner could not positively attribute the physical findings identified during the clinical evaluation to the incident reported by the patient. For example, if the lifting injury resulted from a patient rotating the spine to the right while simultaneously returning to the upright position, the OPT may find that right rotation of the spine or return from a forward-flexed position provides the symptoms. A positive correlation between mechanism of injury and provocation of symptoms with specific test maneuvers will enable the OPT to effectively manage the condition.

Based upon the history provided by the patient, he was undoubtedly reaching. Overhead movements of the upper extremities result in backward bending of the thoracic and lumbar spines. Lowering the object would eventually require spinal forward bending. The assumption made is that the spine was extended and then flexed. The evaluation should therefore include test movements requiring the spine to extend and flex. Further discussion regarding this contention is provided during active motion analysis. The pain diagram and word list recommended by Melzack[2] is utilized to evaluate the patient's perception of pain. The pain diagram requires the patient to draw his pain on a human figure, in addition to requiring a written description. BB localized two major areas: the central low-lumbar region (L5-S1, S1-2) and the left posterior buttock. The two areas were well defined and circular in nature. The buttock area was drawn darker than the lower-lumbar area, signifying that the buttock pain was more intense than the pain felt centrally at L5-S1 and S1-2. The drawing, therefore, is evaluated for the specific or generalized nature of the pain and the intensity of the symptoms in each area marked (noted by the manner in which the markings are drawn—light or dark). The patient's verbal complaint reaffirmed the pain drawing.

In addition, the patient indicated that the pain also radiated into the posterior aspect of the left lower extremity and was most notable in the calf. The use of both the pain drawing and the written description of pain are, therefore, recommended to fully delineate all of the patient's problem areas. According to some authorities,[3] the location of pain may indicate the extent, severity, and type of tissue involvement. For example, hypertonic saline injections into the lumbar interspinous ligaments of people resulted in posterior buttock and central low-lumbar pain according to studies by Kellgren.[4] However, an identical injection technique, to irritate the capsules of the posterior joints in the lumbar spine, resulted in similar pain references and some pain into the posterior thigh.[5,6] The extent, severity, and deviation of the condition may also be inferred by the pain location. Deep, localized, one-sided lumbar discomfort is indicative of irritation to the medial branch of the posterior primary rami. Nerve root irritation, on the other hand, causes segmental pain radiation into the lower extremity. The extent of the radiation into the extremity is determined by the location of the pain source; whereas the severity of the symptoms is related to the amount of irritation. If the symptoms linger, the patient's ability to discriminate exact locations of pain is hindered, and the pain becomes more or less diffuse in nature.[3]

For the OPT to have a complete understanding of the patient's physical source of noxious stimuli, sufficient knowledge of the neurophysiology of pain is required. The referred-pain phenomenon can also be appreciated by the OPT who possesses a fundamental awareness of the embryology of the musculoskeletal system. Therefore, interpretation of pain descriptions and complaints mandates the study of the neurophysiology of pain and musculoskeletal development.

BB's description of pain varied from a deep, dull ache in the lower back to a soreness in the left buttock and a burning in the posterior calf. The words selected from the McGill Pain Questionnaire—dull, ache, burn, and sore—described a physical source of pain, as opposed to words such as terrifying, frightful, unbearable, or torturing, which would have suggested that an emotional component might have been contributing to the patient's pain perception.[7]

The number of words chosen from the questionnaire may indicate the intensity of the symptoms. For example, if three fourths of the words are selected from the questionnaire, the patient is most likely experiencing or perceiving a great deal of pain. Patients selecting only a few words, on the other hand, are probably not in an extremely acute condition. BB selected one word from each of eight columns (maximum possible is 27) to describe the pain. Thus, the OPT felt that the problem was of moderate aggravation and discomfort to the patient. BB's body posture during sitting could best be described as careful and guarded, but fairly comfortable. His movements to and from the chair appeared somewhat protective in nature but were within a normal motion pattern. Thus, the above analysis of the patient's condition was tentatively made. A more accurate identification of the stage of the patient's condition will be made after the entire evaluation is completed.

The patient was asked to answer a number of questions that help the OPT to analyze the condition and determine how to proceed with the physical evaluation. The questions are listed, the patient's answers are provided, and a clinical interpretation is given below.

ASSESSMENT:

1. Q: Where did the pain commence?
   A: Central low back.

   Often, the initial location of the pain is indicative of the area of injury or the primary source of the symptoms. In BB's case, the lumbosacral area was identified. The OPT must remember this piece of information, particularly when the symptoms become diffuse and unlocalized.

2. Q: Where did the pain spread?
A: Left buttock and left calf.

The reference of pain distal from the source is a phenomenon called referred pain. Commonly, the patient with referred pain will be unable to outline a distinct segmental distribution. The clinician attempting to determine the segment or nerve root involved by analyzing the location of the referred-pain pathway becomes frustrated because of the patient's difficulty in delineating a specific pathway. In the case of BB, the pain went into the posterior calf. The OPT interpreted this pain as indicative of the severity of the lesion and did not attempt to correlate the pain to the segmental level. Other examiners may have become suspicious of involvement of the L-5 or S-1 nerve roots on the left side, because the segmental distribution of L-5 and S-1 includes the posterior and posterior lateral calf.[8] The ability to utilize pain as an indicator of the segmental source of the problem is directly related to knowledge of the nature of pain and understanding of the research by Wycke, Kellgren, Mooney and Robertson, and Hutton.

3. Q: What makes the pain worse?
A: Any movement, especially bending (exercises and racquetball), and prolonged sitting or standing (for more than 10 to 15 minutes).

The OPT must know which positions, movements, and activities aggravate the problem. This type of information enables the OPT to determine how to proceed with the examination; that is, how far to stress the spine with movement or manual pressure. Understanding what makes the pain worse also assists the OPT in determining an effective treatment plan.

Knowing the types of positions, movements, and activities that exacerbate pain may also provide additional information about the nature of the problem, the tissue source of irritation, and the severity of the condition. Some authorities[9] claim that pain with prolonged sitting or forward bending movements indicates a disk problem. Other authorities contend that pain during backward bending and side bending of the spine indicates a facet joint lesion.[10] The examiner's purpose for asking the question, "What makes the pain worse?" is twofold: (1) to find out which positions, movements, and activities are not tolerated so that re-evaluation can be done as treatment is given; and (2) to again determine the severity of the problem—how much spinal function has been impaired?

Almost universal in low back histories is the fact that prolonged sitting aggravates the condition. BB's pain was indeed worse when sitting and standing for longer than 10 to 15 minutes. However, BB did admit sitting was worse than standing. In most cases, the reason prolonged sitting is worse than standing is related to poor sitting positions chosen, the design of chairs that usually do not support the lumbar spine adequately, and the fact that intradisk pressures are greater during sitting than when standing.[11]

4. Q: What eases the pain?
   A: Resting on my back, using a heating pad, and taking aspirin.

The answers provided for this question often assist the OPT in correcting the problem and in facilitating the recovery process. The patient often is intuitively assisting the healing process by feeling the body's response to certain positions and movements and reacting accordingly. The OPT needs to be aware of and sensitive to the patient's own analysis of pain-relief methods.

Many low back conditions respond favorably to rest. Forty-four percent of patients with acute low back pain between the ages of 50 and 60 who receive bed rest instruction from a consulting general practitioner as a sole treatment will be able to resume normal activites within 1 week.[12] Back problems that do not react favorably to rest should be regarded as extremely acute conditions. Constant pain unaltered by positional changes, movements, or activities may not be of musculoskeletal origin.

BB said he was better lying on his back with a heating pad, a somewhat typical response by someone suffering from low back pain. Another question that may elicit more information regarding the severity of the condition is, "How long does it take for you to get comfortable after lying down?" Pain that disappears immediately when the patient lies down rather than after 30 or more minutes may suggest a less severe problem.

Some patients with unilateral symptoms discover that side lying on the involved side increases the pain while side lying on the uninvolved side decreases the pain. BB indicated that right side lying (the uninvolved side) with his hips and knees flexed and a pillow placed between his knees was helpful. The pillow assists in preventing hip internal rotation, which theoretically tenses the lumbosacral plexus.[13]

5. To determine if a particular daily pain pattern exists, the following questions are recommended:
   A. Q: Can you get comfortable at night?
      A. Yes.

A patient who is unable to sleep at night because of back pain most probably has considerable spinal pathology. More often than not, the patient who loses sleep because of pain is irritable and physically fatigued. The OPT should be aware of this possibility. BB was able to sleep comfortably, which is a relief not only for the patient, but for the therapist as well. Managing an easily agitated low back patient is usually not a pleasant assignment.

   B. Q: How do you feel when waking up in the morning?
      A: Stiff and sore. It takes a while to loosen up.

Stiffness and soreness upon rising in the morning may be the result of many factors that need to be investigated by the OPT. The following are possibilities:

too hard mattress
too soft mattress
improper sleeping position for that particular condition
prolonged position or inactivity
overextended sexual activity—inappropriate positioning for present condition.

Upon further questioning, the OPT determined that BB's problem in the morning was mainly due to lack of motion and prolonged inactivity during sleep.

C. Q: How do you feel at the end of the day?
A: Worse, especially the leg pain.

The lumbar spine receives many kinds of loading during a day: compression, bending, tension, shear, and torsion. The types of loads imposed on an individual's low back are related to the activities done. For example, a truck driver has high compression loading from sitting and vibration, as well as bending, torsion, and shear loads from lifting. The amount and types of mechanical loads placed upon the lumbar spine may be useful in assessing lumbar spinal pathology.[14]

As an epidemiologist, BB spends his time sitting at a desk, and thus his lumbar spine is under compression load for most of the day. The OPT needs to consider sitting posture, chair selection, and sitting time when planning a treatment approach for BB.

Patients who report a significant decrease or an elimination of symptoms after rest have recuperative abilities. For low back patients, repair of injured tissue is best accomplished in the recumbent position.[15] Patients who report little or no improvement with rest may have limited recuperative abilities. Often, patients with limited healing capacities will have a poor prognosis unless the injury is a first-time injury. The disk, for example, is capable of absorbing fluid at night when the spine is decompressed. However, a degenerated disk is not able to absorb fluid as well as a nondegenerated disk. As a result, it does not receive the nutrients required for repair. A patient with a degenerated disk, therefore, may not recover as fast as a patient without disk degeneration.

6. Q: What is the effect of coughing, laughing, or vibration?
A: Coughing hurts sometimes.

The research regarding the effect of vibration on the spine conducted by the Orthopaedic Department at the University of Vermont indicates that vibrating accelerates degenerative changes in the lumbar spine.[16] Clinical observation supports these studies. Questions such as, "What is the effect of coughing, laughing, or vibration?" are helpful to the OPT in providing advice and counseling on spinal support during those activities.

7. Q: Have you noticed any changes in bladder or bowel function?
A: No.

According to some evidence, lumbar musculoskeletal pain conditions may interfere with bladder or bowel function, especially if the condition is chronic in nature.[17] Somatic dysfunction detected by musculoskeletal examination may reflect visceral disturbances such as constipation, bowel irregularity, or urinary frequency. The nerve pathways responsible for visceral changes that are manifest as somatic dysfunction are called somato-autonomic or somato-visceral reflex arcs.[18] BB had not noticed any alteration in bladder or bowel activity, indicating no significant somato-visceral disturbance.

8. Q: Has the pain become worse recently?
A: Yes. Before, I could get relief by exercise and some activity. Now, exercise has no effect on the pain.

The OPT should know if the problem is worse, unchanged, or improving since the initial onset. Treatment of the condition can be evaluated effectively with knowledge of the pain status and history. For example, a condition that is improving in terms of pain reduction needs to be evaluated in the context of this improvement. A treatment approach cannot necessarily be considered beneficial if the condition was improving spontaneously without treatment, unless a faster recovery is made possible with the treatment.

BB's situation had worsened. He no longer was able to obtain pain relief with exercise or activity. Treatment techniques that prevent the condition from becoming worse or result in a reduction in pain can be considered to have had a beneficial effect.

The extent of the condition can be partially determined by evaluating pain perception in terms of location, frequency, intensity, and type. The condition may be considered worse if the symptoms are becoming diffuse, widespread, constant, and more severe. Some orthopaedic physical therapy practitioners contend that a condition is improving when the symptoms are becoming localized. On the other hand, if the symptoms are becoming diffuse or peripheral in nature, the condition is considered worse.[9]

One must be warned of the tendency to evaluate improvement of a back problem on the basis of pain relief alone. The possibility of a deteriorating nerve condition resulting in motor weakness may not necessarily cause pain. Conceivably, and often realistically, patients report decreasing pain symptoms without awareness of muscle weakness in the foot and/or ankle. OPTs who evaluate a low back condition solely on the basis of pain level may not recognize that the problem is becoming worse.

9. Q: What kinds of testing procedures have been done?
A: X-rays were taken in March 1980 that showed disk degeneration at L5-S1 (Fig. 11-1).

NAME	ROOM NO. 909942-5	SEX M	D.O.B. 1-17-44	X-Ray NO. 47102
CLINICAL HISTORY DEG DISK DISEASE	PHYSICIAN FREEMAN			
EXAMINATION				

Date: ______________________

LUMBAR SPINE:

There is severe disk space narrowing at levels L5-S1. There is also a 5 mm retrolisthesis of L-5 over S-1. There is mobility at the lumbosacral segment on the flexion-extension lateral view. Vertical height of the vertebral bodies is normal. Pedicles are intact. Apophyseal joints and para inter articularis showed no significant radiographic abnormality. There is mild anterior hypertrophic bony spurring lumbar vertebral bodies.

IMPRESSION:

Severe disk space narrowing at levels L5-S1 secondary to disk degeneration with slight retrolisthesis of L-5 over S-1.

RADIOLOGY REPORT ______________________
RADIOLOGIST

FIGURE 11-1. Radiographic report.

The OPT must be fully informed of all radiographic findings. The radiographic findings, however, may not be clinically relevant to the overall condition, according to many authorities.[19] Nonetheless, most physicians utilize roentgenograms as a standard examination procedure for a low back problem. Consequently, the OPT should be fully aware of the radiographic report.

With respect to BB, one study indicates that unisegmental narrowing at the L5-S1 disk space is not pathologically significant in terms of degeneration. Studies such as those done by Kellgren[4] and Mooney and Robertson[5] have helped to focus attention to other potential pain-sensitive tissues in the spine, such as the muscles, posterior joint capsules, and the ligaments. BB's radiographic report of March 1980 suggested L5-S1 disk degeneration because of the narrowing present. Further roentgenograms were not recommended at the time of the initial evaluation on March 16, 1981, because the previous roentgenograms were taken only 1 year previously, and the findings were not considered to be extensive.

The physician involved in BB's case suggested that repeat films with mobility roentgenograms be taken if the patient did not respond to physical therapy. The use of motion roentgenograms enables the radiologist to examine spinal mechanics. The existence of segmental mobility can be assessed by the use of flexion-extension films. An OPT experienced in passive intervertebral motion testing may use motion roentgenogram studies to help support the grades determined by passive motion testing.

10. Q: What past treatments have you had?
A: None, except for the exercise that I do, which consists of knees to chest and sit ups. The exercises used to help, but now they don't.

Previous treatment approaches need to be recorded and noted. More than likely, the patient is coming for another opinion because of past treatment failures. Treatment techniques used before should therefore not be emphasized in the present plan of action unless the previously attempted technique is used to augment another approach. On the other hand, any treatment that the patient did consider helpful should be noted and evaluated to determine if that treatment should be continued. BB indicated that his exercises helped at one time, but not any longer. Such exercises may not be appropriate at the present time.

The patient is also asked whether hospitalization and/or surgery was necessary. A serious back condition may be suspected if either hospitalization or surgery was required. Failed back surgery can be the result of many factors: scar tissue, arachnoiditis, chronic inflammation, post-surgical spinal stenosis, misdiagnosis, posterior joint involvement, or nerve entrapment.[20] Awareness of such factors is imperative for appropriate decision making regarding treatment alternatives. For example, a nerve entrapment problem may be provoked during the evaluation by a straight leg raise test. Flexion movements of the spine, as well as straight leg raise activities, may further irritate the entrapped nerve, and thus the patient should be warned against these motions.

11. Q: Are you presently taking any medications? If so, what are they? How many times a day do you take the medication?
A: Aspirin as needed—about two or three a day.

The amount of medication required for pain control demonstrates the severity of the problem or drug dependency. In monitoring a patient's progress, the amount of medication taken can be used as an indicator. A treatment program that sizably reduces the intake of medication can be considered a successful program.

12. Q: Is there anything else I should know about your condition or your health in general?

A: No.

At this point in the interview, the patient is given full opportunity to give additional information not gathered during the previous questioning. The patient may also wish to stress certain points about the situation that would help the OPT focus during the clinical evaluation. Furthermore, chronic back patients often need to vent some frustrations. The OPT must allow time during the interview for the patient's feelings to be expressed. The patient often wishes the therapist to realize the extent of the problem. The therapist, on the other hand, needs to be aware of how the pain has affected the patient's life.

GENERAL OBSERVATIONS

The overall physical condition of the patient is to be observed during the clinical examination and questioned during the interview. Cardiovascular, cardiopulmonary, and any systemic illnesses that may interfere with the evaluation process or treatment program need to be recorded. For example, a patient with observed shortness of breath and a history of chronic lung disease may not be able to lie prone comfortably for long periods because of increased abdominal pressure and possible interference with diaphragmatic excursion. In addition, a home exercise program should be carefully monitored to determine if the patient can perform it without undue taxation of the cardiopulmonary system.

The OPT sometimes overlooks obvious problems in search of subtle, complex, secondary problems. A grossly overweight patient complaining of low back pain from an insidious, gradual onset needs to be confronted about the weight problem at some time during the treatment. Although no statistical experimental evidence exists to substantiate obesity as a primary cause of low back pain, most clinical authorities believe that overweight individuals place greater loads on the posterior structures of the lumbar spine and thus are susceptible to back pain.[21] Weight was not considered a factor in the case of BB; however, the OPT and the patient did agree that abdominal toning was necessary.

STRUCTURAL EVALUATION

The next part of the examination is a structural inspection of the spine. The OPT observes general physical condition, body type, spinal alignment (in the frontal, horizontal, and sagittal planes), pelvic level, lower-extremity position, muscle contour and development, as well as posture and body image. The examiner is encouraged to observe only and not to palpate. Observation of structure enables the OPT to view the entire patient, and as a result, a holistic approach to the patient is ensured. Palpation for structural alignment is recommended after visual focusing of spinal stress areas.

GENERAL PHYSICAL CONDITION

Observe skin color and texture, particularly in the lower legs, ankles, and feet. Skin dryness and toenail brittleness may indicate interference in neurotrophic protein transport. BB had no evidence of skin dryness or toenail brittleness.

Abdominal weight that accentuates the lumbar lordosis and thus affects anterior-posterior spinal alignment is to be noted. BB was not grossly overweight, but as mentioned previously, he did not have adequate abdominal tone. Excessive weight below the lumbar spine (in the pelvis or hips) does not necessarily increase the compression force on the lumbar spine and therefore may not be a major factor in low back pain. The OPT should also relate body weight to the structural size of the vertebral bodies. Some patients have large vertebral bodies and are more capable of carrying added weight than patients who have small vertebral bodies.

BODY TYPE

BB had a mesomorphic body type. Mesomorphic body types typically have large, strong vertebrae as well as tight, less extensible periarticular (ligaments, capsules) tissues.[22] To confirm the assumption, active spinal movements should be tested and roentgenograms taken. The OPT should not compare the spinal range of motion attained by a mesomorph body type to that attained by an ectomorph body type. The latter typically have smaller, less dense vertebrae and extensible periarticular tissues that allow for greater joint excursion.

SPINAL CURVES

Observation and palpation techniques to detect spinal and pelvic position revealed a left pelvic tilt along with a left compensatory lumbar curve (Fig. 11-2). The pelvic tilt was believed to be the result of a short left lower extremity. The spinal response to this pelvic tilt was deviation to the left. This type of spinal reaction to the pelvic tilt is considered to be a compensatory response. The evaluator also determined that the lumbar spine was shifted to the left in addition to the left compensatory curve. A left shift, by definition, indicates that the vertebral segments have translated (a glide movement) to the left.

The OPT notes if the patient is shifting toward or away from the side of the pain. BB had left-sided symptoms and also shifted to the left. If nerve root irritation was the cause of the symptoms, the problem is likely to be medial to nerve root. Such is the case of a medial disk extrusion, in which the patient shifts to the same side of the injury in an attempt to move the nerve root away from the extrusion.[23]

The anterior-posterior curves of the spine are also to be observed. BB had a relatively straight lumbar spine with normal curves in the thoracic and cervical spines. The OPT is to make a judgment regarding spinal alignment and then evaluate whether the structural alignment has affected spinal motion. Structural malalignment affecting spinal motion is considered to be more significant than structural malalignment that does not affect spinal motion.[24] The peak of the curves is identified, and the type of biomechanical

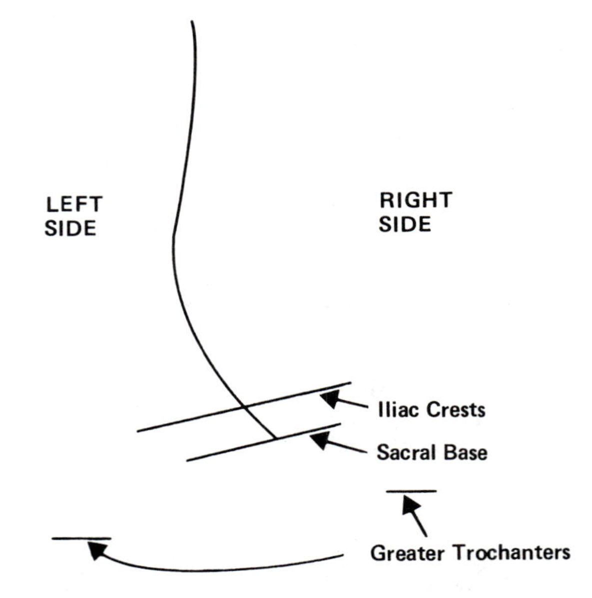

FIGURE 11-2. Spinal alignment of BB—posterior view.

forces is noted at the curve's peak. For example, BB's thoracic posterior curve apex was at T6-7, which as far as location is considered, is within normal limits. The tensional force, however, in the posterior structures of T6-7 is therefore potentially greater than at any other segment in the thoracic posterior curve. With respect to segmental mobility, T6-7 may possibly be hypomobile in the direction of backward bending because of its relative forward-bent position.

ACTIVE SPINAL MOVEMENTS: ANALYSIS

The OPT is to recognize that active spinal movement testing requires the cooperation of the patient. Active spinal motion implies voluntary action—a willingness by the patient to move. Indirectly, therefore, the examiner, in testing active spinal movements, is assessing the patient's pain tolerance. Individuals with a high pain tolerance are likely to move through a greater spinal range than those with low pain tolerance. BB demonstrated active movements suggestive of a person who was willing to move as far as pain allowed. All planes of motion resulted in pain for BB, but especially forward bending and right side bending. The OPT is to examine active spinal movements in terms of range of motion, direction of movement, and motion control. Spinal movements that affect range, direction, and control are considered significantly abnormal. Spinal motions that affect only one parameter are considered only slightly abnormal.

BB's range of motion was most limited in forward bending. The lumbar spine returned to the lordotic position upon forward bending and also deviated to the left. The examiner felt that the retention of the lordotic curve was primarily due to pain. The deviation of the spine to the left upon forward bending is suggestive of a left-sided segmental motion abnormality in the facet joint or joints.[24] The possibility of a left-sided intervertebral disk bulge or nuclear extrusion as a factor resulting in the abnormal motion segment behavior was not ruled out. In addition, forward bending recruitment into the lumbar spine resulted in movement hesitation, which also indicated a motion control problem. Backward bending of the lumbar spine was painful and very restricted in range, especially in the mid- and upper-lumbar segments. The pain location on backward bending, however, differed from the pain location during forward bending. The pain during forward bending was perceived in the lower-lumbar spine, left buttock, and left posterior thigh; whereas the pain during backward bending was confined to the lower-lumbar spine. The OPT is to record the subjective response of the patient during active movements. BB's condition seems more aggravated during forward bending than backward bending, based on pain analysis. Side bending movements were also painful, especially right side bending. Motion direction and control were not visibly affected.

The significant restriction in right side bending was due to pain in the left side of the lower lumbar spine; whereas left side bending was painful at the end range of motion. The results of the side bending tests gave additional support to the possibility of a left-sided facet problem due to the inability of the facet to slide up and forward, as it must during forward and right side bending. The possibility of a left-sided disk lesion also must still be considered. The disk bulge or extrusion is most likely to be positioned medial to the nerve root in this situation, according to DePalma and Rothman[25] (Fig. 11-3). BB, in an attempt to minimize nerve root or tissue irritation, shifts

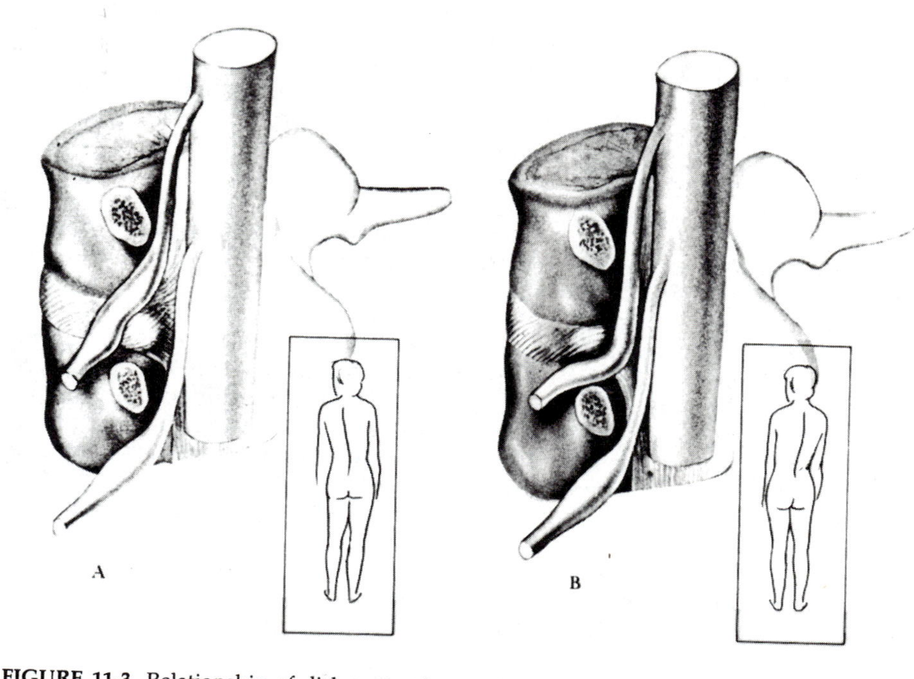

FIGURE 11-3. Relationship of disk protrusion to the nerve root and resultant lateral shift. (From DePalma and Rothman,[25] p. 82, with permission.)

to the left, veers to the left on forward bending, and avoids right side bending.

Active rotation of the spine produced pain and was restricted in both directions. The demonstrated rotational movements did not help the OPT to differentially diagnose between facet dysfunction and a disk lesion. In summary, BB's active movement pattern was limited due to pain and segmental restriction, particularly in forward bending and right side bending. Other motions were also painful and restricted, but not as much as forward and right side bending. The range of motion obtained and the manner in which the motion was produced suggest two possible lesions: (1) facet joint dysfunction, or (2) disk lesion. Further testing may help to differentiate between these possibilities.

NEUROLOGIC TESTING

The OPT is to include manual clinical tests to determine neurologic involvement. The purpose of neurologic tests is to help differentiate nerve root compression from nerve root irritation and to rule out significant nerve root involvement from referred pain syndromes due to tissue irritation. The extent, severity, and stage of the condition is then appreciated by the OPT.

The first part of the exam consists of manual muscle testing of the lower extremity musculature. Manual muscle testing will hopefully screen those patients with significant muscle weakness suggestive of motor nerve conduction interference. Any questionable finding during manual muscle testing, particularly in patients with extensive referred-pain patterns, should be recorded and the test repeated. If the symptoms are worse at the end of the day, the OPT may request that the patient return to the clinic at that time to be retested. The results of manual muscle testing may be more conclusive at the end of the day when the condition worsens rather than at the beginning of the day when the problem is not as bad. In cases where significant numbness, tingling, or severe pain are perceived in the lower extremities, the OPT should request an electromyogram (EMG) to determine the nature of the nerve interference.

In the case of BB, no demonstrable difference was noted in muscle strength between left and right lower extremities. However, the examiner felt that this was not conclusive and that an EMG would possibly show evidence of nerve root involvement. An EMG was ordered and performed by the clinic's physical medicine specialist. The results of the EMG testing (Fig. 11-4) confirmed the OPT's speculation. An early left S-1 motor nerve root denervation was determined. The OPT is to be reminded that manual muscle testing is not as specific or accurate as EMG testing, particularly in the early stages of motor nerve root involvement. Thus, any suspicions of a nerve root problem during the history or structural or active movement examinations should be followed up by manual muscle testing and EMG analysis.

The use of EMG testing to demonstrate left S-1 motor nerve involvement helps to locate the source of the pain. The S-1 nerve root is in close proximity to the intervertebral disk of L5-S1 as it descends obliquely to exit the S-1 foramen. The L5-S1 facet joint is located posterior to the nerve root of S-1. Thus, the possible pain source is the L5-S1 intervertebral disk and/or the facet joint.

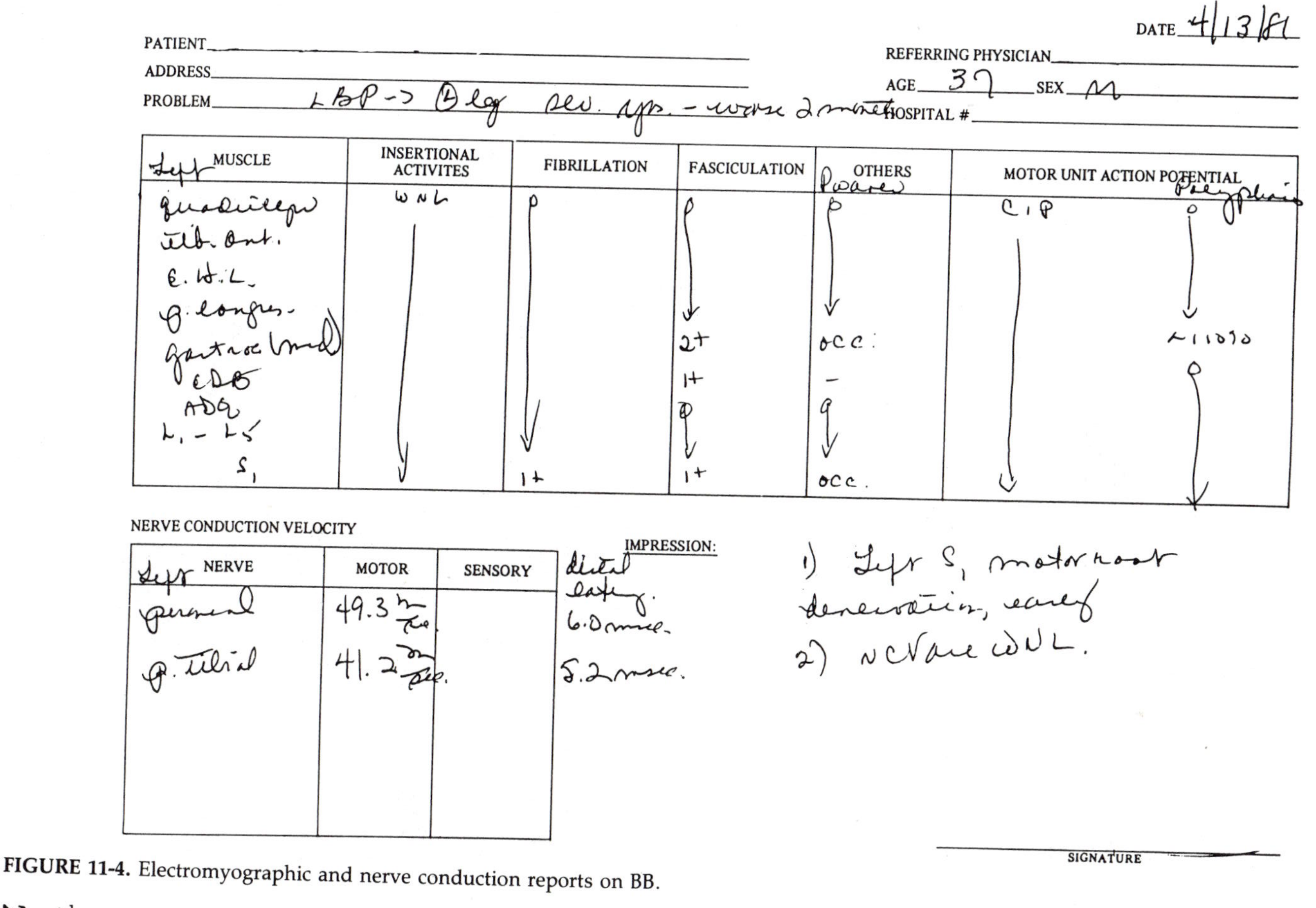

DATE 4/13/81

PATIENT
ADDRESS
PROBLEM LBP → (L) leg sev. sx. – worse 2 months

REFERRING PHYSICIAN
AGE 37 SEX M
HOSPITAL #

Left MUSCLE	INSERTIONAL ACTIVITES	FIBRILLATION	FASCICULATION	OTHERS	MOTOR UNIT ACTION POTENTIAL
quadriceps	WNL	0	0	0 (waves)	C.I.P. / 0 (Polyphasic)
tib. ant.	↓	↓	↓	↓	↓
E.H.L.	↓	↓	↓	↓	↓
p. longus	↓	↓	↓	↓	↓
gastroc (med)	↓	↓	2+	occ.	↓ / ~10%
EDB	↓	↓	1+	–	↓ / 0
ADQ	↓	↓	0	0	↓
L1 – L5	↓	↓	↓	↓	↓
S1	↓	1+	1+	occ.	↓

NERVE CONDUCTION VELOCITY

Left NERVE	MOTOR	SENSORY	distal latency
peroneal	49.3 m/sec		6.0 msec.
p. tibial	41.2 m/sec.		5.2 msec.

IMPRESSION:
1) Left S1 motor root denervation, early
2) NCV are WNL.

SIGNATURE

FIGURE 11-4. Electromyographic and nerve conduction reports on BB.

Reflex testing of the knee and ankle yielded bilateral, equal, and symmetrical responses. Impairment of the ankle jerk response is often related to S-1 nerve root conduction interference.[25] However, in the case of BB, no evidence of reflex alteration was found. Studies by Brown and Pont[26] show that 50 percent of patients with known lumbar disk lesions at L5-S1 have no change in the Achilles tendon reflex. Therefore, the lack of any appreciable correlation between ankle jerk reflex and muscle strength should not confuse the examiner.

The above neurologic tests are, for the most part, objective in nature. The results of manual muscle, reflex, and EMG testing are based on clinical judgments by the examiner according to measurable data. Provocation testing of the low back pain patient requires the testimony of the patient and thus is subjective in nature. The OPT is to be fully aware of the type of testing being undertaken so that appropriate analysis and interpretation can be done.

Straight leg testing is considered a provocation test and is commonly used to determine the irritability of lumbar nerve roots. Straight leg raise mechanical studies by Goodard and Reid[27] demonstrate downward movement and tension development in the sciatic nerve complex, the L-4, L-5, and S-1 nerve roots, and the dura. The greatest amount of motion was found in the first sacral nerve during straight leg raising. Movements of the L-5 lumbar nerve root were 3 mm; whereas the S-1 nerve root averaged 4 to 5 mm of movement. In addition, at the intervertebral foramen, movement was not apparent until 20 degrees to 30 degrees of straight leg raising occurred. The greatest amount of nerve root movement occurs from 35 degrees to 70 degrees of straight leg raising. Goodard and Reid[27] point out that when nerve movement is restricted, tension in the nerve and nerve pressure over bony prominences increase.

BB had bilateral limitation in straight leg raising due to pain in the left thigh and buttock as well as hamstring tightness. Thirty-five degrees of straight leg raising was tolerated on the left side before left thigh and buttock pain prohibited further movement. Excessive tension was palpated in the left hamstrings during the straight leg raise test. The right lower extremity tolerated 45 degrees of straight leg raising before low back pain and hamstring tightness prevented further movement. Based on the results of the straight leg raise and previous testing, the examiner concluded that moderate nerve root involvement most probably existed. In addition, the patient had tight hamstring muscles bilaterally.

LOWER-QUARTER AND PELVIC EXAMINATION

Evaluation of the lower extremities and pelvis revealed no significant biomechanical positional or motion abnormality aside from an adduction and internal rotation limitation of the left hip joint. Palpation of the left piriformis muscle revealed increased tension, which is a common clinical finding among patients with acute low back pain episodes or in patients with chronic low back involvement. Hyperactivity of the piriformis may eventually lead to adaptive shortening. The result of increased tone and tightness in the left piriformis may be a restriction in left hip internal rotation and adduction. The reason for piriformis hyperactivity in BB may be due to the involvement of the S-1 motor nerve fibers, which, in part, innervate the piriformis. Another possible explanation may lie in the phasic/postural muscle dysfunction theory proposed by Vladimir Janda.[28] The basic contention of this muscle dysfunction theory is that postural muscles will tighten and phasic muscles will weaken in response to dysfunction. The piriformis muscle is classified as a postural muscle because of its histologic properties. Therefore, the piriformis may contract and tighten in a possible attempt to stabilize the lumbosacral complex.

One additional finding in the lower-quarter and pelvic evaluation having possible clinical relevance concerned bilateral iliopsoas muscle tightness. The iliopsoas is also a postural muscle, according to Janda's[28] histologic classification scheme, and therefore also tends to shorten during dysfunction. A modified form of the Thomas test,[29] used to determine iliopsoas tightness, revealed bilateral shortening. An increased compression load on the posterior elements of the lumbar spine is possibly exerted by the vertebral portion of the psoas muscle as a result of this shortening (bilateral contraction of the psoas causes backward bending of the lumbar spine).

PALPATION TESTING

Condition

A layer palpation method was used to assess the condition of the involved tissues. In the layer palpation technique, the examiner evaluates each tissue layer from superficial to deep for tissue tone. Areas of somatic dysfunction, detected by palpation techniques, are correlated with the previous findings on structural evaluation, lower-quarter and pelvic assessment, and active movements.

Skin

Skin temperature and moisture were cool and dry in the left lower lumbar paraspinals when compared to the right side. Cool and dry skin in the involved area is consistent with BB's recurrent chronic low back problems. Vasomotor disturbance as a result of sympathetic involvement may explain temperature and moisture changes in the skin.

Further indication of sympathetic disturbance was revealed through the scratch test. Very little skin response was elicited following a scratch to the paraspinals in the low-lumbar area on the left side. A light skin reaction to a scratch is characteristic of a chronic condition, which was elicited in the history reported by BB.

Subcutaneous—Fascia

No evidence of swelling or subcutaneous nodule formation was found by palpation in the involved region. However, compression and shear testing for fascial mobility revealed hypoextensibility in both lumbar paraspinal areas, especially in the lower-lumbar spine. Further evidence of fascial mobility restriction was seen in the subcutaneous tissue rolling test.

Muscle

Compression of the left lower lumbar paraspinal musculature and the left piriformis muscle elicited reflex muscle contractions. A reflex muscle contraction or twitch in response to a slowly applied compression force indicates a lower threshold level of motor excitation. Lower excitation of muscle may indicate a segmental facilitation because lesioned segments are characterized by lowered motor reflex thresholds.[30] Weak stimuli applied to the lesioned segment may elicit a muscle contraction; whereas the same intensity stimuli applied to a nonlesioned segment is unlikely to produce a muscle response.

Light pressure to the lower-lumbar paraspinals on both sides revealed exaggerated muscle activity bilaterally when compared to the upper-lumbar and low-thoracic paraspinal musculature. Increased activity in the lower-back extensors suggests a protective muscle-guarding state. Protective muscle guarding is the body's attempt to stabilize or splint to avoid pain and allow for repair.

Further evaluation of BB's muscle condition revealed a marked imbalance of muscle tone between the abdominals and back extensors. The back extensors had an increased activity level; whereas the abdominals were noticeably weak. Manual muscle examinations of both groups were not done on the initial visit because of the pain profile. Moreover, when studying the sequence in which the lumbar extensors contracted upon hip extension, the examiner learned that the patient's muscle-firing pattern was abnormal. EMG studies by Janda[28] showed contralateral extensor contraction before ipsilateral extensor contraction when hip extension is performed on one side.

BB had the correct sequence of muscle-firing with right hip extension, but left hip extension resulted in ipsilateral erector spinae activity before contralateral contraction. The degree of activity on the left side was much greater than on the right side. The OPT is to be aware of faulty muscle-firing patterns because of the possible asymmetric force transmissions into the lumbar spine. Left-sided paraspinal activity that is greater than the right and that occurs before the right side, as in the case of BB, may eventually result in greater compression loading on the left side of the lumbar spine.

The possibility of earlier degenerative changes occurring on the left side of the spine due to the excess stress imposed by the aberrant muscle behavior must be considered. Overactivity of the left paraspinals may result in an extensor, left side bending and left rotation movement on the lumbar spine that is not being counter-opposed by equal activity on the right side. Ultimately, this muscle imbalance may affect the position of the lumbar spine. Spinal alignment change may, in turn, affect spinal mechanics.

In previous analysis of the active motion pattern, the restrictive barriers to movement were determined to be pain, abnormal facet mechanics, and/or an intervertebral disk problem. By analyzing muscle tone through palpation and observing the firing sequence of the paraspinals, an additional restrictive barrier was determined—muscle. The OPT is to examine all possible motion-restriction barriers and then determine which are the primary and secondary factors producing abnormal mechanical activity.

Ligaments

The superficial and palpable posterior longitudinal ligaments of the spine are the supraspinous and interspinous ligaments. Palpation of the supraspinous and interspinous ligaments for trophic change, increased tone, reduced elasticity, and tenderness is done to assess the ligamentous condition. Thickening of a ligament may occur in response to excessive stress. A ligament that thickens and hardens may eventually lose elasticity and impair segmental motion.

BB had ligamentous hypertrophy of the supraspinous and interspinous ligaments at L1-2 and L2-3. Springing over the ligaments at L1-2 and L2-3 revealed a loss of normal mobility and less elasticity. Palpation of the L4-5 and L5-S1 interspaces elicited a pain response from BB. The same pressure at the L1-2 and L2-3 interspaces did not evoke pain. The segmental facilitation concept proposed by Korr[30] suggests that a lowered reflex response to a sensory stimulus is characteristic of a lesioned segment. The trophic changes in the superficial posterior lumbar ligaments at the L1-2 and L2-3 interspaces that resulted in thickening may also explain the loss of motion evidenced in the active motion examination.

SUMMARY OF CONDITION

The palpation tests that assess tissue-texture abnormality suggest soft-tissue facilitation secondary to a biomechanical segmental dysfunction. The extent of involvement is assessed by evaluating the types and amount of tissues affected. Abnormal findings were demonstrated throughout all low-lumbar tissue layers: skin, fascia, muscle, and ligament. The OPT therefore felt significant somatic dysfunction existed in the lower-lumbar spine, especially on the left side.

POSITION

Vertebral position by palpation is performed to determine if any gross positional disturbances have occurred. Vertebral position is palpated by identifying the relative positions of adjacent spinous processes. Only abrupt changes in position are considered significant. The most obvious finding on BB occurred between L-4 and L-5. The OPT determined that L-4 was anterior to L-5, or L-5 was posterior to L-4. A positional change such as described above suggests increased segmental stress. The examiner is to make note of positional disturbances to determine if segmental motion is affected.

Congenital anomalies in the development of spinous processes may result in misinterpretation of suspected positional disturbances. For example, if the spinous process of BB's L-5 was unusually large, the OPT may be misled in believing that a positional fault existed between L-4 and L-5. The OPT needs to be aware of the fact that bony anomalies exist in the spine, particularly in the lower-lumbar spine. In one study by Farfan,[31] congenital bony anomalies were found in the lower lumbar spine in 23 percent of a sample population of normal people (without back pain). Another study, by Brailsford,[32] reported asymmetric facet joints in 32 percent of a sample population of 3000 individuals with backaches.

MOBILITY

Passive segmental mobility tests are used by the OPT to analyze intervertebral motion at each level of the spine. The purpose is to identify specific

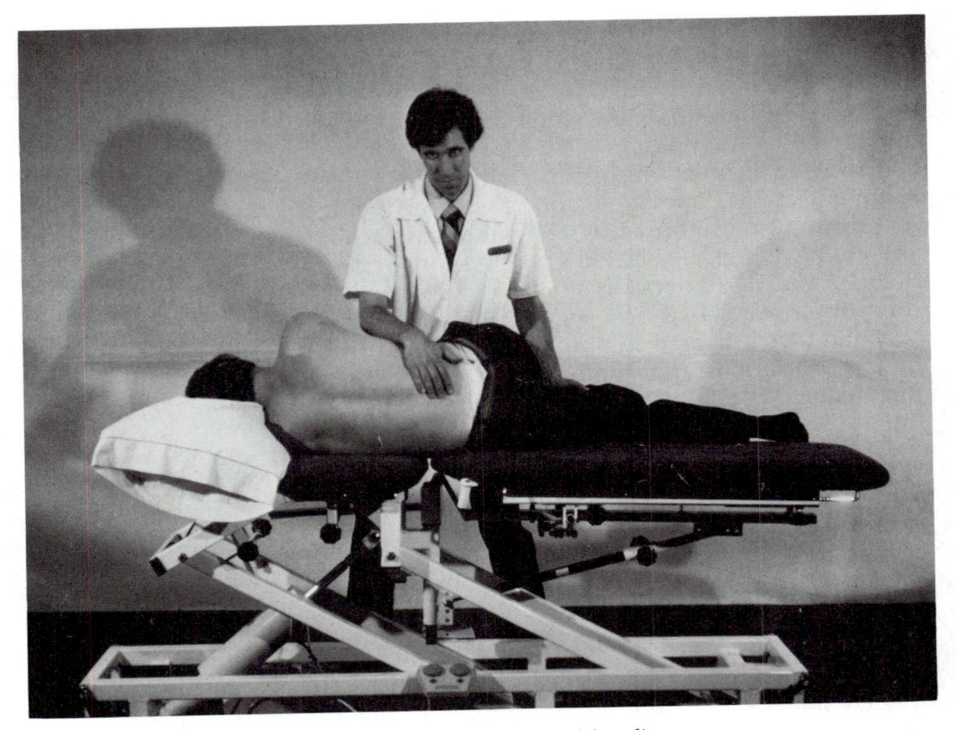

FIGURE 11-5. Passive segmental mobility test—forward bending.

segmental motion to determine motion abnormalities. Biomechanical information of this nature is believed to be of significant value to the OPT in determining a management plan.

Various techniques are utilized by OPTs. However, two essential criteria are necessary for the OPT to reliably evaluate segmental mobility: (1) patient relaxation: the test procedure requires passive induction of a specific motion by the therapist; the patient is to be totally relaxed so that muscle interference is negligible; and (2) therapist concentration: the perception of segmental motion by means of palpation is subtle indeed. The OPT must totally focus into receiving motion activity by finger palpation. Both range of motion and motion ease or resistance are to be analyzed. Figure 11-5 illustrates a passive segmental test for forward bending in the lumbar spine. All directions of motion can be passively induced and tested.

Intra-rater reliability of passive segmental testing has been determined to be acceptable according to a study by Gonnella, Paris, and Kutner.[33] The same study indicated poor inter-rater reliability correlation. Further standardization of technique and redefinition of grading scale is believed to be essential in improving inter-rater reliability. Segmental mobility testing of BB proved to be of value in assessing the overall condition. The grading scale utilized to detect segmental range of motion was devised by Paris, Grieve, and Kaltenborn.[33] The key is illustrated in Table 11-1. Table 11-2 illustrates the segmental grades of BB's lumbar spine from T12-L1 to L5-S1, as determined by the evaluator.

TABLE 11-1. Rating System for Evaluating Passive Mobility of the Spine*

GRADE	DESCRIPTION	CRITERIA
0	Ankylosed	No detectable movement within the segment. Requires stress film radiology for confirmation.
1	Considerable restriction (hypomobility)	Significant decrease in expected range. Significant resistance to movement.
2	Slight restriction (hypomobility)	Limitation expected in range. Some resistance to movement.
3	Normal	Expected range for body type. Uniform movement throughout range.
4	Slight increase (hypermobility)	Some increase expected in range. Less than normal resistance to movement.
5	Considerable increase (hypermobility)	Excessive range (but eventually restricted by capsular and ligamental structure).
6	Unstable	Excessive range (as in Grade 5) but without the restraint of capsular and ligamental structure.

*From Gonnella, Paris, and Kutner,[33] p 438, with permission.

By referring to Figure 11-1, one is able to identify that BB had a considerable motion restriction at L5-S1, particularly in forward and right side bending. The L4-5 segment was slightly hypermobile in all planes of movement. Above L4-5 either slight motion limitations or normal motion was detected. The motion throughout the lumbar spine was, therefore, not evenly distributed at each segment. The existence of a significant segmental motion restriction adjacent to a segmental hypermobility is a common spinal biomechanical phenomenon.[34] Segmental motion imbalance is perhaps one of the biomechanical factors that contribute to tissue deformation and, eventually, painful irritation.

An experienced OPT will correlate the results of the active movement examination with the segmental grades determined by passive motion testing. In the case of BB, a direct positive correlation existed between active and passive movements, which most likely implicates L5-S1 mechanical involvement. Active motion testing revealed a left-sided motion restriction in the lumbar spine. Passive motion testing indicated restriction in forward bend-

TABLE 11-2. BB's Segmental Grades Determined by Passive Segmental Testing

LEVEL	FB	BB	RSB	LSB	RR	LR
L5-S1	1	2	1	2	2	2
L4-5	4	4	3+	3+	3	3
L3-4	2	2−	2−	2+	2	2
L2-3	2+	2−	2−	2+	2	2
L1-2	2	2−	2	2	2+	2+
T12-L1	3	3	3	3	3	3

ing and right side bending at L5-S1. (Left-sided facet movement is essential for right side bending.) The L5-S1 limitation is therefore calculated to be the major culprit in affecting active spinal movements. The slight instability detected at L4-5 by passive motion testing was not reflected in the active motion patterns. Segmental instabilities frequently are exhibited during active forward bending in the form of muscle fasciculations or spinal juddering (vibration). The indication for passive segmental testing is demonstrated in the case of BB, in whom segmental instability was not apparent in active movements, but was determined passively. Passive segmental test results, in addition, help to determine if joint manipulation is necessary. The type of joint manipulation to be used is also partly determined by passive segmental test grades.

RADIOGRAPHIC REPORT

Routine lumbar spine roentgenograms were taken following the clinical examination by the OPT. Routine roentgenograms of the lumbar spine should include anterior-posterior, lateral, oblique, and flexion-extension mobility films. Roentgenogram impressions should be made following the clinical examination to avoid potential bias during the evaluation procedures. The radiology report on BB's lumbar spine revealed severe disk-space narrowing at L5-S1, which the radiologist believed to be secondary to disk degeneration. In addition, a 5-mm retrolisthesis of L-5 over S-1 was reported. This 5-mm backward displacement of L-5 was considered a slight retrolisthesis according to the radiologist.

Other than mild anterior hypertrophic bony spurring of the lumbar vertebral bodies, no other significant bony radiographic abnormalities were demonstrated. The flexion-extension mobility films were basically unremarkable. However, the radiologist did report that motion existed at the lumbosacral segment. Thus, mobility roentgenogram films are helpful in clarifying the results of passive segmental testing. No attempt to quantify segmental range of motion at L5-S1 was done by radiographic measurements in the case of BB. Utilizing the segmental measuring technique of Tanz,[35] the OPT was able to determine that the L5-S1 level was most restricted in motion compared to the remaining lumbar levels. Thus, a positive correlation exists between segmental range of motion at L5-S1, as determined by passive motion tests and flexion-extension mobility films.

One should be cautious in relating disk degeneration to disk narrowing, as suggested within the above radiographic report. Disk height may not necessarily be related to the degree of disk degeneration, according to a study by Nachemson, Schultz, and Berkson.[36] Appreciable disk histopathology in the presence of normal or increased disk heights when measured by roentgenogram has been demonstrated in a number of selected cases. Therefore, a prediction of the degree of disk degeneration by disk height determination through roentgenogram is not possible. Furthermore, speculation arises about the accuracy of standard lateral roentgenogram films in measuring intervertebral disk height. A study by Andersson, Schultz, Nathan, and Irstam[37] suggested that intervertebral disk height cannot be reliably determined by lateral radiographs, especially if only L5-S1 is involved.

The general consensus among the radiologist, physiatrist, and OPT was that BB did indeed have significant L5-S1 intervertebral narrowing.

TABLE 11-3. Summary of Significant Findings

1. A considerable left L5-S1 motion restriction
2. Slight motion restrictions at L3-4, L2-3, and L1-2
3. An L4-5 slight segmental instability
4. A left S-1 nerve root irritation
5. L5-S1 intervertebral disk narrowing
6. A left pelvic tilt; a short left lower extremity
7. A slight left lateral shift
8. Protective muscle guarding in both iliopsoas muscles, the left lower lumbar paraspinals, and left piriformis muscle
9. Poor abdominal tone

Other clinical data such as the existence of an S-1 nerve root irritation and the detection of a motion restriction at L5-S1 seemed to lend support to the contention that the intervertebral space at L5-S1 was narrow. The demonstration of a backward displacement of L-5 on S-1 is sometimes related to segmental instability at the lumbosacral junction.[38] In the case of BB, L5-S1 was hypomobile according to motion studies; therefore, the positional change could be considered a more stable situation.

CORRELATION OF SIGNIFICANT FINDINGS

A thorough clinical evaluation of the chronic low back problem requires numerous testing procedures. The data collected from the examination is to be reviewed, analyzed, and correlated. No one test or procedure can be expected to give the OPT the entire pathomechanical problem or provide all the information for the solution. Significant data are largely the result of a number of positive test correlations. A list of significant clinical findings for BB is provided in Table 11-3.

PLANNED TREATMENT

Planning a treatment approach is based upon obtaining knowledge of the potential pain sources as well as determining the specific biomechanical problem areas. The evidence for L5-S1 being the segment responsible for giving rise to BB's pain is quite strong based on radiographic reports, EMG analysis, clinical motion studies, and the subjective report during the history. One could also contend that L4-5 is partly responsible for the pain reported by BB on the basis of passive segmental motion testing, which demonstrated slight hypermobility. Capsular and ligamentous irritation as a result of excessive motion at L4-5 could indeed contribute to pain perception.

The biomechanical analysis reveals disproportionate motion in the lumbar spine suggestive of a regional mechanical motion imbalance. Motion restrictions exist at L2-3, L3-4, and most notably, at L5-S1; whereas L4-5 exhibits a slight increase in motion.

If the motion restrictions at L5-S1, L3-4, and L2-3 are largely the result of facet dysfunctions, then the facets at these levels are less capable of serving as force attenuators. Greater load is then possibly transferred to the disk, which ultimately may lead to premature wear and tear.

An OPT adopting this theoretical biomechanical analysis of lumbar mobility would perhaps suggest that the treatment approach include improving the range of motion at the restricted segmental levels. In the case of BB, the evaluator decided on using specific joint manipulation techniques to restore segmental range at the involved levels.

Since discogenic involvement has not been ruled out because of a left lateral shift, positive neurologic signs, active movement results, and pain with prolonged sitting, the OPT must take special precautions in the choice of manipulative technique. The results of active movement testing suggest that forward bending movements result in a more distal pain reference than backward bending, in which the pain is confined to the low back. The use of the extension principle in correction of suspected lumbar disk derangements was suggested by McKenzie.[9] The OPT needs to consider the extension approach as a possible means of promoting healing, reducing pain, and increasing range of motion of the lumbar spine whenever a disk lesion is hypothesized. The sequencing of specific manipulative therapy and self-mobilization exercises is a critical step for the OPT to achieve optimal results and avoid possible adverse reactions.

The evaluator for BB decided that specific manipulative treatment to L5-S1, L3-4, and L2-3 was necessary first. As range of motion improved at these levels, the patient would then better tolerate passive self-mobilization exercise in extension. The existence of a hypermobile segment at L4-5 was an additional factor in the OPT's decision to use specific manipulation treatment first. Establishing increased motion in the mid-lumbar segments and at the lumbosacral junction may prevent additional strain on the already hypermobile L4-5 segment.

As in many cases of low back pain, BB's symptoms were not severe enough or sufficiently disabling for him to consider taking time off from work. The symptoms are certainly annoying and did interfere with his normal everyday functional activities, but he preferred to go to work. As an epidemiologist, his work activities require him to be seated. Unfortunately, as we are already aware, there is considerable intradisk pressure in the sitting position. The OPT, therefore, is to instruct BB on the best sitting positions possible and the best choice of chair designs. BB also needs to be instructed in positions of rest and in rest periods for the low back when not at work.

The hypertonic muscle behavior in the lower-lumbar paraspinals, left piriformis, and iliopsoas is believed to be a secondary response to the underlying mechanical pathology. Chronically facilitated muscle states may eventually become another problem. The muscle is deprived of an adequate blood supply and retains metabolic waste products, which lead to muscle irritability and lost extensibility. The OPT must regain proper muscle tone to reduce pain, which possibly may arise from chemically irritated sensory nerve endings. The OPT must also improve extensibility so that the elongation properties are returned. Therefore, a program of soft-tissue inhibition, soft-tissue mobilization, and stretching is to be included in the management plan.

The left pelvic tilt, believed to be the result of a short left lower extremity, is also to be considered as part of the biomechanical problem because of the potential asymmetrical force distribution at L5-S1 that the pelvic tilt may cause. Detailed consideration is to be given about when such a correction of

TABLE 11-4. Summary of Treatment Plan

1. Instruction in erect, supportive sitting and proper rest positions when lying down.
2. Instruction in activity pacing, types of functional activities.
3. Soft-tissue inhibition (relaxation) and mobilization to the involved tissues.
4. Specific therapeutic manipulation to restricted lumbar segments.
5. Self-mobilization exercise.
6. Lift therapy to correct leg length discrepancy and pelvic imbalance.
7. Muscle re-education toning and elongation.
8. Prevention through back-school education in lifting, body mechanics, posture, general exercise, and nutrition.

pelvic height should be made. At present, the mechanical restrictions in the lumbar spine may not permit adjustment to a change in pelvic position. Therefore, in treatment sequencing, the OPT must put the steps in priority. Table 11-4 summarizes the treatment plan.

PROGNOSIS AND GOALS

The existing nerve involvement and impairment in BB's function caused the OPT to be cautiously guarded in terms of a speedy recovery. The OPT's prognosis for recovery was 2 months. The immediate goal was to reduce pain and promote healing. After significant pain relief and the initiation of a repair process, the OPT is to improve biomechanical function through therapeutic manipulation of soft tissues and joints. Restoration of normal spinal mechanics will reduce the likelihood of reinjury.

TREATMENT APPROACH AND MANAGEMENT

The treatment plan for BB commenced in March 1981. He was seen on a fairly regular basis for physical therapy from March until June of 1981. BB returned in July of 1982 for a re-evaluation of his condition. He had no major complaints. An additional three visits in 1982 were basically for some minor problems. In November of 1982, however, BB experienced severe left-sided pain in the low back and left lower extremity. An intense outpatient physical therapy program was initiated without a significant reduction in pain. BB was subsequently hospitalized on bed rest with further diagnostic testing for 2 weeks. Improvement in the condition was noted after hospitalization. BB is currently being monitored by the OPT and is doing satisfactorily.

The specifics of the treatment approach and management plan as the plan occurred on a weekly basis will now be identified. The rationale is provided for the techniques chosen and the decisions made. Additional testing is described, and the results are identified. SOAP progress report notes are used to clearly follow the physical therapy course of action and the patient's condition.

WEEK 1—TWO TREATMENTS

S— The initial evaluation temporarily aggravated the condition. The patient noticed an increase in left leg symptoms following the examination;

these gradually disappeared overnight. The pain this week was moderate (average) and existed in the left buttock and posterior thigh. The treatments had a temporary effect on the pain level. During the week, BB played racquetball one night after work, and the pain in the low back increased.

O—Structure

The lateral shift was corrected during both treatment sessions, but there appeared to be poor carryover. Forward bending and right side bending continued to be the most painful active movements. A slight improvement was observed in lumbar backward bending after the second treatment session.

—Palpation

The muscle tone remained hyperactive. The activity of the left piriformis increased significantly after racquetball. L4-5 and L5-S1 interspinous spaces continued to be sensitive to palpation. Passive segmental tests revealed improvement at L2-3 and L3-4 for mobility. Test grades of 2+ and 2+, respectively, were given to L2-3 and L3-4 after the second treatment session.

—Neurologic Findings

Nerve root tension signs were still present based on straight leg raise testing.

A—Stage of condition was unsettled; nerve and tissue irritability were present. Lumbar biomechanical improvement at L2-3 and L3-4, but no appreciable difference in active movements. Muscle tone demonstrates protective guarding response.

P—Moist heat, muscle stimulation, and manual soft-tissue inhibition to the paraspinals, piriformis, and iliopsoas were effective in reducing the muscle tone so that joint manipulation could be effective. Joint manipulation for the purpose of mechanical correction of position and mobility is more effective and longer lasting when the soft-tissue environment in the involved region is normalized with respect to activity states.

Gentle forms of joint manipulation, such as stretch mobilizations, were utilized at L2-3 and L3-4 to increase range of motion. Sacral repositioning by the manual technique to restore biomechanical equilibrium at L5-S1 was also done. L5-S1 mobility, however, did not improve this week. In fact, sacral pressures were not tolerated well by BB—the technique caused an increase in left leg symptoms. The dural membrane system, because of its attachment to the posterior aspect of the sacrum and coccyx,[39] was stretched with posterior-anterior (P/A) pressures on the base of the sacrum. Increasing dural tension on an irritable dural membrane may explain the accentuation of pain felt by BB with P/A pressure to the base of the sacrum.

BB was instructed in supine Fowler's and semi-Fowler's rest positions to help reduce pain and expedite the healing process. Intradisk pressure studies provide supportive evidence for reduced disk pressures in the Fowler's and semi-Fowler's positions. BB, incidently, felt quite comfortable in these positions.

BB was also instructed in right side lying over a bolster that was placed under the right waist line. The patient is advised to flex the hips and knees so that the lumbar spine is flexed. The bolster is used to create right side bending of the lumbar spine. Positioning in this manner has been advocated by Paris[40] as a means to decompress the involved portion of the disk and open the intervertebral foramen. For BB, the left posterior lateral aspect of the disk is unloaded and the left intervertebral foramen opened as the spine is positioned in flexion and right side bending. The OPT is encouraged to maximize the decompression and opening at the intervertebral foramen at the involved level by palpation. BB found that positioning his back in this manner, a technique described as positional distraction by Paris,[40] was very helpful in reducing the pain in the left leg.

WEEK 2—THREE TREATMENTS

S— BB reported that the instructions given to him for rest positions were helpful in decreasing the pain. He also stated that an erect, supportive sitting posture was better than slouched, flexed sitting, but that prolonged sitting was uncomfortable. The left leg pain was worse this week, but BB did not report any increase in activity. The treatments provided temporary relief from pain. The pain relief between treatments was negligible.

O—Structure

The lateral shift remained and, before one treatment session, was noted to have increased slightly.

—Active Movements

Forward bending continued to be the most painful and restricted active motion. Right side bending range increased, especially in the mid-lumbar spine, as did backward bending. The OPT related this improvement in active movements to the improvement in segmental range at L2-3 and L3-4.

—Palpation

The tone in the lower-lumbar region and left piriformis responded favorably to soft-tissue inhibition and mobilization, but the effects were not long lasting.

—Segmental Mobility

Segmental range of motion at L2-3 and L3-4 continued to improve. A noted change at the right L5-S1 facet was palpated during segmental motion testing. The major restriction at the left L5-S1 facet was still apparent.

—Neurologic Findings

The results of straight leg raise testing indicated continued nerve root irritability. Manual muscle testing, however, did not reveal lower-extremity motor weakness.

A—Based on the symptoms and the continued presence of positive neurologic findings, the condition was still considered unsettled. An improvement in mid-lumbar mobility helped to establish and maintain biomechanical motion balance in the lumbar spine. The mobility at L5-S1 had also improved in the right facet joint, but the major restriction on the left remained. As a result, lumbosacral biomechanical stress distribution remained asymmetric.

P— The mechanical correction techniques were preceded by preparatory soft-tissue inhibition and mobilization procedures. The evaluator felt that the myofascial tone responded well to the soft-tissue mobilization techniques. Less time was required to inhibit the tone and obtain sufficient relaxation for joint mechanical stretching. The OPT was not encour-

TABLE 11-5. Manipulation Types

General	Specific
Indirect	Direct
Noncontact	Contact
Cyclic Loading	Sustained Loading
Non-Thrust	Thrust
Graded Oscillation—1–4	Surgical
Progressive Stretch	General
Continuous Stretch	Specific
Muscle Energy Technique	High Velocity
Functional Technique	Overpressure
Counterstrain	Locking
Distraction Types	
Mechanical	
Positional	
Manual	
Inhibitory	
Oscillatory	
Progressive	
Continuous	

aged by the limited carryover of change in myofascial tone between treatments.

An example of the types of decision-making processes that the OPT undergoes when working with a patient such as BB now follows. The first decision the OPT faces is in choosing an appropriate technique. Many medical practitioners and physical therapists are unaware of the numerous types of manipulative procedures. A brief list of the various manipulative techniques is given in Table 11-5. A basic understanding of the operational definitions for each manipulative technique is necessary. The OPT must choose the most appropriate manipulative technique for the problem, mechanical dysfunction, and stage of the condition. In the case of BB, the OPT chose a stretch mobilization maneuver, which is a non-thrust procedure involving a slow, gradual, continuous pressure performed within the patient's pain tolerance. The rationale for choosing a stretch mobilization technique for BB is related to the fact that the evaluator can continually monitor tissue response. Slow, gradual, continuous pressures allow for instantaneous sensory feedback from the patient's tissues. BB tolerated the stretch mobilizations to L2-3 and L3-4 well. No signs of protective muscle guarding or reflex muscle contractions were present during the application of the technique to L2-3 and L3-4.

The criteria for effective manipulation are listed in Table 11-6. The direction of motion during performance of a manipulation is one factor that needs to be considered. Manipulations can be performed into the direction of the motion restitution (direct technique) or away from the motion restitution (indirect technique). In the direct technique, if the motion restriction is right side bending, the manipulation is performed in right side bending. For the indirect technique, the manipulation is done in a direction other than right side bending; that is, left side bending. Direct techniques are more likely to produce immediate adverse reactions, such as a temporary increase in pain. Indirect techniques are often necessary before direct techniques can be effec-

TABLE 11-6. Criteria for Manipulation Technique

Appropriate choice of technique
Rationale for chosen technique
Appropriate sequencing of techniques
Appropriate adjustments of technique
Appropriate time length
Evaluation of effect of technique
Technique criteria
Patient position
Therapist position
Specificity of locking
Hand placement
Recruitment of tissue (force velocity or development)
Sensitivity to tissue response
Force direction
Force control
Amount of force
Force amplitude

tive. The risk of adverse reactions with indirect techniques is less than with direct techniques. The stretch mobilization techniques used by the OPT on BB were direct. The OPT decided that a direct technique would be tolerated by BB and would produce the quickest biomechanical improvement. BB did, indeed, tolerate the direct technique well. Improvement in segmental movement at L2-3 and L3-4 occurred within five treatment sessions.

The sequencing of manipulative therapeutic techniques is another concern of the OPT. Due to the possible disk involvement at L5-S1, the OPT initially decided not to use rotary manipulation techniques because of the potential increase in torsional force on the intervertebral disks. Instead, side bending stretch mobilizations were performed first. Also note that in the treatment plan, the OPT preceded mechanical manipulation with soft-tissue inhibition and mobilization. The effects of gentle forms of joint manipulation are enhanced whenever the soft-tissue tension in the surrounding environment is reduced. Joint excursion is, in part, determined by periarticular soft-tissue structures and muscle tone. Joint manipulation without adequate preparation of the myofascial tissues is not likely to result in permanent change.

The OPT must be able to appropriately adjust a technique when necessary. The patient's reaction to a manipulation must be assessed by the OPT. The OPT evaluates a patient's response by observation of facial expression, inspection of body parts for tension, and by palpation of tissue tone. Adjustment in technique can be made in many ways. The OPT can adjust patient position, hand placement, the direction of force application, the force amplitude, and the amount, velocity, and development of force.

A technique may not be tolerated because of position. Some patients cannot tolerate a prone position because of inadequate backward bending. Prone techniques, therefore, may not be desirable until an increase in backward bending has been achieved.

Often, the involved spinal levels are sensitive to palpation. Noncontact manipulation techniques are therefore necessary to avoid pressure on tender tissue or bone structures. If a contact technique is used, the OPT must learn how to dissipate manipulation pressure. Force development and control are essential elements in force dissipation. BB tolerated contact techniques without difficulty.

The amount of force is largely determined by the type of problem, the stage of the condition, and the manipulative style of the OPT. In general, the greater the force used, the greater the chance for an adverse reaction. One philosophy concerning force amount is best expressed by the following saying: "Use as much force as is required, but as little as necessary." The above philosophic approach to manipulative management contends that the body is able to tolerate and adjust to slowly applied gentle forces better than quickly applied strong forces. A natural, safe, physiologic tissue change will therefore occur. The possibility of discogenic involvement in BB caused the OPT to choose the conservative, gentle form of manipulation. In terms of biomechanical change in tissue length, the OPT must be able to sense when the plastic portion of the length tension curve of a biologic tissue has been obtained during a stretch manipulation. This sort of sensory discrimination ensures an effective treatment result and safeguards against creating tissue failure or permanent weakening.

The length of time necessary to obtain an effective result is variable. In general, if the OPT does not sense a favorable response to a specific joint manipulation technique within 2 to 3 minutes, then a different technique should be attempted. To gain optimal soft-tissue and joint function may require anywhere from 10 to 45 minutes of treatment during a session. A 50 percent change in function is considered a significant change. Full restoration of function is not recommended during one treatment session for the chronic low back problem because of the possibility of an adverse reaction.

A summary of the types of considerations an OPT faces when working with the spinal orthopaedic musculoskeletal problem has been provided. The decision-making skills of the OPT are an important aspect of clinical maturity and effectiveness. Appropriate management is dependent on the exercise of excellent clinical judgment.

WEEK 3

S— The treatments continued to offer temporary relief from pain, but no significant pain relief was noticed between treatments. Postural instruction and advice for sitting and resting continued to be beneficial. The pain intensity in the left leg was relatively unaltered.

O—Structure

An improvement in the lateral shift was noticed. Correction of the lateral shift was made easier by working in the hands-and-knees position. The resistance of the spine to shift correction was considerably less in this position. The lumbar spine returned and remained in the midsagittal position this week.

—Active Movements

Lumbar backward bending was also enhanced in the hands-and-knees position. BB's range of motion in lumbar extension increased by 50 percent once the OPT began working the patient in the all-four position. The all-four position is decompressive, so the spine can move more easily. The all-four position also permits motion in all directions. Thus, spinal range of motion can be improved. Active lumbar motion tests demonstrated an increase in extension. The joint manipulation efforts at L2-3 and L3-4 continued to be beneficial in improving and maintaining mid-lumbar mobility.

—Palpation

The myofascial tone in the lower lumbar paraspinals and left piriformis continued to respond to soft-tissue mobilization. In fact, a greater carryover occurred between sessions.

—Segmental Mobility

Segmental mobility at the left L5-S1 facet remained the major obstacle to establishing regional mechanical balance. Attempts to mobilize the sacrum on L-5 were not tolerated. The L2-3 and L3-4 segmental levels, however, were now within normal range of motion limits.

—Neurologic Findings

Straight leg raising remained limited to 33 degrees because of pain in the left thigh.

A—S-1 nerve irritation continued. With the exception of L5-S1, biomechanical improvement was made at all involved levels. The OPT should note that biomechanical changes do not always result in immediate symptomatic improvement. In the case of BB, significant impairment to nerve conduction at the left S-1 nerve root persisted despite a demonstrable mechanical improvement. The use of the all-four position provided a breakthrough in normalizing mechanical function and in correcting the lateral shift.

P—After consultation with the physiatrist, a plan was initiated to attempt a facet injection at the left L5-S1 joint. The injection solution consisted of Marcaine and Depo-Medrol (a local anesthetic and a steroid). The rationale for this effort was to desensitize the facet capsule and reduce any swelling or fluid congestion that possibly could be causing nerve root irritation. The OPT should be reminded of the superior position of the lumbar nerve roots within the intervertebral foramen and their close relationship with the posterior aspect of the facet joints.

Unfortunately, BB did not have a pleasant experience with this injection technique. The leg symptoms were exacerbated for 2 days after the injection. The reaction confirmed the belief that the left L5-S1 facet was involved. The results of joint manipulation are often improved after steroid injection because of the softening effect the steroid has on periarticular tissues. The OPT therefore planned a series of manipulative techniques to the left L5-S1 facet post-injection in an attempt to improve range. In addition, the patient was instructed in reverse pelvic tilting (anterior pelvic tilting) in the all-four position to facilitate lumbar backward bending range.

WEEK 4—THREE SESSIONS

S— As mentioned, the injection seemed to have irritated the condition. BB experienced an increase in symptoms during the early part of the week. The symptoms were gradually reduced by the end of the week and, in fact, seemed to become more localized. BB stated that the pain in the left posterior thigh had decreased. The pain now seemed focused in the left buttock.

O—Structure

No evidence of a lateral shift this week. A slight return of the lower-lumbar lordosis was observed. This observation was encouraging because it possibly indicated that the extension exercises were having a positive effect.

—Active Movements

Forward bending was restricted and painful. Less deviation to the left was noted during forward bending, but the motion range and control were still abnormal.

—Palpation

An increase in myofascial activity was noted after the injection, which perhaps interfered with the manipulation attempts early in the week.

—Segmental Mobility

The movement at L5-S1 improved at the end of the week, particularly on the left side. Sacral pressure was tolerated for the first time. The evaluator was encouraged by what appeared to be a minor joint release at the left L5-S1 facet.

—Neurologic Findings

Straight leg raising improved at the end of the week. Buttock pain developed at 50 degrees of straight leg raising, as compared with the previous posterior thigh pain at 35 degrees.

A—The condition at this stage was settling. Nerve root irritation was less intense; and for the first time, L5-S1 appeared to be normal for functional mobility. The difficulty one has in analyzing the effects of treatment is due to the multiplicity of effects from the treatment procedures. For example, is the facet injection alone responsible for the improvement noted at the end of the week? Did the facet injection just aggravate the condition? Were the manipulation techniques responsible for the reduction in pain noted? If so, which manipulation technique provided the best result? Was the combined injection and manipulation approach effective, or was perhaps just time (45 days at this point) responsible for the improvement? These questions cannot be fully explained in the case of BB. Nonetheless, problem and solution analyses such as these are important. The OPT should endeavor to use a scientific inquiry approach so that improved understanding of the problem confronting the examiner is possible.

P—The plan was to continue working on mechanical correction of L5-S1 until the left facet has full mobility restored. The all-four extension exercises have been effective and therefore have been encouraged by the OPT through administration of a home program.

WEEKS 5 TO 8

S—BB progressed slowly but gradually from the fifth to the eighth weeks. The pain gradually subsided and became less intense and more focused to the left lower lumbar region and left buttock. A few minor episodes occurred during this period, but each time the pain went away within 2 days. BB reported that he was sleeping better, sitting for longer periods without pain, and tolerating more activity. The pain still seemed to increase slightly at the end of the day.

O—The most dramatic change during this period occurred at the L5-S1 level. Sacral position and mobility were restored and seemed to have a favorable biomechanical impact at the lumbosacral junction. L-5 was manipulated on S-1 with left rotation, forward bending, and right side bending stretch techniques. Active range of motion of the lumbar spine increased in all planes, especially in forward bending. Straight leg raising on the left side was tolerated at 65 degrees. Then hamstring tightness developed.

A—The condition during this time period had definitely settled. Minor setbacks occurred but were tolerated well. Recovery took only 2 days. Objective improvement in active range, myofascial tone, segmental mobility, and straight leg raising were apparent.

P— A full program of exercises was initiated to maintain function and prevent reinjury. Education in self-reliance is perhaps the most important aspect of managing the spinal orthopaedic related dysfunction. Without adequate knowledge of the problem and without a home program of proper spinal posture and exercise, the patient is susceptible to reinjury. Reoccurrence is a major problem in the orthopaedic handling of a back condition. The severity of symptoms and the mechanical problems usually became worse with each reinjury. Most back conditions have a self-limiting nature. The problems tend to go away with time alone. So regardless of which method of corrective intervention is chosen, the condition, in most cases, will get better in time. The major problem, however, is reoccurrence. Thus, it behooves the OPT to instruct the patient in spinal anatomy, mechanics, proper rest positions, postures for sitting, use of correct chair designs, exercise, body mechanics with lifting, daily functional activities, and in sports endeavors. BB's exercise program consisted of:

1. all-four flexion-extension
2. side lying gentle rotation
3. supine—hooklying—knee drop to floor and return
4. supine—knees to chest
5. hamstring stretching
6. calf stretching
7. axial distraction of head and neck.

All exercises were done three times a day, with 10 to 12 repetitions per session. BB was encouraged in short walking activities and in swimming. He was advised not to play racquetball. Pacing of weekend activities was recommended. Short rest periods were encouraged to allow the low back to relax. Non-weight-bearing positions were suggested during the rest times.

BB was seen on a follow-up basis three times the following year and was doing well. He seemed satisfied with his present condition, and the appointment session was used for re-evaluation purposes, minor mechanical adjustment, and home program review and revision.

FOLLOW-UP—1 YEAR

S— Following the third month of treatment, BB was relatively pain free. On a 0 to 10 pain scale (10 being the severest pain), BB identified his pain level as ranging from 1 to 3. He reported returning to almost all of his daily, routine functional activities, such as gardening, swimming, and racquetball. Occasionally, after prolonged, heavy–labor type activities, BB would feel stiff and sore the following morning. The stiffness and soreness eventually subsided during the day as activity increased. Overall, no major symptoms occurred for a 12-month period.

O—BB returned for re-evaluation and monitoring purposes on several occasions during the year.

—Structure

Spinal alignment was within normal limits. No evidence of lateral shift.

—Active Movements

Within normal limits in all planes. Forward bending especially improved in terms of range of motion, direction of motion, and movement control. No signs of instability were observed.

—Palpation

Muscle tone varied on each occasion; an accentuation in tone was palpated during two sessions. Prior to each session, BB was involved in some heavy work that required bending and lifting. Passive segmental testing revealed a normalization of L5-S1 mobility and improvement in motion in the upper-lumbar segments.

—Neurologic Findings

No signs of nerve irritation with dural stretch or straight leg raise tests. Normal muscle strength returned in extensor hallucis longus and flexor hallucis longus of the left foot.

A—The condition was stabilized. Mechanical function in the lumbar spine was significantly improved for position, motion, and overall function. Some precautions were necessary in avoiding prolonged work activities that require bending, lifting, or sitting.

P— Patient was encouraged to continue with self-mobilization exercises. Patient was reminded to maintain proper spinal posture when standing and sitting, and was cautioned with regard to strenuous lifting, repeated bending, and prolonged sitting and semi-flexed positions. Monitor condition on an as-needed basis.

FOLLOW-UP—18 MONTHS

S— BB returned to the Atlanta Back Clinic with severe left posterior thigh and leg pain after having worked in his backyard the previous day raking leaves. The symptoms were quite intense (rated 9 on the 0 to 10 pain scale) and were *not* appreciably reduced in non–weight-bearing lying positions. BB was having difficulty sleeping at night because of the pain.

O—Structure

A significant right lateral shift was present. The lumbar lordosis was relatively flat, and the trunk was inclined forward.

—Active Movements

They were significantly reduced in all directions due to pain. Forward bending resulted in an immediate discomfort in the posterior left thigh. The lateral shift was extremely resistant to correction in the standing position.

—Palpation

The temperature of the lumbosacral area was elevated. The lumbar paraspinals were in muscle spasm, as were the left piriformis and left quadratus lumborum. The hyperactive musculature did not readily change activity states with changes in position. Passive segmental testing of the lumbar spine demonstrated a considerable limitation in motion at L5-S1 and generalized restrictions in the upper-lumbar segments.

—Neurologic Findings

SLR testing elicited pain in the left-lower extremity upon 30 degrees of elevation of either leg, indicating signs of nerve irritation.

A—BB had suffered a major episode of low back pain and sciatica. The chronic condition had become, for the time being, acute. BB was not comfortable, and lying positions did not afford significant relief.

P— An orthopaedic medical consultation was required to evaluate the need for further diagnostic testing and to determine if medication for pain would be necessary. Correct the lateral shift condition and restore normal spinal mechanics. Utilize therapeutic modalities such as ice, muscle stimulation, and TENS to reduce muscle spasm and decrease pain.

WEEK 2

S— BB's subjective report of pain did not appreciably change during 2 weeks of orthopaedic physical therapy. The left posterior–lower extremity pain continued. The pain intensity began to subside in non–weight-bearing positions but did not substantially change in upright positions. Bending to put on shoes and pants was extremely difficult.

O—Structure

The lateral shift was eventually corrected during the second week of treatment. The hands-and-knees position was the easiest position in which to make the lateral shift correction. Prolonged upright positions resulted in reappearance of the lateral shift within 2 minutes. The lumbar curve returned within 5 days. This allowed BB to obtain a more vertical, upright position.

—Active Movements

Forward bending remained considerably restricted due to pain in the left posterior thigh and leg. BB's ability to move his lumbar spine in the all-four position improved. Side bending and backward bending movements increased in range and became less painful. Spinal movements from the standing upright position were still significantly restricted.

—Palpation

The motion at L5-S1 did not change during the 2-week period of treatment with the use of specific joint and soft-tissue manipulation techniques.

—Neurologic Findings

Remained positive.

A—Condition remained acute. A neurologic and orthopaedic consult was arranged at the University Hospital. No appreciable gains were made with physical therapy intervention except for greater comfort while sleeping.

P— Provide temporary pain relief. Monitor condition and prevent further symptoms. See patient on an as-needed basis.

WEEK 3

S— BB was hospitalized for bed rest and further diagnostic tests. After 10 days of enforced bed rest and immobilization, BB felt better. The pain radiation extending into the left lower extremity was significantly less in terms of frequency and intensity.

O—CAT scan demonstrated evidence of a large disk protrusion at L5-S1 just left of the midline. Disk-space narrowing and posterior joint degenerative changes at the same level were also noticed. Thus, the CAT scan findings provided support and further documentation of the clinical findings and radiographic report.

A—Surgeons discussed the various options, which are listed below, with BB:

1. Continue bed rest, immobilization, and restricted activity.
2. Perform a diskogram to determine if chymopapain injection is a possible choice.
3. Prepare BB for lumbar surgery. The two procedures discussed were as follows:
   A. L5-S1 disk excision and foraminotomy (posterior-lateral approach).
   B. L5-S1 disk excision and foraminotomy (posterior laminotomy approach).

The surgeons discussed the possible choices with BB and allowed BB to decide which option to take.

P— BB discussed the situation with the OPT. After a day of deliberation, BB decided to avoid surgery for the time being, recognizing that surgery is a real possibility at some time in the future. BB also decided to learn more about chemonucleolysis and, as a result, did his own literature review on the subject. BB also wished to return for further physical therapy. The OPT agreed to continue with treatment and obtained verbal consent from the orthopaedist to treat accordingly.

2 MONTHS LATER

S— BB had minimal symptoms. The pain radiation extending into the left lower extremity had been eliminated during 2 months of treatment. BB occasionally would feel some left buttock discomfort with associated muscle tension, especially after prolonged sitting or semi-flexed functional activity.

O—Structure

Lateral shift corrected. Lumbar anterior curve returned.

—Active Movements

All lumbar spinal motions except for backward bending were within normal limits. Backward bending was still noticeably more restricted than the other spinal motions, with the most notable limitations being in the upper-lumbar spine. Pain was *not* a factor in any of the lumbar movements.

—Palpation

Occasional evidence of increased muscle activity in the left piriformis, which was usually associated with an increase in physical activity or prolonged sitting. Lumbar segmental mobility at L5-S1 improved to a grade 3— (refer to Fig. 11-5) when tested on two separate sessions. On the average, L5-S1 graded 2+ and 2, indicating that total correction would probably not be attainable. The OPT is to note that late-stage degenerative segmental conditions will most likely restrict motion at the involved level.

—Neurologic Findings

No clinical evidence of nerve irritation during straight leg raise and dural stretch tests. Muscle strength of the extensor hallucis longus and flexor hallucis longus of the left foot had not fully returned to normal.

A—BB was satisfied with the progress he had made while in the hospital and following his hospitalization. BB was warned by the OPT that despite the symptoms being almost negligible, a fair amount of repairing and healing was still occurring. Patients and therapists often mistake recovery, healing, and spinal health as being synonymous with pain relief. Provided that BB does not reinjure himself, complete healing with scar formation may take up to 3 years. The OPT was also satisfied with the improvement made by BB, but cautioned BB against returning to normal functional everyday duties that require bending, lifting, twisting, or prolonged sitting. The condition can be labeled at this time as settled.

P—BB is to be monitored on an as-needed basis. The OPT recommended that BB be seen in 6 months to check on BB's home program, activity status, spinal alignment and mechanics, and pain level.

SUMMARY

A case study of a patient with chronic low back pain and sciatica was presented. The evaluation methodology was reviewed, and a correlative analysis of the evaluative data was discussed. Evaluative judgments were made and rationale given to support the various contentions. Scientific evidence was provided, whenever possible, to justify the decisions made. The role of the OPT in the clinical examination of a chronic low back pain patient was identified. The clinical skills and knowledge level of the OPT were also discussed to provide insight into the requirements necessary to do an adequate job.

The management of BB was outlined in SOAP progress report form. The criteria for manipulation and the decision-making process that accompanies manipulation were presented. A multiple-treatment approach was utilized, and the integration of techniques was analyzed. Many ways of managing a condition such as BB's could be used. The method chosen by one OPT was identified, and the rationale for the techniques employed was offered.

Overall, the case study has attempted to demonstrate and discuss the complexities of evaluating and treating the chronic low back pain patient. Unfortunately, no easy solution was provided. Difficult problems require a high level of expertise and sensitivity for effective management. The case study of BB is an example of how the OPT must strive to maintain a high level of clinical competence to remain an effective health care provider. The challenge presented and the information provided hopefully will assist in leading us, as physical therapists, toward excellence in clinical practice.

REFERENCES

1. Sternbach, R: *Psychological aspects of pain and the selection of patients.* Clin Neurosurg 21:323–333, 1974.
2. Melzack, R: *The McGill Pain Questionnaire: Major properties and scoring methods.* Pain 1:277–299, 1975.
3. Wycke, B: *The neurology of low back pain.* In Jayson, M (ed): *The Lumbar Spine and Back Pain.* Pitman Publishing, Marshfield, Mass, 1976, pp 265–339.
4. Kellgren, JH: *On the distribution of pain arising from deep somatic structures with charts of segmental pain areas.* Clin Sci 4:35–46, 1939.
5. Mooney, V and Robertson, J: *The facet syndrome.* Clin Orthop 115:149–156, 1976.
6. McCall, I, Park, W, and O'Brien, J: *Induced pain referral from the posterior lumbar elements in normal subjects.* Spine 4(5):441–446, 1979.
7. Melzack, R: *The Puzzle of Pain.* Basic Books, New York, 1973.
8. Hoppenfeld, S: *Physical Examination of the Spine and Extremities.* Appleton-Century-Crofts, New York, 1976.
9. McKenzie, R: *The Lumbar Spine: Mechanical Diagnosis and Therapy.* Spinal Publications Limited, Waikanae, New Zealand, 1981.
10. Kirkaldy-Willis, WH and Hill, RJ: *A more precise diagnosis for low back pain.* Spine 4(2):102–109, 1979.
11. Nachemson, A and Morris, JM: *In vivo measurements of intradiscal pressure: Discometry, a method for the determination of pressure in the lower lumbar discs.* J Bone Joint Surg 46A:1077, 1964.
12. Fry, J: *Back Pain and Soft Tissue Rheumatism.* Advisory Services Collequium Proc. (Advisory Services (Clinical and General) LLD, London), 1972.
13. Bries, A and Troup, JOG: *Biomechanical considerations in the straight leg raising test: cadaveric and clinical studies of the effects of medial hip rotation.* Spine 4(3):242–250, 1979.
14. Schultz, AB, et al: *Mechanical properties of human lumbar spine motion segments. I. Responses in flexion, extension, lateral bending and torsion.* J Biomech Eng 101:46–52, 1979.
15. Fahrni, W: *Conservative treatment of lumbar disc degeneration: Our primary responsibility.* Orthop Clin North Am 6(1):93–103, 1975.
16. Troup, JDG: *Driver's back pain and its prevention: A review of the postural, vibratory and muscular factors, together with the problem of transmitted road shock.* Ergonomics 9:207–214, 1978.
17. Hix, EL: *Viscerovisceral and Somatovisceral Reflex Communication.* The Physiologic Basis of Osteopathic Medicine, Postgraduate Institute of Osteopathic Medicine and Surgery, 1970.
18. Koizumi, K: *Autonomic system reactions caused by excitation of somatic afferents: A study of cutaneo-intestinal reflex.* In Korr, I (ed): *Neurobiologic Mechanisms of Manipulative Therapy.* Plenum Press, New York, 1978, pp 219–227.
19. Cyriax, J: *Textbook of Orthopaedic Medicine,* Vol 1, *Diagnosis of Soft Tissue Lesions.* Williams & Wilkins, Baltimore, 1975.
20. Mooney, V: *The Role of Spine Fusion: Question 7.* Spine 6(3):304–305, 1981.
21. Mennell, J: *Back Pain.* Little, Brown & Co, Boston, 1960.
22. Goldthwaitt, JE, et al: *Body Mechanics in the Study and Treatment of Disease.* JB Lippincott, Philadelphia, 1934.
23. *Les Attitudes Antalgiques Dans La Sciatique Discoradiculaire Commune. Etude Cunique Et Radiologique-Interpretation Pathogenique.* Sem Hop Paris, Desezé, 31:2291, 1955.
24. Stoddard, A: *Manual of Osteopathic Practice.* Hutchinson Medical Publications, London, 1959.
25. DePalma, AF and Rothman, R: *The Intervertebral Disc.* WB Saunders, Philadelphia, 1970.
26. Brown, HA and Pont, MA: *Disease of lumbar discs: Ten years of surgical treatment.* J Neurosurg 20:410–417, 1963.
27. Goodard, MD and Reid, JD: *Movements induced by straight leg raising in the lumbo-sacral roots, nerves and plexus, and in the intrapelvic section of the sciatic nerve.* J Neurol Neurosurg Psychiatry 28:12–17, 1965.
28. Janda, V: *Muscles, central nervous motor regulation and back problems.* In Korr, I (ed): *Neurobiologic Mechanisms of Manipulative Therapy.* Plenum Press, New York, 1978, pp 27–41.
29. Kendall, F and Kendall, H: *Muscle Testing with Function,* ed 2. Williams & Wilkins, Baltimore, 1971.
30. Korr, I: *Symposium on the functional implications of segmental facilitation. I. The concept of facilitation and its origins.* Journal of the American Osteopathic Association 54(5):265–268, 1955.

31. FARFAN, HF: *Mechanical Disorders of the Low Back.* Lea & Febiger, Philadelphia, 1973.
32. BRAILSFORD, JF: *Deformities of the lumbosacral region of the spine.* Br J Surg 16:562, 1929.
33. GONNELLA, C, PARIS, S, AND KUTNER, M: *Reliability in evaluating passive intervertebral motion.* Phys Ther 62(4):436–444, 1982.
34. FRONING, EC AND FROHMAN, B: *Motion of the lumbosacral spine after laminectomy and spine fusion: Correlation of motion with the result.* J Bone Joint Surg 50-A:896, 1968.
35. TANZ, S: *Motion of the lumbar spine: A roentgenologic study.* American Journal of Roentgenology 69(3):399–412, 1953.
36. NACHEMSON, A, SCHULTZ, A, AND BERKSON, M: *Mechanical properties of human lumbar spine motion segments: Influences of age, sex, disc level and degeneration.* Spine 4(1):1–8, 1979.
37. ANDERSSON, G, ET AL: *Roentgenographic measurement of lumbar intervertebral disc height.* Spine 6(2):154–158, 1981.
38. KNUTSSON, F: *The instability associated with disk degeneration in the lumbar spine.* Acta Radiol 25:593–609, 1944.
39. WILLIAMS AND WARWICK: *Gray's Anatomy,* 36th British Edition. WB Saunders, Philadelphia, 1980.
40. PARIS, S: *Mobilization of the spine.* Phys Ther 59(8):988–995, 1979.

Chapter 12

CLINICAL DECISION MAKING: MANAGEMENT OF THE NEONATE WITH MOVEMENT DYSFUNCTION

SUZANN K. CAMPBELL, Ph.D., L.P.T.

The development of a physical therapy program for neonates involves a number of decisions regarding the selection of appropriate clients. These decisions include: (1) whom to evaluate, (2) with which assessment tools, (3) criteria for initiating treatment, and (4) identification of appropriate goals for newborn treatment.

When attempting to identify children who will later have handicaps, an important question is where to start—what population will form the base from which to establish a group at high risk for developing central nervous system (CNS) dysfunction? If one starts with 58,000 pregnancies sampled from the general population, as the Collaborative Perinatal Project[1] did, one finds that about half of the 128 survivors with cerebral palsy were never at high risk during the antepartum, intrapartum, or neonatal periods and would thus escape detection or attention in any preventive program. On the other hand, it is also important to note that many, many so-called high-risk infants will turn out to be perfectly normal. In fact, most of the large-scale studies of outcome morbidity in high-risk infants show very low incidences of serious dysfunction and, furthermore, demonstrate that specific risk factors are not adequate predictors of who will be normal and who will be abnormal.[1]

The literature on outcome prediction has been discouraging to those wishing to perform early identification and diagnosis of neuromotor dysfunction. Nonetheless, investigators have continued to search for the formula for predicting long-term morbidity. The focus of recent research on long-term outcome has been on two particular types of infants: the very low birthweight ($\leq$ 1000 grams) infant with asphyxia and/or intracranial hemorrhage, and the full-term asphyxiated infant—two groups that continue to have both high mortality and large proportions of handicapped survivors.

THE VERY LOW BIRTHWEIGHT INFANT

The incidence of handicaps in very low birthweight survivors has been studied extensively during the past 40 to 50 years. A relatively low incidence of major neurologic complications (4 percent to 15 percent) was reported in the period from the early 1920s through the 1940s. In this period, however, mortality was high, and neonatal management was not aggressive.[2] The survivors, therefore, were undoubtedly a select, vigorous group with few iatrogenic problems. The incidence of significant handicaps increased during the 1950s and 1960s, before the establishment of more modern perinatal care systems and coincident with the time during which oxygen concentrations were kept low to avoid retrolental fibroplasia and when delayed initial feeding was routine. The incidence of permanent handicaps decreased during the late 1960s and 1970s, so that in recent reports, the rates of neurologic, intellectual, and developmental handicaps averaged well under 20 percent.[3]

Still, specific groups of very low birthweight infants appear to have higher risk for permanent handicaps when compared with their cohorts. These include infants with clinical evidence of birth asphyxia, intracranial hemorrhage, severe respiratory failure, and, perhaps, those who are both very premature and who have a head size small for gestational age.[2,4,5] Those at highest risk for defects of the CNS are the very premature babies with significant intraventricular or periventricular bleeding. As a result of advances in neonatal care in recent years, however, asphyxiated preterm infants in high-technology intensive care settings have the same chance for intact survival as asphyxiated full-term infants.[5]

THE ASPHYXIATED FULL-TERM INFANT

The incidence of major neurologic and intellectual handicaps in the survivors of perinatal asphyxia is relatively low in recent studies; but it is also quite variable, ranging from as low as 1.8 percent up to a high of about 28 percent.[2] In the asphyxiated full-term infant, several CNS-related clinical findings seem related to the severity of the insult and, possibly, to the ultimate prognosis; antepartum and intrapartum variables are relatively unrelated to both mortality and morbidity.[5-7] Hypotonia lasting for over 5 days of life, or changing to extensor hypertonia within the first 24 hours, Apgar scores of 0 to 3 at 5 minutes, early or constant seizures, delay of more than 1 minute in onset of spontaneous respiration at birth, abnormal levels of consciousness, and a suppressed electroencephalogram are associated with the likelihood of cerebral damage.

NEUROPATHOLOGY AND PATHOKINESIOLOGY OF CNS DYSFUNCTION

Perinatal hypoxic-ischemic brain injury is an important cause of cerebral palsy. It is defined as asphyxia followed by abnormal neonatal behavior, including movement dysfunction.[8] The main causes of hypoxemia in the perinatal period are as follows: (1) intrauterine asphyxia with respiratory failure at the time of birth, (2) postnatal respiratory insufficiency secondary

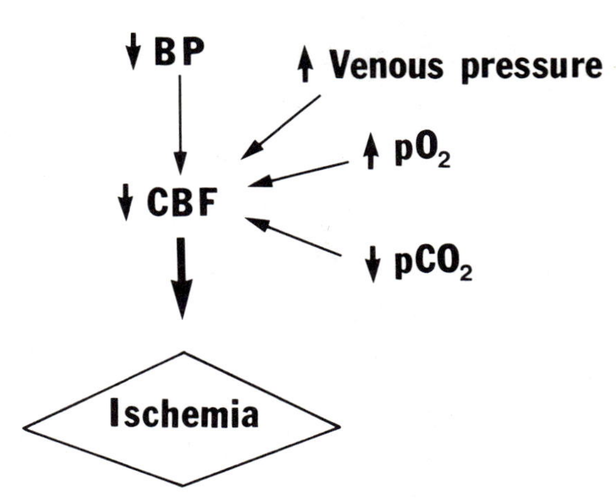

FIGURE 12-1. Model for the production of cerebral ischemia after Pape and Wigglesworth.[4] Decreased blood pressure (BP) is thought to lead to decreased cerebral blood flow (CBF) and ischemia. If respiratory distress and its management cause an increase in venous pressure or PO_2, or decreased PCO_2, these events will contribute to decreasing CBF.

to severe hyaline membrane disease with recurrent apnea, and (3) severe right-to-left shunting secondary to cardiovascular disease or persistent fetal circulation.[8] The main causes of cerebral ischemia are as follows: (1) intrauterine asphyxia with cardiac insufficiency, or (2) postnatal cardiac insufficiency secondary to congenital heart disease or recurrent apnea.[8] Clinically important hypoxemia and ischemia typically occur together, with one or the other mechanism predominating.

A model for the production of brain ischemia from the work of Pape and Wigglesworth[4] is presented in Figure 12-1. The major precipitating event is thought to be a drastic decrease in blood pressure resulting in decreased cerebral blood flow and ischemia. Following significant ischemia affecting brain tissues, typical clinical features include coma, seizures, apnea, hypotonia, and feeding difficulties. Proximal muscle weakness is usual in full-term newborns; while premature infants demonstrate primarily lower-extremity muscle weakness.[8]

Five types of neuropathology are recognized as typical outcomes.[8] They include: (1) selective neuronal necrosis, (2) status marmoratus, (3) parasagittal cerebral necrosis, (4) periventricular leukomalacia, and (5) focal ischemic brain injury.

Selective neuronal necrosis has a characteristic distribution, including the cerebral cortex, cerebellar cortex, thalamus, and brain stem. Damage to the latter area is frequently reflected in poor sucking and swallowing, which is presumed to be due to lesions of the cranial nerve nuclei involved in those functions. The long-term sequelae of selective neuronal necrosis types of lesions include mental retardation, seizures, hypertonic motor dysfunction, and bulbar deficits.

Status marmoratus is a condition resulting in damage to the basal ganglia. No specific behavioral correlates have been identified during the newborn period. The long-term outcomes include choreoathetosis and rigidity.

Parasagittal cerebral necrosis is necrotic white matter in the parasagittal areas of the cerebral convexities, typically coinciding with the boundary zone

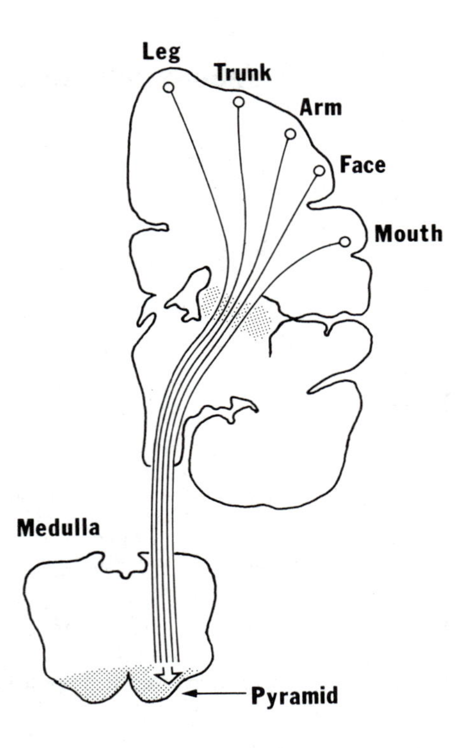

FIGURE 12-2. Typical lesion affecting descending motor pathways to lower-extremity muscles from periventricular leukomalacia.

areas between cerebral artery distributions. The typical neonatal picture is of weakness of proximal extremity musculature, which is more pronounced in the upper extremities than in the lower.

Periventricular leukomalacia is the typical lesion of the preterm brain.[4] It consists of necrosis of periventricular white matter in a distribution that affects the descending motor pathways from the cerebral cortex to the motoneurons of the lower-extremity musculature (Fig. 12-2). Thus, the principal long-term neurologic outcome is spastic diplegia with relative sparing of intellectual function. Visual-perceptual and language deficits are common, however, because of damage to other pathways in the internal capsule subserving these functions.

Focal ischemic brain injury is more typical of the full-term infant than of the preterm infant and is often associated with cardiovascular instability resulting in cerebral artery obstructions. The long-term deficits include psychomotor retardation if many lesions are present, or spastic hemiplegia in the case of more limited focal lesions.

In addition to hypoxic-ischemic lesions caused by birth asphyxia, the preterm infant is especially susceptible to intracranial hemorrhages. The primary types of intracranial hemorrhage in the newborn are subdural, primary subarachnoid, intracerebellar, and periventricular/intraventricular (PVH/IVH).[4,8] PVH/IVH is the most common type and accounts for a large percentage of mortality and morbidity in neonatal intensive care units. Ap-

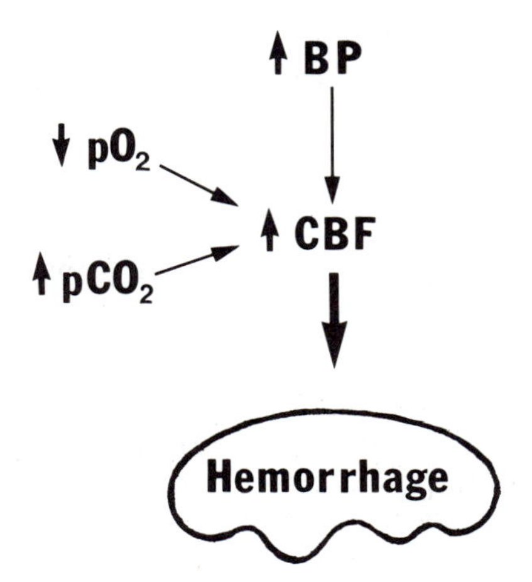

FIGURE 12-3. Model for the production of periventricular/intraventricular hemorrhage after Pape and Wigglesworth.[4] Increased blood pressure (BP), decreased Po_2, and increased Pco_2 lead to increased cerebral blood flow (CBF) resulting in hemorrhage.

proximately 80 percent of PVH/IVHs originate in the subependymal germinal matrix, the source of cerebral neurons and glia; IVH results when the initial bleeding extends into the ventricular system. The main correlate of PVH/IVH, in addition to prematurity, is the presence of a hypoxic-ischemic event such as perinatal asphyxia or severe respiratory distress syndrome.

Pape and Wigglesworth[4] presented a model for the production of PVH/IVH that postulates that the precipitating condition is an increase in blood pressure that along with the presence of decreased Po_2 and increased carbon dioxide retention, leads to increased cerebral blood flow and hemorrhage into the subependymal germinal matrix (Fig. 12-3). The clinical course may include catastrophic deterioration or a more saltatory course resulting from a series of small lesions.[8]

The typical lesions in the brain include (1) destruction of periventricular white matter, (2) destruction of germinal matrix, and (3) post-hemorrhagic hydrocephalus.[8]

RATIONALE FOR TREATMENT OF NEONATES[9]

Psychologists and a few nurses have studied the impact of early supplemental stimulation on growth and development, weight gain, visual responsiveness, and other sensorimotor functions. Some of these results were only short term, but several researchers have been able to demonstrate effects at 1 year of age, especially if intervention extended beyond the neonatal period. Despite suggesting an overall positive influence of intervention, considerable work remains to be done in order to clarify the details regarding how and why intervention works, with whom, and on which aspects of development. Infants who may need intervention the most, such as asphyxiated newborns, do not appear to have been studied at all; most research involves the relatively healthy premature infant weighing more than 1000 grams at birth.

Global intervention studies provided a program that took place several times a day and consisted of tactile and kinesthetic inputs such as stroking and massaging the body, and holding, cradling, and rocking the infants in imitation of normal maternal behaviors.[9-12] The effects of global intervention programs can be summarized as follows:

1. Mental Development: Of six studies using standardized tests of mental development during the first year, five demonstrated significant effects from intervention.[13-17]
2. Motor Development: Of five studies evaluating gross motor development on the Bayley Scales of Infant Development, only two reported significant results in favor of the experimental group.[13,16] One of the negative reports demonstrated differences in developmental reflex achievement despite nonsignificant results on the Bayley Motor Scale.[15] Two of the intervention studies report significant differences on *neonatal* tests of motor functioning,[17,18] but two also report negative findings.[13,19]
3. Weight Gain: Four of seven studies reported significant effects on weight gain.[14-16,20]
4. Visiting: Both of the studies in which maternal visits to the nursery were assessed reported positive effects,[19,21] but in one study, the effect was not sustained after the mothers themselves left the hospital.[19]

The bulk of the studies, then, support the effectiveness of intervention in positively influencing weight gain and mental development test scores during the first year of postnatal life. Long-term benefits have not been demonstrated. The lack of solid support for effects on gross motor development is somewhat puzzling, but may be due to the relatively more genetically preprogrammed nature of neuromuscular development or to the fact that none of the reported studies were specifically designed to influence motor development and were not conducted with infants with movement dysfunction.

Research on the characteristics of the high-risk infant reveals a picture of an immature organism attempting to deal with certain types of overstimulation in the nursery environment (especially auditory, visual, and nociceptive) with compromised physiologic survival mechanisms, weak signaling devices, and aberrant state control and behavior.[22-24] A dearth of helpful assists such as cuddling, soothing touch, movement, or positioning are available, and a partially responsive caretaker may or may not provide a modicum of skillfully administered social stimulation at a time when the infant is in an optimal state to receive and respond to it. If this picture is accepted as a model of the system with which we desire to intervene, the design of an intervention program should have the following characteristics:[9]

1. modification of the environment to decrease overstimulation
2. avoidance of unnecessary handling during periods of quiet sleep
3. introduction of diurnal rhythms to promote behavioral organization
4. provision of contingent tactile and kinesthetic responses to stress signals

5. provision of social interaction stimuli (auditory, visual, tactile, kinesthetic) during alert periods
6. immediate termination of or alterations in stimulation producing avoidance responses
7. establishment of individualized programs based on assessed needs for prevention or amelioration of movement dysfunction—the primary role of the physical therapist.

GOALS FOR THERAPY IN THE NEONATAL PERIOD

The goals of physical therapy for neonates with movement dysfunction include: (1) establishment of a fund of normal perceptual and motor experience upon which later learning can build; (2) facilitation of interaction skills, such as visual and auditory orientation to the human face and voice; and (3) inhibition of abnormal postural tone and movement patterns. Specific objectives include:

1. Free active head movement from side to side and ability to hold the head briefly in midline in the supine position while maintaining tucked chin.
2. Ability to perform antigravity movements of the arms and legs with appropriate levels of postural tone in the supine position. Posterior pelvic tilt produced by abdominal muscle contraction should accompany hip flexion. Shoulder girdle should maintain normal depression and protraction during arm movements.
3. Hand-to-mouth pattern; hands together pattern.
4. Coordinated sucking.
5. Tolerance of side lying in a relaxed posture with protracted shoulders and head aligned with trunk.
6. Ability to roll from supine to either side lying or semi–side lying.
7. Visual and auditory orientation to faces, bright objects, voices, and rattles, without extraneous body movement or excessive effort, and with smooth eye-head coordination.

Each of these activities can be done by the full-term newborn;[25-27] hence, the goals of therapy are to make it possible for the high-risk neonate to accomplish the normal developmental agenda for his age. In addition, the therapist should seek to prevent the development of abnormal patterns, such as neck retraction, scapular elevation and retraction, and lack of abdominal muscle tone, typical of the child with CNS dysfunction, while preparing the child for the developmental stages ahead.

THE EVALUATION PROCESS

Given the identification of infants at high risk for movement dysfunction and a frame of reference for establishing treatment goals for the neonatal period, the therapist must decide when and how to initiate the evaluation process. The baby should be assessed at the earliest possible moment to facilitate early treatment; however, the assessment process should not contribute to the infant's risk for mortality or morbidity and should yield useful, reliable data for planning intervention.[28] That is, the baby should be sufficiently medically stable to tolerate the stress of evaluation and to respond appropriately to the stimulation provided by the therapist. Als[29] developed a hierarchical model of neurobehavioral organization in the neonate that suggests that the stressed infant cannot progress to achievement of competency in motor control until physiologic homeostasis has been attained. Too early an assessment, therefore, may be unreflective of the baby's future capacity for organizing motor responses for feeding, self-comforting, position changing, and interacting with a caretaker.

During this period of acute illness, the high-risk baby can be provided with positioning, stroking, gentle range of motion, and facilitation of sucking to prevent development of contractures, hypersensitivity to touch, and disuse weakness. The baby's reaction to this intervention is part of the evaluation process. The therapist should observe the baby for hypersensitivity to stimulation, respiratory incoordination, seizure activity, abnormal tone, and color changes, as well as alerting to stimulation and attempts at self-control and organization. During this period, the therapist should carefully review the medical record and discuss the baby's condition with other staff members to gain adequate knowledge of the baby's medical and behavioral problems, whether the baby's course is unusual, special concerns such as feeding or need for postural drainage, and the types of equipment, such as ventilator or intravenous line, the baby needs. The therapist must become skilled in handling this equipment appropriately and recognize personal limitations in knowledge and ability so that the baby's safety is guaranteed. Limitations on handling, such as the need to maintain a horizontal position when a shunt for hydrocephalus has been inserted without a valve until the baby has attained a certain size, must be observed. Obtaining information from the social worker or nurses regarding parental visiting patterns in preparation for planning parent education programs is also useful at this time. The therapist should become aware of exactly what information the parents have been given by physicians and nurses.

L. and V. Dubowitz[30] developed a neurobehavioral assessment for the premature or full-term infant that allows assessment of the infant's neurologic development from the early stages of acute illness until the end of the perinatal period. This scale can be used to document increasing maturity of the premature infant on a weekly basis: identification of developing postural tone and primitive reflexes, presence of abnormal neurologic signs, quality of shutdown of responsiveness to disturbing stimulation during sleep, and ability to alert and orient to visual and auditory stimuli. For the purposes of planning a physical therapy program, the therapist can also document the presence or absence of the movement patterns previously listed as goals for therapy. A simple checklist can be used to indicate the conceptual age at which the infant was able to perform each movement pattern independently, whether the pattern could be attained with handling, or whether the infant was totally unable to move in a given pattern. When repeated weekly, this checklist also provides a record of progress in achieving therapy goals.

Whatever format for assessment is used, the Neonatal Behavioral Assessment Scale of Brazelton[25] and the hierarchical model of Als[29] provide a useful frame of reference for evaluating the overall quality of the baby's ability to organize behavior and interact with caretakers. The therapist must assess the infant's ability to attain and maintain behavioral state organization, the use of hand-to-mouth and rolling to the side for self-comforting, the reflex threshold, the degree of sensitivity to stimulation, and the ability to organize responsiveness to social cues. This information will assist the therapist in deciding where to begin in treatment. For example, if the infant is found to be hypersensitive to handling and intolerant of changes in position, acceptance of handling must be achieved before facilitation of active movement patterns can be initiated in therapy. Oral motor dysfunction that interfers with adequate nutritional intake by mouth should also receive a high priority.

CASE HISTORIES

The following case histories illustrate the goals and treatment, with their rationale, of two newborns with movement dysfunction.

CASE 1

Baby girl Evelyn was born on 2/11/82 at 29 weeks gestation, weighing 1350 grams, to a primigravida in whom labor was induced prematurely because of severe preeclampsia evidenced by a blood pressure of 160/100, 3+ proteinuria, and a 14-pound weight gain over a 4-week period (Fig. 12-4). At birth, the baby was limp, blue, and without spontaneous respirations; Apgar scores were 2 and 6 at 1 and 5 minutes, respectively. A summary of Evelyn's perinatal problems is provided in her POPRAS form in Figure 12-5. Evelyn was ventilated for 11 days after birth, as well as periodically at several later points, and she required oxygen therapy until 6/18/82. In addition to perinatal asphyxia, bronchopulmonary dysplasia, hyperbilirubinemia requiring phototherapy, and a patent ductus arteriosus, she suffered a subependymal hemorrhage, which was diagnosed by ultrasound scan of the head.[31]

Evelyn was seen for initial physical therapy evaluation on 5/26/82 because of irritability and hypertonicity. Her problems included extensor muscle hypertonicity expressed in the presence of shoulder elevation and retraction, inability to flex hips and posteriorly rotate pelvis to lift legs from the supporting surface, poor head control with head preference to the right side and complete lack of head righting when pulled up to sit, intolerance for the side lying position, general irritability with movement, and uncoordinated visual and auditory orientation.

Table 12-1 illustrates the identified problems, therapeutic goals, intervention techniques, and methods of assessment suggested for Evelyn's physical therapy. The first problem to be considered in treatment must be the irritability. Because Evelyn is intolerant of position change and handling, highly sensitive intervention is necessary to help her become able to participate in a therapy program. Assessment of her ability to tolerate the movements and positions imposed by the therapist must be done continually during a therapy session through observation of respiration, color, tone, and facial expression. With increasing tolerance for therapy, the second target should be improving abdominal muscle strength and tone as support for movement of more distal parts. Progress toward goals should be evaluated in 7 to 14 days after institution of the treatment program, although changes

PATIENT WEIGHT	AGE	TERM	PREMI	Ab	LIVE	PRENATAL CARE ☐ NO ☐ YES	CLINIC OR PHYSICIAN	CODE
	20	0	0	0	0			

ADMISSION DATE	TIME	LMP		CONDENSED PRENATAL PROBLEM LIST	PROB.NO.		PROB.NO.
__/__/__	----						
MEMBRANES RUPTURED	TIME	EDC	GEST. AGE				
__/__/__	----	4/9/82	29				
ONSET LABOR	TIME						
__/__/__ 1	----						

PRENATAL HOSPITALIZATION ☐ No ☐ Yes PRENATAL SCORE ▶ 10

PATIENT TRANSFERRED FROM ANOTHER HOSPITAL ☐ NO ☐ YES - specify:

	+ −	Risk Value	Prob. No.	
EARLY PROBLEMS	10	10	101	PREMATURE LABOR <37 ▶ Lung Maturity: ☐ Immature ☐ Interm. ☐ Mature Treatment: ☐ Alcohol ☐ B-Mimetic ☐ Other:
		10	102	HYDRAMNIOS – A clinical estimate of excessive amniotic fluid.
		10	103	MULTIPLE PREGNANCY
		10	104	ABN PRESENTATION ☐ Breech ☐ Face ☐ Brow ☐ Compound ☐ Transverse Lie ☐ Other
	10	10	105	MODERATE SEVERE PRE-ECLAMPSIA - B.P ≥ 160/110 or Proteinuria > 2 + after 26 wks Gest. Age
		5	106	MILD PRE-ECLAMPSIA #1 required for the Diagnosis ☐ 1 BP ≥ 140/90 or + 30mm in systolic or 15 mm in diastolic ☐ 2 Proteinuria 1 + or 2 + ☐ 3 – Persistent edema of Hands or Face
	5	5	107	INDUCTION ☐ Medical ☐ Elective ☐ Amniotomy ☐ Oxytocin
		5	108	PREMATURE RUPTURE OF MEMBRANES – Rupture 12 hours or more prior to labor onset.
		5	109*	C-SECTION ☐ Primary ☐ Repeat
		10	110	HEAVY MECONIUM – Dark stained Amniotic Fluid – usually dark green and tenacious
		5	111	LIGHT MECONIUM – Light stained Amniotic Fluid – yellow or greenish
		5	112	PROLONGED LATENT PHASE – Over 13 hours Multipara, over 20 hours Nullipara
INTERIM PROBLEMS		5	113	PRIMARY DYSFUNCTIONAL LABOR - W/O Oxytocin after 4 cm dilatation ☐ 1 - Nullipara - at least 1 cm per hour ☐ 2 - Multipara - 1.5 cm per hour
		1	114	SECONDARY ARREST OF DILATATION – Failure to progress after 5 cm Cervical Dilatation
		5	115	PITOCIN AUGMENTATION OF LABOR – Use of Oxytocin to improve uterine contractions
		10	116	CORD PROLAPSE
		10	117*	UTERINE BLEEDING ☐ Abruption ☐ Previa ☐ Marginal Separation
		10	118	FETAL TACHYCARDIA > 160 beats per minute lasting more than 30 minutes.
		10	119	AMNIONITIS ☐ Mat. Temp. ≥ 100.4° ☐ Bacteria in Amniotic Fluid
		10	120	FETAL BRADYCARDIA – < 120 Beats/min. or abnormal heart rate patterns (HRP) persisting over 30 min ☐ Mild ☐ Mod ☐ Sev cord comp. or ☐ Mild ☐ Mod ☐ Sev late decel. HRP
		10	121	DECREASE BASE LINE VARIABILITY DUE TO ☐ Medication ☐ Acidosis ☐ Unknown

MONITORED			☐ EXTERNAL ☐ INTERNAL SCALP SAMPLE? ☐ YES
COMPLETE DILATION DATE TIME __/__/__ 2 ____		5	122 EXCESSIVE MEDICATION ☐ Demerol, greater than 150 mg ☐ Phenobarbitol, greater than 60 mg ☐ Magnesium Sulfate, greater than 25 grams ☐ Other
		10	123 SEIZURE ☐ Eclampsia ☐ Previous Seizure Disorder ☐ Unknown
LATE PROBLEMS		10	124 * BREECH DELIVERY (VAGINAL) METHOD: ☐ Spontaneous ☐ Assisted ☐ Breech Ext. TYPE: ☐ Single Footling ☐ Double Footling ☐ Frank
		10	125 SHOULDER DYSTOCIA
		5	126 * ☐ OPERATIVE FORCEPS ☐ VACUUM EXTRACTION ☐ FAILED VACUUM
		1	127 * OUTLET FORCEPS ☐ Simpson ☐ Tucker McLane ☐ Luikart ☐ Other
		5	128 LATE PASSAGE OF MECONIUM - Any stained fluid after previously clear fluid
		10	129 COMPLICATIONS OF ANESTHESIA ☐ Convulsion ☐ Fetal Bradycardia ☐ Hypotension ☐ Other:
		5	130 SECOND STAGE > 2.5 HOURS
DELIVERY DATE TIME __/__/__ 3 ____		5	131 PRECIPITOUS LABOR < 3 HOURS TOTAL
		5	132 LABOR > 20 HOURS TOTAL
PLACENTA DATE TIME __/__/__ 4 ____			133 MOTHER-INFANT BONDING ☐ Excellent ☐ Good ☐ Poor
			134 DELIVERED ☐ Home ☐ In Transit ☐ Elsewhere in Hospital
			135 STILLBIRTH ☐ Antepartum ☐ Intra-partum

	HOURS	MIN
STAGE I 1 (-2)	--	--
STAGE II 2 (-3)	--	--
STAGE III 3 (-4)	--	--
TOTAL LABOR TIME		

25 **FINAL SCORE**

HOSPITAL BIRTH DATE

SHARON H.

SIGNATURES

1-

2-

3-

COPYRIGHT © POPRAS, 1975, 1976

4 B R INTRAPARTUM PROBLEM LIST

FIGURE 12-4. Problem Oriented Perinatal Risk Assessment System (POPRAS) summary of maternal labor and delivery problems for Case 1, baby girl Evelyn.

CODE = SHADED AREAS
A = Date Active R = Date Resolved

+	Val	GENERAL
	5	1) Hypothermia ≤ 97°F. or 36.2°C. ®
10	10	2) Prenatal Score ≥10 10
10	10	3) Intrapartum Score ≥10 25
5	5	4) Apgar 1 min ≤5 2
	10	5) Apgar 5 min ≤5 6
10	10	6) Asphyxia
10	10	7) Resuscitation
	5	8) Neg Foam Test or L/S < 1.5
	1	9) Intermed. F.T. or L/S 1.5-2.0
10	10	10) Preterm ≤37 wks. 29 wKs
	1	11) Term 38-42 wks.
	5	12) Post Term >42 wks.
	10	13) SGA <10% ile
1	1	14) AGA 1350 gms
	5	15) LGA >90% ile
		SKIN
	1	16) Positive Finding
		Type Code
		A R
		HEAD-NECK
	5	17) Low set ears
	10	18) Cleft Palate
	10	19) Choanal Atresia
	10	20) Retrolental Fibroplasia
		A R
	10	21) Retinoblastoma
		22) Other

+	Val	CARDIOVASCULAR
	10	36) Congenital Heart Disease
		A R
		Type
10	10	37) Patent Ductus Arteriosus
		A R
	10	38) Persistent Fetal Circulation
		A R
	10	39) Congestive Heart Failure
		A R
	5	40) Heart Murmur
		A R
		Type
✓		41) Persistent Cyanosis
		42) Other
		GASTRO-INTESTINAL
	5	43) Distended Abdomen
		A R
5	5	44) Vomiting
		A R
	10	45) Diarrhea/Gastroenteritis
		A R
	5	46) Blood in stool
		A R
	10	47) Bowel obstruction
		A R
	10	48) Pyloric Obstruction
		A R
	5	49) Meconium Plug

+	Val	GENITO-URINARY
	10	62) Renal Failure
		A R
		63) Anomaly
		Type
		64) Other
		HEMATOLOGICAL
	5	65) Isoimmunization
		A R
		☐ Rh ☐ ABO ☐ Other
	10	66) Hyperbilirubinemia
5	5	☐ Indirect
		☐ Direct
		Highest value _____ mg %
	10	67) Hemorrhagic Diathesis
		A R
		Type
	5	68) Anemia
		A R
		Type
	5	69) Polycythemia
		A R
		Highest Hct
		70) Other
		INFECTION
	1	71) Scalp Abscess
		A R
	5	72) Eye Infection
		A R

+	Val	NEUROLOGICAL
		83) Abnormal Head
		☐ Micro ☐ Hydro ☐ Anen.
	5	84) CNS Depression < 24 hrs.
		A R
10	10	85) CNS Depression >24 hrs.
		A R
	10	86) Seizure
		A R
		Type
10	10	87) Jittery-Hyperactive
		A R
	10	88) Withdrawal Symptoms
		A R
		Type
	10	89) Paralysis
		A R
		Type
10	10	90) Other IVH
		ORTHOPEDIC
	10	91) Fracture
		Type
	10	92) Hip Dislocation R L
		93) Other
		GENETIC/ENDOCR.
	10	94) Downs Syndrome
	10	95) Other
		SPECIAL TREATMENT
		Pulmonary

		RESPIRATORY	
	10	23) Meconium Aspiration	
		A	R
	5	24) Aspiration (other)	
		□ Am. Fl. □ Blood □ Formula	
		A	R
	5	25) Mild respiratory distress (T.T.N.)	
		A	R
	5	26) Mild RDS (Syndrome)	
		A	R
10	10	27) Severe RDS (Syndrome)	
		A	R
	10	28) Congenital Pneumonia	
		A	R
10	10	29) Apnea	
		A	R
	10	30) Pneumothorax	
		A	R
	10	31) Pneumomediastinum	
		A	R
	10	32) Interstitial Emphysema	
		A	R
10	10	33) Broncho-pulm. dysplasia	
		A	R
	10	34) Anomaly	
		Type	
		35) Other	

		A	R
	10	50) Necrotizing Enterocolitis	
		A	R
	10	51) Tracheo-Esophageal Fistula	
		52) Other	
		METABOLIC	
	10	53) Hypoglycemia	
		A	R
		Lowest Value	
	10	54) Hypocalcemia	
		A	R
		Lowest Value	
	5	55) □ Hypo □ Hypermagnesemia	
		A	R
		Low/High Value	
	10	56) □ Hypo □ Hyperthyroidism	
		A	R
		Low/High Value	
	10	57) □ Hypo □ Hypernatremia	
		A	R
		Low/High Value	
	10	58) Inappropriate ADH	
		A	R
	10	59) Persistent Metabolic Acidosis	
		A	R
5	5	60) Failure to Gain	
		A	R
		61) Other	

1	73) Monilia	
	A	R
5	74) Omphalitis	
	A	R
10	75) Sepsis	
	A	R
10	76) Meningitis	
	A	R
10	77) □ T □ O □ R □ C □ H	
	A	R
5	78) Urinary Tract Infection	
	A	R
10	79) Syphilis	
	A	R
5	80) Elevated IgM	
	81) Other	
Code	82) List Organisms	
	1-	
	2-	
	3-	

1. X O_2 >1 day	5. □ Chest Tube
2. □ Ambu Bag	6. □ Chest X-Ray
3. □ C-PAP	7. □ Other
4. X Respirator	8. □
HEMATOLOGIC	
9. X Phototherapy	11. □ Transfusion
10. □ Exch. Trans.	12. □
SPECIAL TESTS	
13. □ Biopsy - Type	16. □ Spinal Tap
14. □ Cardiac Cath	17. □ Other
15. □ EKG	18. □
OPERATIONS — PROCEDURES	
19. □ PDA Ligation	22. □ UV Cath.
20. □ UA Cath.	23. X LUNG
21. □ Circumcision	24. □ BIOPSY-OPEN
DRUGS	
25. X Antibiotics	29. □ Digitalis
26. □ Bicarb	30. X MORPHINE
27. □ Calcium	31. □
28. □ Glucose	32. □

FINAL NEWBORN SCORE ▶ 141

EVELYN· H.

B.D. 2/11/82

9 B R NEWBORN PROBLEM LIST

MOTHER: SHARON H.

FIGURE 12-5. Neonatal POPRAS form summary of medical problems of Case 1, baby girl Evelyn.

TABLE 12-1. Case Study: Neonate with Movement Dysfunction—Evelyn

PROBLEM	GOAL	INTERVENTION STRATEGIES	ASSESSMENT
1. Irritability	Normalize physiologic and affective response to being moved and placed in different positions	a. Slow, rhythmical movements and gradual position changes b. Swaddling c. Neutral warmth	a. Irritability, behavioral state, and postural tone items on the Brazelton scale b. Color changes with movement and positioning c. Facial expression with movement and positioning d. Length of crying during treatment e. Care giver comments about child's irritability
2. Lack of neck rotation to the (L)	Active neck rotation from midline to 45° toward (L)	a. Inhibition of extensor tone by swaddling, controlling shoulders in protraction and neck in flexion, and positioning baby in semi-reclining position b. Use visual and auditory stimulation to facilitate eye tracking and head turning c. While infant sucks on nipple, move it toward (L), facilitating head and mouth to follow	a. Degrees of neck rotation toward (L) with visual or auditory stimulation b. Frequency of spontaneous neck rotation toward (L) c. Alertness and orientation items on Brazelton scale
3. Scapular retraction and elevation	Antigravity arm movements	a. Positioning in side lying, prone, and supported sitting b. Swaddling with neck, trunk, hip, and knee flexion and scapular protraction—activities in this position include sucking, neck rotation, assisted or independent hands-to-mouth or midline, or rolling to side lying	a. Frequency of hand-to-mouth behavior in supine, side lying, prone, and supported sitting with or without swaddling or controls by therapist b. Frequency of hands to midline in supine, side lying, and supported sitting with or without scapular control or swaddling
4. Lack of hip and trunk flexion	Ability to maintain posterior pelvic tilt while flexing hips and knees in supine	a. Positioning in side lying or semi-reclining supine position (sometimes head up, sometimes down) with neck, trunk, and hip flexion b. Decrease extensor tone by handling techniques such as pressure on sternum, tactile contact with abdominal muscles, scapular protraction, gentle approximation through shoulder or hip area	a. Frequency of hip flexion with posterior pelvic tilt in supine b. Ability to maintain side lying position c. Rolling from supine to side lying

in the program would be considered earlier if no response or adverse reactions were noted at any time.

The rationale for the choice of goals for Evelyn is that all movement patterns selected are in the repertoire of the full-term neonate. Because Evelyn was 1 month corrected age and physiologically stable at the time of initial evaluation, these were appropriate goals for her therapy. The treatment techniques selected were designed to facilitate the movement goals while normalizing tone and preventing the influence of abnormal patterns; they are believed to be effective on the basis of empirical evidence. Unfortunately, no research support is available to justify the selection of treatment techniques, or even, as demonstrated earlier, the provision of treatment for stressed neonates per se.

CASE 2

Baby girl Cornelia was born on 3/20/82 at 36 to 37 weeks gestation, weighing 2860 grams, the second born of twins to a primigravida with a normal pregnancy other than late hydramnios and threatened early delivery that was suppressed at 33 weeks gestation (Fig. 12-6). After the birth of the first twin, who weighed 2360 grams, the cervix closed down and Cornelia was not born until 2 hours later, with the aid of low forceps. Her Apgar scores were 7 and 9 at 1 and 5 minutes, respectively; however, about 1 hour after birth, she experienced severe respiratory difficulty and cardiac arrest requiring prolonged resuscitation efforts. Sepsis was suspected in the mother but never confirmed. Cornelia's perinatal problems are summarized in her POPRAS form in Figure 12-7. Cornelia was treated with prophylactic antibiotics; her cultures were negative, so the cause of her problem was never discovered. Subsequent ultrasound scan of the head was normal, and no seizures were noted despite an abnormal electroencephalogram; however, Cornelia's muscle tone was extremely low, and spontaneous movement was sluggish and infrequent for more than a week. Cornelia was on a respirator until 4/3/82 and required oxygen therapy until 4/20/82.

She was seen for initial physical therapy evaluation on 4/15/82 because of poverty of movement. Figure 12-8 shows the results of The Neurological Assessment of the Preterm and Full-Term Newborn Infant of Dubowitz and Dubowitz[30] performed on 4/20/82, when Cornelia was 1 month old. This test revealed the presence of poor head control in all positions, sluggish or absent limb recoil responses, and generalized poverty of movement. The right side of the body was more involved than the left. Visual orientation was present (Fig. 12-9) but accomplished despite strabismus and uncoordinated eye movements (Fig. 12-10). Auditory orientation was limited to shifting of the eyes toward the sound source; head turning was incomplete. Also noted during the examination were persistent shoulder retraction and elevation (Figs. 12-11 through 12-13), increased extensor tone during movements of the legs, preference for head to the left posture, and intolerance of side lying position.

Although the movement *goals* for this child would be strikingly similar to those outlined for Evelyn, the *causes* of Cornelia's movement dysfunction were quite different. Cornelia did not demonstrate irritability upon movement except that she disliked being placed in the side lying position because of lack of experience with it. Her poverty of movement was related to under-

PATIENT WEIGHT	AGE	TERM	PREMI	Ab	LIVE	PRENATAL CARE	CLINIC OR PHYSICIAN	CODE
	19	0	0	0	0	☐ NO ☐ YES		

ADMISSION DATE	TIME	LMP	CONDENSED PRENATAL PROBLEM LIST	PROB NO.		PROB NO.
__/__/__	____					
MEMBRANES RUPTURED	TIME	EDC / GEST. AGE				
__/__/__	____	3/25/82 / 36-37				
ONSET LABOR	TIME					
__/__/__ 1	____					

PRENATAL HOSPITALIZATION ☐ No ☐ Yes PRENATAL SCORE ▶ 20

PATIENT TRANSFERRED FROM ANOTHER HOSPITAL ☐ NO ☐ YES - specify:

	+ −	Risk Value	Prob. No.	
SUPPRESSED AT 33 weeks **EARLY PROBLEMS**	10	10	101	PREMATURE LABOR <37 ▶ Lung Maturity: ☐ Immature ☐ Interm. ☐ Mature Treatment: ☐ Alcohol ☐ B-Mimetic ☐ Other:
	10	10	102	HYDRAMNIOS – A clinical estimate of excessive amniotic fluid.
	10	10	103	MULTIPLE PREGNANCY
		10	104	ABN PRESENTATION ☐ Breech ☐ Face ☐ Brow ☐ Compound ☐ Transverse Lie ☐ Other
		10	105	MODERATE SEVERE PRE-ECLAMPSIA - B.P ≥ 160/110 or Proteinuria > 2 + after 26 wks Gest. Age
		5	106	MILD PRE-ECLAMPSIA #1 required for the Diagnosis ☐ 1 BP ≥ 140/90 or + 30mm in systolic or 15 mm in diastolic ☐ 2 Proteinuria 1 + or 2+ ☐ 3 – Persistent edema of Hands or Face
		5	107	INDUCTION ☐ Medical ☐ Elective ☐ Amniotomy ☐ Oxytocin
		5	108	PREMATURE RUPTURE OF MEMBRANES – Rupture 12 hours or more prior to labor onset.
		5	109 *	C-SECTION ☐ Primary ☐ Repeat
		10	110	HEAVY MECONIUM – Dark stained Amniotic Fluid – usually dark green and tenacious
		5	111	LIGHT MECONIUM – Light stained Amniotic Fluid – yellow or greenish
		5	112	PROLONGED LATENT PHASE – Over 13 hours Multipara, over 20 hours Nullipara
INTERIM PROBLEMS		5	113	PRIMARY DYSFUNCTIONAL LABOR - W/O Oxytocin after 4 cm dilatation ☐ 1 - Nullipara - at least 1 cm per hour ☐ 2 - Multipara - 1.5 cm per hour
		1	114	SECONDARY ARREST OF DILATATION – Failure to progress after 5 cm Cervical Dilatation
		5	115	PITOCIN AUGMENTATION OF LABOR – Use of Oxytocin to improve uterine contractions
		10	116	CORD PROLAPSE
		10	117 *	UTERINE BLEEDING ☐ Abruption ☐ Previa ☐ Marginal Separation
		10	118	FETAL TACHYCARDIA > 160 beats per minute lasting more than 30 minutes.
		10	119	AMNIONITIS ☐ Mat. Temp. ≥ 100.4° ☐ Bacteria in Amniotic Fluid
		10	120	FETAL BRADYCARDIA – < 120 Beats/min. or abnormal heart rate patterns (HRP) persisting over 30 min ☐ Mild ☐ Mod ☐ Sev cord comp. or ☐ Mild ☐ Mod ☐ Sev late decel. HRP
		10	121	DECREASE BASE LINE VARIABILITY DUE TO ☐ Medication ☐ Acidosis ☐ Unknown

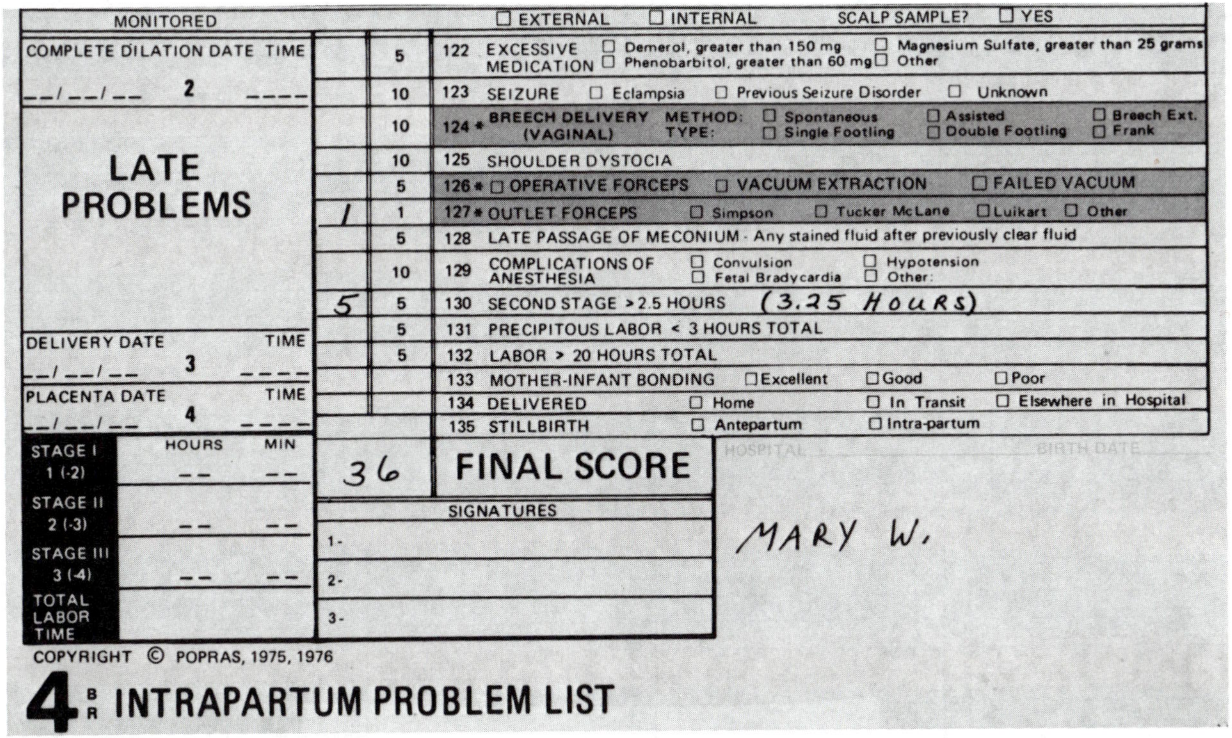

MONITORED ☐ EXTERNAL ☐ INTERNAL SCALP SAMPLE? ☐ YES

COMPLETE DILATION DATE __/__/__ 2 TIME ____

LATE PROBLEMS

DELIVERY DATE __/__/__ 3 TIME ____

PLACENTA DATE __/__/__ 4 TIME ____

Checked	Points	No.	Problem	Options
	5	122	EXCESSIVE MEDICATION	☐ Demerol, greater than 150 mg ☐ Phenobarbitol, greater than 60 mg ☐ Magnesium Sulfate, greater than 25 grams ☐ Other
	10	123	SEIZURE	☐ Eclampsia ☐ Previous Seizure Disorder ☐ Unknown
	10	124*	BREECH DELIVERY (VAGINAL)	METHOD: ☐ Spontaneous ☐ Assisted ☐ Breech Ext. TYPE: ☐ Single Footling ☐ Double Footling ☐ Frank
	10	125	SHOULDER DYSTOCIA	
	5	126*	☐ OPERATIVE FORCEPS	☐ VACUUM EXTRACTION ☐ FAILED VACUUM
1	1	127*	OUTLET FORCEPS	☐ Simpson ☐ Tucker McLane ☐ Luikart ☐ Other
	5	128	LATE PASSAGE OF MECONIUM - Any stained fluid after previously clear fluid	
	10	129	COMPLICATIONS OF ANESTHESIA	☐ Convulsion ☐ Fetal Bradycardia ☐ Hypotension ☐ Other:
5	5	130	SECOND STAGE >2.5 HOURS	(3.25 HOURS)
	5	131	PRECIPITOUS LABOR < 3 HOURS TOTAL	
	5	132	LABOR > 20 HOURS TOTAL	
		133	MOTHER-INFANT BONDING	☐ Excellent ☐ Good ☐ Poor
		134	DELIVERED	☐ Home ☐ In Transit ☐ Elsewhere in Hospital
		135	STILLBIRTH	☐ Antepartum ☐ Intra-partum
36			FINAL SCORE	

	HOURS	MIN
STAGE I 1 (-2)	--	--
STAGE II 2 (-3)	--	--
STAGE III 3 (-4)	--	--
TOTAL LABOR TIME		

SIGNATURES

1-

2-

3-

HOSPITAL BIRTH DATE

MARY W.

4 B R INTRAPARTUM PROBLEM LIST

FIGURE 12-6. POPRAS form summary of maternal labor and delivery problem for Case 2, baby girl Cornelia.

CODE = SHADED AREAS
A = Date Active R = Date Resolved

+	Val	GENERAL
5	5	1) Hypothermia ≤ 97°F. or 36.2°C. ®
10	10	2) Prenatal Score ≥10 20
10	10	3) Intrapartum Score ≥10 36
	5	4) Apgar 1 min ≤5
	10	5) Apgar 5 min ≤5
10	10	6) Asphyxia CARDIAC ARREST
10	10	7) Resuscitation
	5	8) Neg Foam Test or L/S < 1.5
	1	9) Intermed. F.T. or L/S 1.5-2.0
10	10	10) Preterm ≤37 wks. 36-37 wks
	1	11) Term 38-42 wks.
	5	12) Post Term > 42 wks.
	10	13) SGA <10% ile
1	1	14) AGA 2860 gms
	5	15) LGA > 90% ile
		SKIN
	1	16) Positive Finding
		Type Code
		A R
		HEAD-NECK
	5	17) Low set ears
	10	18) Cleft Palate
	10	19) Choanal Atresia
	10	20) Retrolental Fibroplasia
		A R
	10	21) Retinoblastoma
		22) Other

+	Val	CARDIOVASCULAR
	10	36) Congenital Heart Disease
		A R
		Type
	10	37) Patent Ductus Arteriosus
		A R
10	10	38) Persistent Fetal Circulation
		A R
	10	39) Congestive Heart Failure
		A R
	5	40) Heart Murmur
		A R
		Type
		41) Persistent Cyanosis
	✓	42) Other VENT. TACH.
		GASTRO-INTESTINAL
	5	43) Distended Abdomen
		A R
5	5	44) Vomiting
		A R
	10	45) Diarrhea/Gastroenteritis
		A R
	5	46) Blood in stool
		A R
	10	47) Bowel obstruction
		A R
	10	48) Pyloric Obstruction
		A R
	5	49) Meconium Plug

+	Val	GENITO-URINARY
	10	62) Renal Failure
		A R
		63) Anomaly
		Type
		64) Other
		HEMATOLOGICAL
	5	65) Isoimmunization
		A R
		☐ Rh ☐ ABO ☐ Other
	10	66) Hyperbilirubinemia
	5	☐ Indirect
		☐ Direct
		Highest value _____ mg %
10	10	67) Hemorrhagic Diathesis
		A R
		Type
5	5	68) Anemia
		A R
		Type
	5	69) Polycythemia
		A R
		Highest Hct
		70) Other
		INFECTION
	1	71) Scalp Abscess
		A R
	5	72) Eye Infection
		A R

+	Val	NEUROLOGICAL
		83) Abnormal Head
		☐ Micro ☐ Hydro ☐ Anen.
	5	84) CNS Depression < 24 hrs.
		A R
10	10	85) CNS Depression > 24 hrs.
		A R
	10	86) Seizure
		A R
		Type
	10	87) Jittery-Hyperactive
		A R
	10	88) Withdrawal Symptoms
		A R
		Type
	10	89) Paralysis
		A R
		Type
	✓	90) Other ABNORMAL EEG
		ORTHOPEDIC
	10	91) Fracture
		Type
	10	92) Hip Dislocation R L
		93) Other
		GENETIC/ENDOCR.
	10	94) Downs Syndrome
	10	95) Other
		SPECIAL TREATMENT
		Pulmonary

RESPIRATORY

Score	Code	Problem	
	10	23) Meconium Aspiration	
		A	R
	5	24) Aspiration (other)	
		☐ Am. Fl. ☐ Blood ☐ Formula	
		A	R
	5	25) Mild respiratory distress (T.T.N.)	
		A	R
	5	26) Mild RDS (Syndrome)	
		A	R
10	10	27) Severe RDS (Syndrome)	
		A	R
	10	28) Congenital Pneumonia	
		A	R
10	10	29) Apnea	
		A	R
	10	30) Pneumothorax	
		A	R
	10	31) Pneumomediastinum	
		A	R
	10	32) Interstitial Emphysema	
		A	R
	10	33) Broncho-pulm. dysplasia	
		A	R
	10	34) Anomaly	
		Type	
		35) Other	

Score	Code	Problem	
		A	R
	10	50) Necrotizing Enterocolitis	
		A	R
	10	51) Tracheo-Esophageal Fistula	
		52) Other	

METABOLIC

Score	Code	Problem	
	10	53) Hypoglycemia	
		A	R
		Lowest Value	
	10	54) Hypocalcemia	
		A	R
		Lowest Value	
	5	55) ☐ Hypo ☐ Hypermagnesemia	
		A	R
		Low/High Value	
	10	56) ☐ Hypo ☐ Hyperthyroidism	
		A	R
		Low/High Value	
10	10	57) ☐ Hypo ☐ Hypernatremia	
		A	R
		Low/High Value	
	10	58) Inappropriate ADH	
		A	R
10	10	59) Persistent Metabolic Acidosis	
		A	R
5	5	60) Failure to Gain	
		A	R
		61) Other	

Code	Problem	
1	73) Monilia	
	A	R
5	74) Omphalitis	
	A	R
10	75) Sepsis	
	A	R
10	76) Meningitis	
	A	R
10	77) ☐ T ☐ O ☐ R ☐ C ☐ H	
	A	R
5	78) Urinary Tract Infection	
	A	R
10	79) Syphilis	
	A	R
5	80) Elevated IgM	
	81) Other	
Code	82) List Organisms	
	1-	
	2-	
	3-	

1. X O_2 >1 day	5. ☐ Chest Tube
2. ☐ Ambu Bag	6. X Chest X-Ray
3. ☐ C-PAP	7. ☐ Other
4. X Respirator	8. ☐
HEMATOLOGIC	
9. ☐ Phototherapy	11. X Transfusion
10. ☐ Exch. Trans.	12. ☐
SPECIAL TESTS	
13. ☐ Biopsy - Type	16. ☐ Spinal Tap
14. ☐ Cardiac Cath	17. X Other EEG
15. X EKG	18. X US-HEAD
OPERATIONS — PROCEDURES	
19. ☐ PDA Ligation	22. ☐ UV Cath.
20. X UA Cath.	23. ☐
21. ☐ Circumcision	24. ☐
DRUGS	
25. X Antibiotics	29. ☐ Digitalis
26. X Bicarb	30. X PAVULON
27. ☐ Calcium	31. X MORPHINE
28. ☐ Glucose	32. X DOPAMINE

FINAL NEWBORN SCORE ▶ 141

CORNELIA W.
B. D. 3/20/82

MOTHER: MARY W.

9 B R NEWBORN PROBLEM LIST

FIGURE 12-7. Neonatal POPRAS form summary of medical problems of Case 2, baby girl Cornelia.

A

NAME	D.O.B./TIME	WEIGHT	E.D.D. L.N.M.P.	E.D.D. U/snd.
CORNELIA W.	3/20/82	2860		
HOSP. NO.	DATE OF EXAM	HEIGHT		
	4/20/82			
RACE SEX	AGE	HEAD CIRC.	GESTATIONAL ASSESSMENT	SCORE WEEKS
♀	1 mo CA			36-37

STATES

1. Deep sleep, no movement, regular breathing.
2. Light sleep, eyes shut, some movement.
3. Dozing, eyes opening and closing.
4. Awake, eyes open, minimal movement.
5. Wide awake, vigorous movement.
6. Crying.

						STATE	COMMENT	ASYMMETRY
HABITUATION (≤state 3)								
LIGHT Repetitive flashlight stimuli (10) with 5 sec. gap. Shutdown = 2 consecutive negative responses	No response	A. Blink response to first stimulus only. B. Tonic blink response. C. Variable response.	A. Shutdown of movement but blink persists 2-5 stimuli. B. Complete shutdown 2-5 stimuli.	A. Shutdown of movement but blink persists 6-10 stimuli. B. Complete shutdown 6-10 stimuli.	A. Equal response to 10 stimuli. B. Infant comes to fully alert state. C. Startles + major responses throughout.			
RATTLE Repetitive stimuli (10) with 5 sec. gap.	No response	A. Slight movement to first stimulus. B. Variable response.	Startle or movement 2-5 stimuli, then shutdown	Startle or movement 6-10 stimuli, then shutdown	A. B. C. Grading as above			
MOVEMENT & TONE	Undress infant							
POSTURE * (At rest — predominant)			(hips abducted)	(hips adducted)	Abnormal postures: A. Opisthotonus. B. Unusual leg extension. C. Asymm. tonic neck reflex			
ARM RECOIL Infant supine. Take both hands, extend parallel to the body; hold approx. 2 secs. and release.	No flexion within 5 sec. R L	Partial flexion at elbow >100° within 4-5 sec. R L	Arms flex at elbow to <100° within 2-3 sec. R L (L) FASTER	Sudden jerky flexion at elbow immediately after release to <60° R L	Difficult to extend; arm snaps back forcefully			
ARM TRACTION Infant supine; head midline; grasp wrist, slowly pull arm to vertical. Angle of arm scored and resistance noted at moment infant is initially lifted off and watched until shoulder off mattress. Do other arm.	Arm remains fully extended R L	Weak flexion maintained only momentarily R L	Arm flexed at elbow to 140° and maintained 5 sec. R L	Arm flexed at approx. 100° and maintained R L	Strong flexion of arm <100° and maintained R L			
LEG RECOIL First flex hips for 5 secs, then extend both legs of infant by traction on ankles; hold down on the bed for 2 secs. and release.	No flexion within 5 sec. R L	Incomplete flexion of hips within 5 sec. R L	Complete flexion within 5 sec. R L	Instantaneous complete flexion R L	Legs cannot be extended; snap back forcefully R L			
LEG TRACTION Infant supine. Grasp leg near ankle and slowly pull toward vertical until buttocks 1-2" off. Note resistance at knee and score angle. Do other leg.	No flexion R L	Partial flexion, rapidly lost R L	Knee flexion 140-160° and maintained R L	Knee flexion 100-140° and maintained R L	Strong resistance; flexion <100° R L			

POPLITEAL ANGLE Infant supine. Approximate knee and thigh to abdomen; extend leg by gentle pressure with index finger behind ankle.	180-160° R L	150-140° R L	130-120° R L	110-90° R L	<90° R L			
HEAD CONTROL (post. neck m.) Grasp infant by shoulders and raise to sitting position; allow head to fall forward; wait 30 sec.	No attempt to raise head	Unsuccessful attempt to raise head upright	Head raised smoothly to upright in 30 sec. but not maintained.	Head raised smoothly to upright in 30 sec. and maintained	Head cannot be flexed forward			
HEAD CONTROL (ant. neck m.) Allow head to fall backward as you hold shoulders; wait 30 secs.	Grading as above	Grading as above	Grading as above	Grading as above				
HEAD LAG * Pull infant toward sitting posture by traction on both wrists. Also note arm flexion.								
VENTRAL SUSPENSION * Hold infant in ventral suspension; observe curvature of back, flexion of limbs and relation of head to trunk.								
HEAD RAISING IN PRONE POSITION Infant in prone position with head in midline.	No response	Rolls head to one side	Weak effort to raise head and turns raised head to one side	Infant lifts head, nose and chin off	Strong prolonged head lifting			
ARM RELEASE IN PRONE POSITION Head in midline. Infant in prone position; arms extended alongside body with palms up.	No effort	Some effort and wriggling	Flexion effort but neither wrist brought to nipple level	One or both wrists brought at least to nipple level without excessive body movement	Strong body movement with both wrists brought to face, or 'press-ups'			
SPONTANEOUS BODY MOVEMENT during examination (supine). If no spont. movement try to induce by cutaneous stimulation.	None or minimal Induced	A. Sluggish. B. Random, incoordinated. C. Mainly stretching.	Smooth movements alternating with random, stretching, athetoid or jerky	Smooth alternating movements of arms and legs with medium speed and intensity	Mainly: A. Jerky movement. B. Athetoid movement. C. Other abnormal movement.	1 2		
TREMORS Mark: Fast (>6/sec.) or Slow (<6/sec.)	No tremor	Tremors only in state 5-6	Tremors only in sleep or after Moro and startles	Some tremors in state 4	Tremulousness in all states			
STARTLES	No startles	Startles to sudden noise, Moro, bang on table only	Occasional spontaneous startle	2-5 spontaneous startles	6+ spontaneous startles			
ABNORMAL MOVEMENT OR POSTURE	No abnormal movement	A. Hands clenched but open intermittently. B. Hands do not open with Moro.	A. Some mouthing movement. B. Intermittent adducted thumb	A. Persistently adducted thumb B. Hands clenched all the time.	A. Continuous mouthing movement. B. Convulsive movements.			

FIGURE 12-8. Neurological Assessment of the Preterm and Full-Term Newborn Infant for Case 2, baby girl Cornelia. (Reprinted from Dubowitz, L. and Dubowitz, V.: *The Neurological Assessment of the Preterm and Full-term Newborn Infant.* Spastics International Medical Publications, 5A Netherhall Gardens, London NW3 5RN, 1981.)

B

REFLEXES						STATE	COMMENT	ASYMMETRY
TENDON REFLEXES Biceps jerk Knee jerk Ankle jerk	Absent		Present	Exaggerated	Clonus			
PALMAR GRASP Head in midline. Put index finger from ulnar side into hand and gently press palmar surface. Never touch dorsal side of hand.	Absent	Short, weak flexion	Medium strength and sustained flexion for several secs.	Strong flexion; contraction spreads to forearm	Very strong grasp. Infant easily lifts off couch			
ROOTING Infant supine, head midline. Touch each corner of the mouth in turn (stroke laterally).	No response	A. Partial weak head turn but no mouth opening. B. Mouth opening, no head turn.	Mouth opening on stimulated side with partial head turning	Full head turning, with or without mouth opening	Mouth opening with very jerky head turning			
SUCKING Infant supine; place index finger (pad towards palate) in infant's mouth; judge power of sucking movement after 5 sec.	No attempt	Weak sucking movement: A. Regular. B. Irregular.	Strong sucking movement, poor stripping: A. Regular. B. Irregular.	Strong regular sucking movement with continuing sequence of 5 movements. Good stripping.	Clenching but no regular sucking.			
WALKING (state 4, 5) Hold infant upright, feet touching bed, neck held straight with fingers.	Absent		Some effort but not continuous with both legs	At least 2 steps with both legs	A. Stork posture; no movement. B. Automatic walking.			
MORO One hand supports infant's head in midline, the other the back. Raise infant to 45° and when infant is relaxed let his head fall through 10°. Note if jerky. Repeat 3 times.	No response, or opening of hands only	Full abduction at the shoulder and extension of the arm	Full abduction but only delayed or partial adduction (R) DELAYED	Partial abduction at shoulder and extension of arms followed by smooth adduction A. Abd>Add B. Abd=Add C. Abd<Add	A. No abduction or adduction; extension only. B. Marked adduction only.		J S	
NEUROBEHAVIOURAL ITEMS								
EYE APPEARANCES	Sunset sign Nerve palsy	Transient nystagmus. Strabismus. Some roving eye movement	Does not open eyes	Normal conjugate eye movement	A. Persistent nystagmus. B. Frequent roving movement C. Frequent rapid blinks.			
AUDITORY ORIENTATION (state 3, 4) To rattle. (Note presence of startle.)	A. No reaction. B. Auditory startle but no true orientation.	Brightens and stills; may turn toward stimuli with eyes closed	Alerting and shifting of eyes; head may or may not turn to source	Alerting; prolonged head turns to stimulus; search with eyes	Turning and alerting to stimulus each time on both sides		S	

VISUAL ORIENTATION (state 4) To red woollen ball	Does not focus or follow stimulus	Stills; focuses on stimulus; may follow 30° jerkily; does not find stimulus again spontaneously	Follows 30-60° horizontally; may lose stimulus but finds it again. Brief vertical glance	Follows with eyes and head horizontally and to some extent vertically, with frowning	Sustained fixation; follows vertically, horizontally, and in circle			
ALERTNESS (state 4)	Inattentive; rarely or never responds to direct stimulation	When alert, periods rather brief; rather variable response to orientation	When alert, alertness moderately sustained; may use stimulus to come to alert state	Sustained alertness; orientation frequent, reliable to visual but not auditory stimuli	Continuous alertness, which does not seem to tire, to both auditory and visual stimuli			
DEFENSIVE REACTION A cloth or hand is placed over the infant's face to partially occlude the nasal airway.	No response	A. General quietening. B. Non-specific activity with long latency.	Rooting; lateral neck turning; possibly neck stretching.	Swipes with arm	Swipes with arm with rather violent body movement			
PEAK OF EXCITEMENT	Low level arousal to all stimuli; never > state 3	Infant reaches state 4-5 briefly but predominantly in lower states	Infant predominantly state 4 or 5; may reach state 6 after stimulation but returns spontaneously to lower state	Infant reaches state 6 but can be consoled relatively easily	A. Mainly state 6. Difficult to console, if at all. B. Mainly state 4-5 but if reaches state 6 cannot be consoled.			
IRRITABILITY (states 3, 4, 5) Aversive stimuli: Uncover — Ventral susp. Undress — Moro Pull to sit — Walking reflex Prone	No irritable crying to any of the stimuli	Cries to 1-2 stimuli	Cries to 3-4 stimuli	Cries to 5-6 stimuli	Cries to all stimuli			
CONSOLABILITY (state 6)	Never above state 5 during examination, therefore not needed	Consoling not needed. Consoles spontaneously	Consoled by talking, hand on belly or wrapping up	Consoled by picking up and holding; may need finger in mouth	Not consolable			
CRY	No cry at all	Only whimpering cry	Cries to stimuli but normal pitch	Lusty cry to offensive stimuli; normal pitch	High-pitched cry, often continuous			

NOTES * If asymmetrical or atypical, draw in on nearest figure

Record any abnormal signs (e.g. facial palsy, contractures, etc.). Draw if possible.

Record time after feed: 1 HR.

EXAMINER: SKC

FIGURE 12-8. *Continued.*

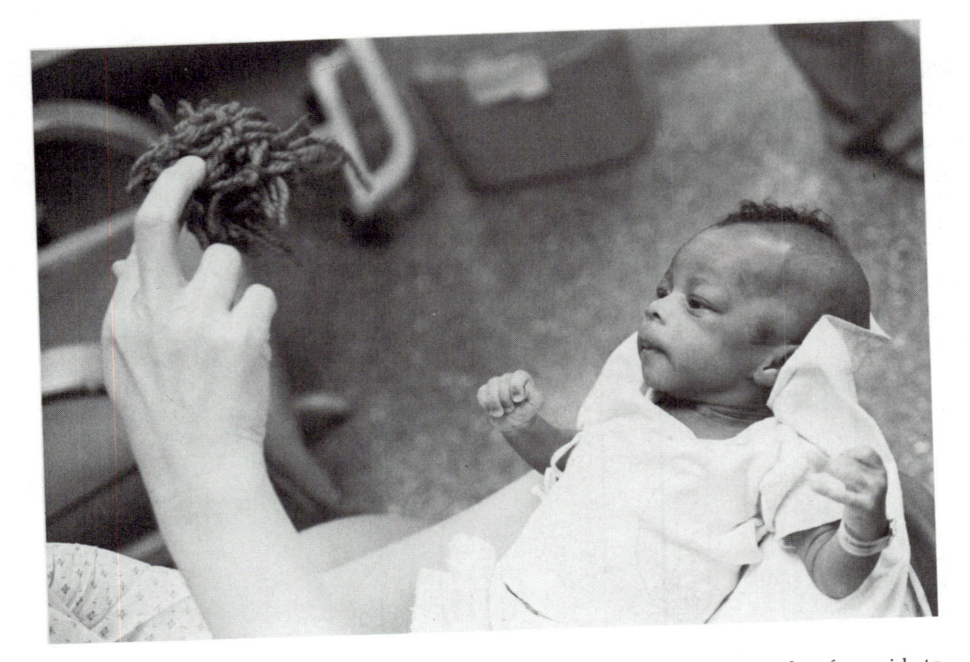

FIGURE 12-9. Visual orientation performance of baby girl Cornelia was complete from side to side but evoked increased tension in arms and trunk.

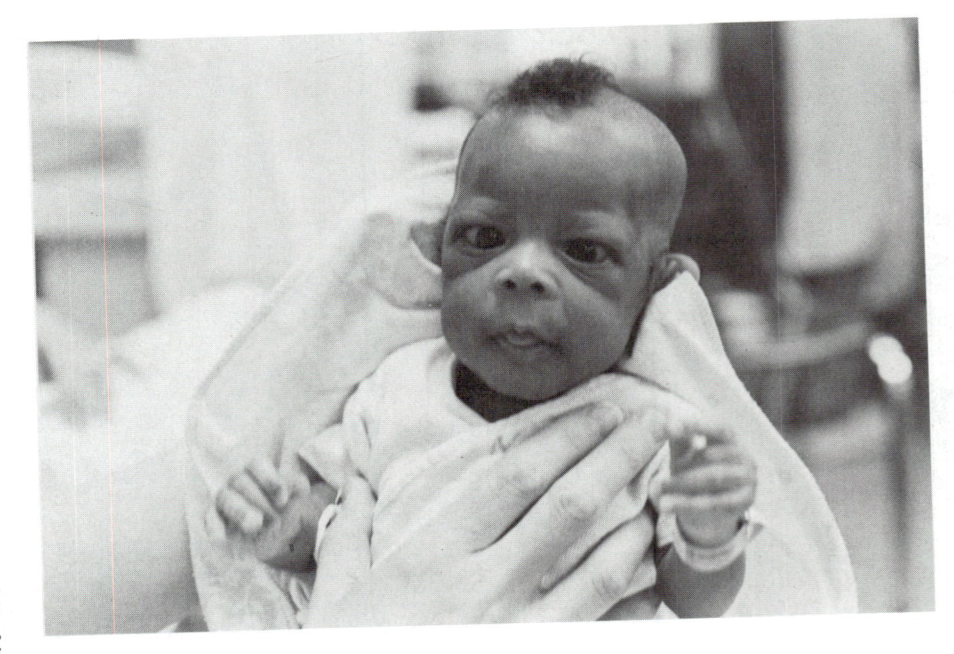

FIGURE 12-10. Eye coordination of baby girl Cornelia was poor, with frequent strabismus accompanying attempts to fixate on objects.

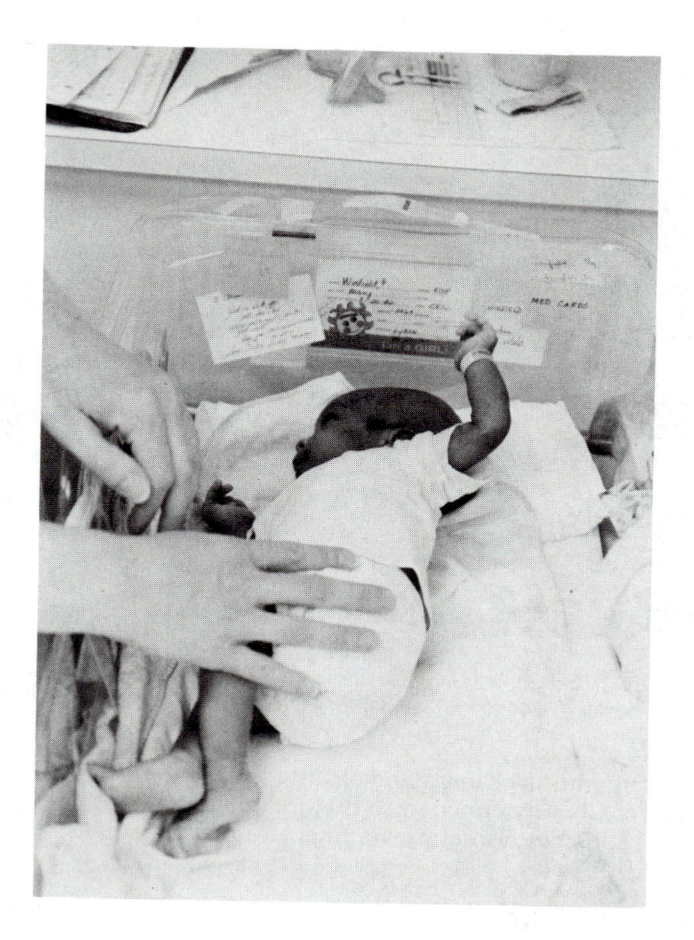

FIGURE 12-11. Baby girl Cornelia was intolerant of positioning in side lying and demonstrated scapulohumeral retraction and elevation.

lying low postural tone, although increased extensor tone developed when she attempted to move her legs, and increased deep tendon reflexes in the leg muscles gave other evidence that tone might be increasing. Her handling, again with similar movement goals in mind, must be oriented to: raising her underlying tone without creating increased tone in the hip extensors or elsewhere; stimulating more active, spontaneous movement; and helping her to prolong her states of alertness. In addition to using some of the treatment techniques outlined for Evelyn, one might consider vestibular stimulation from gentle movement in one's arms, in a hammock, or in a partially deflated small beach ball, and the use of one's voice to alert Cornelia and raise her underlying postural tone. In so doing, the therapist must remain alert to the signs of overstimulation, such as color changes, hiccuping, yawning, gaze aversion, emesis, and trunk arching. The therapist must also remember the possibility that a child with these types of problems could be on the way to developing overall hypertonicity.

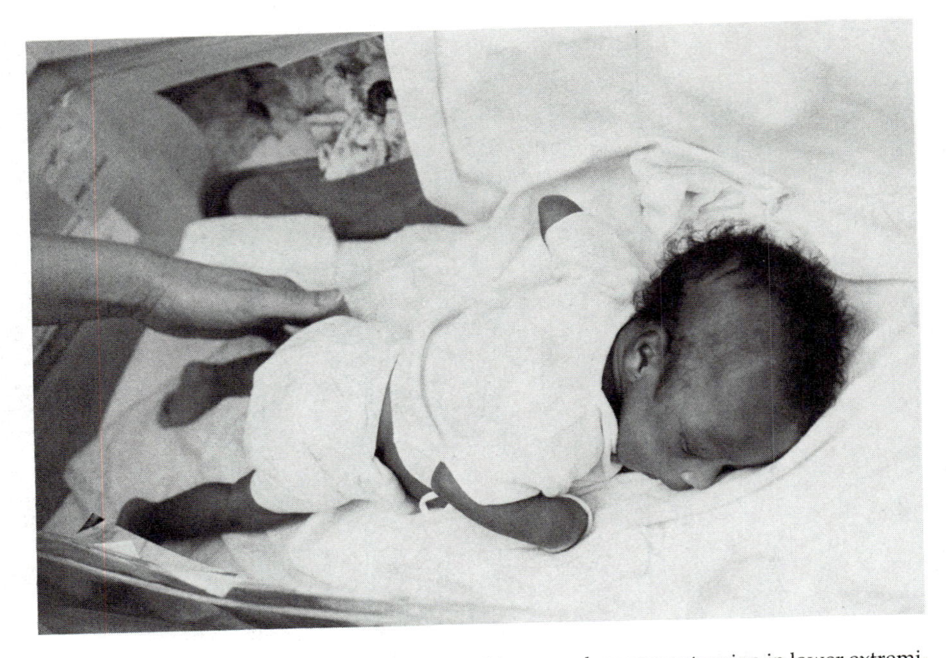

FIGURE 12-12. Baby girl Cornelia in prone position reveals excess extension in lower extremities, retracted, elevated scapulae with inability to release hands, and poor ability to lift head.

Handling must be careful and always done with recognition of the natural history of CNS dysfunction so that treatment will not only be aimed at present problems but also at preventing future eventualities.

ACCESS TO PRACTICE IN THE SPECIAL CARE NURSERY

Suggested steps in establishing a nursery service have been reviewed by Campbell and Wilhelm.[2] The ability of physical therapists to gain acceptance and recognition for their services for infants with movement dysfunction depends on the following: (1) knowledge of the medical conditions and management of high-risk infants, (2) personal interaction skills that provide the basis for learning from and teaching other members of the special care nursery team, (3) establishment of a dialogue with nursery personnel leading to acceptance of a standard protocol for types of patients and services to be provided, (4) competencies in assessment and treatment of newborns, and (5) parent education skills.

Each therapist must examine his or her capabilities in establishing a list of services that might be offered. These could include some or all of the following:

1. pulmonary physical therapy
2. positioning, splinting, and range of motion
3. facilitation of movement and postural adaptations

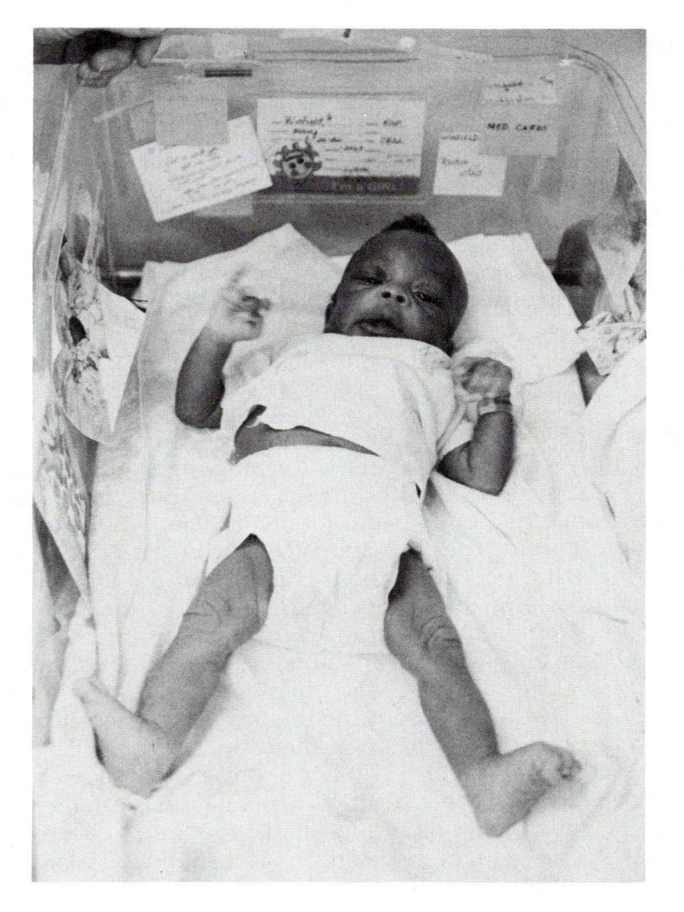

FIGURE 12-13. Baby girl Cornelia in supine position demonstrates increased extensor tone in lower extremities, retracted scapulae, and head preference to left.

4. intervention to promote cognitive and affective development as well as parent-infant attachment
5. oral/feeding programs
6. parent and staff consultation or education
7. planning for referrals and follow-up care in developmental assessment and treatment
8. electromyography and electrotherapy for care of brachial plexus injuries.

In developing a protocol, examination of personal competencies as well as the perceived needs and special interests of nursery personnel should be considered so that the initial impact of the program is rapid, powerful, and effective. For example, if nursery personnel are convinced that postural drainage is an effective treatment for infants with respiratory distress syndrome but are overburdened with the time demands of this service, beginning a nursery physical therapy service by offering this treatment may establish an immediate sense of value and appreciation of the therapist. On the other hand, it would hardly be the place to start if postural drainage is not already recognized as valuable. Individual evaluation of each work environment is necessary.

In areas that are novel for nursery personnel, such as movement therapy, it is highly effective to demonstrate what therapy can do, such as with a videotape showing initial assessment, treatment, and outcome, or with a case study documenting treatment of a special child or problem. As with entering any new area of practice, large amounts of both teaching and learning are essential to success.

SUMMARY

Management of the neonate with movement dysfunction requires decisions regarding which infants to evaluate and treat, when and how to assess neonatal movement dysfunction, and how to plan, implement, and monitor a therapy program based on a sound rationale. The format suggested in this chapter is one of basing the evaluation and treatment of movement dysfunction in the neonatal period on three goals: (1) to aid stressed neonates in attaining the developmental movement agenda for their conceptual ages, (2) to prevent common muscular and movement problems that result from inactivity and postures imposed by immaturity and medical procedures, and (3) to avoid increasing the risk of mortality and morbidity in the acutely ill neonate. Evaluation and therapy methods that are sensitive to both the physiologic responses and the movement and behavioral patterns of the neonate should be successful in attaining these goals; however, clinical research to demonstrate the effects of neonatal physical therapy is sorely needed. A personal continuing education program for developing knowledge of this special patient population and continual dialogue with other professionals working in the intensive care nursery are essential aspects of achieving higher levels of competency in decision making for management of neonates with movement dysfunction.

REFERENCES

1. Nelson, KB and Ellenberg, JH: *Neonatal signs as predictors of cerebral palsy.* Pediatrics 64:225, 1979.
2. Campbell, SK and Wilhelm, IJ: *Physical therapy in the special care nursery.* In Pearson, PH and Fieber, N (eds): *Physical Therapy Services in the Developmental Disabilities.* Charles C Thomas, Springfield. (in press)
3. Hack, M, Fanaroff, AA, and Merkatz, IR: *Current concepts: The low birthweight infant: Evolution of a changing outlook.* N Engl J Med 301:1162, 1979.
4. Pape, K and Wigglesworth, JS: *Haemorrhage, Ischaemia and the Perinatal Brain.* Clinics in Developmental Medicine, No. 69/70. JB Lippincott, Philadelphia, 1979.
5. Mulligan, JC, et al: *Neonatal asphyxia. II. Neonatal mortality and long-term sequelae.* J Pediatr 96:903, 1980.
6. Brann, AW and Dykes, FD: *The effects of intrauterine asphyxia on the fullterm neonate.* Clin Perinatol 4:1249, 1978.
7. Finer, NN, et al: *Hypoxic-ischemic encephalopathy in term neonates: Perinatal factors and outcome.* J Pediatr 98:112, 1981.
8. Hill, A and Volpe, JJ: *Seizures, hypoxic-ischemic brain injury, and intraventricular hemorrhage in the newborn.* Ann Neurol 10:109, 1981.

9. Campbell, SK: *Effects of developmental intervention in the special care nursery.* In Wolraich, ML and Routh, D (eds): *The Advances in Developmental and Behavioral Pediatrics.* JAI Press, Greenwich, 1983.
10. Cornell, EH and Gottfried, AW: *Intervention with premature human infants.* Child Dev 47:32, 1976.
11. Field, T: *Supplemental stimulation of preterm neonates.* Early Hum Dev 4:301, 1980.
12. Masi, W: *Supplemental stimulation of the premature infant.* In Field, TM, et al (eds): *Infants Born at Risk: Behavior and Development.* SP Medical and Scientific Books, New York, 1979.
13. Leib, SA, Benfield, DG, and Guidabbaldi, J: *Effects of early intervention and stimulation on the preterm infant.* Pediatrics 66:83–90, 1980.
14. Field, TM, et al: *Teenage, lower-class, black mothers and their preterm infants: An intervention and developmental follow-up.* Child Dev 51:426–436, 1980.
15. Rice, RD: *The effects of the Rice Sensorimotor Stimulation Treatment on the development of high-risk infants.* Birth Defects 15:7–26, 1979.
16. Powell, LF: *The effect of extra stimulation and maternal involvement on the development of low-birth-weight infants and on maternal behavior.* Child Dev 45:106–113, 1974.
17. Scarr-Salapatek, S and Williams, ML: *The effects of early stimulation on low-birth-weight infants.* Child Dev 44:94–101, 1973.
18. Neal, MV: *Organizational behavior of the premature infant.* Birth Defects 15:43–60, 1979.
19. Brown, JV, et al: *Nursery based intervention with prematurely born babies and their mothers: Are there effects?* J Pediatr 97:478–481, 1980.
20. White, JL and Labarba, RC: *The effects of tactile and kinesthetic stimulation on neonatal development in the premature infant.* Dev Psychobiol 9:569–577, 1976.
21. Rosenfield, AG: *Visiting in the intensive care nursery.* Child Dev 51:939–941, 1980.
22. Long, JG, Philip, AGS, and Lucey, JF: *Excessive handling as a cause of hypoxemia.* Pediatrics 65:203, 1980.
23. Prechtl, HFR, Theorell, K, and Blair, AW: *Behavioral state cycles in abnormal infants.* Dev Med Child Neurol 15:606, 1973.
24. Prechtl, HFR, et al: *Postures, motility and respiration of low-risk pre-term infants.* Dev Med Child Neurol 21:3, 1979.
25. Brazelton, TB: *Neonatal Behavioral Assessment Scale.* Spastics International Medical Publications Monograph No. 50. William Heinemann, London, 1973.
26. Casear, P: *Postural Behavior in Newborn Infants.* Clinics in Developmental Medicine, No. 72. JB Lippincott, Philadelphia, 1979.
27. Saint-Anne Dargassies, S: *Neurological Development in the Full-Term and Premature Neonate.* Excerpta Medica, New York, 1977.
28. Wilhelm, IJ: *The neurologically suspect infant.* In Campbell, SK (ed): *Clinics in Physical Therapy: Pediatric Neurologic Disorders.* Churchill Livingstone, New York. (in press)
29. Als, H: *Assessing an assessment: Conceptual considerations, methodological issues, and a perspective on the future of the Neonatal Behavioral Assessment Scale.* In Sameroff, AJ (ed): *Organization and Stability of Newborn Behavior: A Commentary on the Brazelton Neonatal Behavior Assessment Scale.* Monogr Soc Res Child Dev 43:14, 1978.
30. Dubowitz, L and Dubowitz, V: *The Neurological Assessment of the Preterm and Full-term infant.* Clinics in Developmental Medicine, No 79. JB Lippincott, Philadelphia, 1981.
31. Bejar, R, et al: *Diagnosis and follow-up of intraventricular and intracerebral hemorrhages by ultrasound studies of infant's brain through the fontanelles and sutures.* Pediatrics 66:51, 1980.

BIBLIOGRAPHY

Avery, G: *Neonatology,* ed. 2. JB Lippincott, Philadelphia, 1981.

Brierley, JB and Meldrum, BS (eds): *Brain Hypoxia.* JB Lippincott, Philadelphia, 1971.

Campbell, SK and Wilhelm, IJ: *Developmental sequences in infants at high risk for central nervous system dysfunction: The recovery process in the first year of life.* In Stack, JM (ed): *The Special Infant: An Interdisciplinary Approach to the Optimal Development of Infants.* Human Sciences Press, New York, 1982.

Connolly, KJ and Prechtl, HFR (eds): *Maturation and Development: Biological and Psychological Perspectives.* Clinics in Developmental Medicine #77/78. William Heinemann, London, 1981.

Feldman, RG, Young, RR, and Koella, WP: *Spasticity: Disordered Motor Control.* Year Book Medical Publishers, Chicago, 1980.

PRECHTL, HFR: *The behavioral states of the newborn infant (a review).* Brain Res 76:184, 1974.

PRECHTL, HFR: *Assessment methods for the newborn infant: A critical evaluation.* In STRATTON, P (ED): *Psychobiology of the Human Newborn.* John Wiley & Sons, Chichester, 1982.

ST. JAMES-ROBERTS, I: *Neurological plasticity, recovery from brain insult, and child development.* Adv Child Dev Behav 14:253, 1979.

Chapter 13

CLINICAL DECISION MAKING: NEUROLOGIC DYSFUNCTION IN INFANCY

JANET E. YOUNG, M.D., P.T.

The spectrum of diagnosing, evaluating, and treating infants is a broad one, and I will not even attempt to cover all aspects of the subject. This chapter will focus on one rather specific etiologic consideration, albeit an increasingly common one: the at-risk premature infant.

Many infants who suffer apparently significant central nervous system (CNS) insults in the newborn period go on to develop with no apparent problems. Others may manifest a variety of mild or even questionable findings, many of which resolve over the next 12 to 18 months. Some of these infants may develop behavioral, learning, and/or coordination problems during the school years. The correlation between their early and later problems is just beginning to be examined.

The case to be examined in this chapter is a premature infant with documented significant CNS insult. The child manifested a variety of indicators of neurologic dysfunction in the first 6 months of life. These indicators included: (1) delayed disappearance of primitive reflexes, (2) tonal abnormalities, (3) asymmetries, (4) increased deep tendon reflexes, and (5) delayed appearance of postural mechanisms.

First, I will present some general diagnostic and etiologic considerations. Then, I will develop an operating framework for evaluation based on physiologic and developmental concepts. I will then examine the evaluation process and apply it to a case, and finally, I will begin to develop some treatment approaches based on this process.

DEFINITIONS

We are dealing with a spectrum of manifestations of insult to the very young nervous system. The actual nature of the insult can vary, partly depending on the infant's age at the time of the insult and partly depending on the specificity of the insult. The timing and duration of the insult may also play a role in determining the nature of the outcome. Toward one end of the spectrum of manifestations lies the clustering of symptoms and signs we typically associate with the static encephalopathies or cerebral palsy: abnormal deep tendon reflexes (DTRs); fixed abnormalities of tone, usually imbalance of flexor and extensor tone; fixed asymmetries; and movement disorders. These findings are permanent and do not disappear with age or even with treatment. At the other end of the spectrum are those symptoms or signs that may be called neurologic dysfunction or disorganization: transient tonal abnormalities, typically hypotonia; delayed integration of primitive reflexes; delayed emergence of postural mechanisms; and brisk DTRs. These findings are often transient and may disappear with maturation or treatment.

To make a firm diagnosis of cerebral palsy in the first year of life is often quite difficult because one cannot always be certain which infants will fall in the dysfunction category and which in the static encephalopathy, or truly abnormal, category. Even infants who manifest true tonal abnormalities or increased DTRs can show complete resolution of these findings. Perhaps true neurologic asymmetry, not to be confused with functional asymmetry, is the best indicator, but it may not always be present even in cases that eventually can be labeled as static encephalopathy.

ETIOLOGY

As noted above, we are talking about infants who were at risk in the perinatal period and who now manifest some degree of neurologic dysfunction. Prematurity is most certainly one of the more common causes. One of the biggest difficulties with premature infants illustrates the point:

> A newborn infant at 32 weeks of gestation had a relatively benign hospital course, requiring oxygen by hood for 3 to 4 days and gavage feeding for 1 week. The infant went home at 2 weeks of age, an apparently intact, healthy premature grower. At 10 months and 18 months, the child was noted to have significant neurologic abnormalities and developmental delays in all areas consistent with the diagnoses of severe cerebral palsy and severe mental retardation.
>
> Another infant born at 28 weeks of gestation had a complicated neonatal course that included a CNS bleed intubation and respirator support for 6 weeks. Total hospital time was 3 months. This infant was neurologically and developmentally normal in all areas at ages 9 months and 18 months.

Other etiologic factors may include birth complications, illnesses in early infancy, rare genetic factors, and unknown factors. Any factor that can influence the development of the brain prenatally, natally, or postnatally may have an effect on the neurologic function and organization of the young infant. It appears that the nature and degrees of the problems are not easily predicted.

PHYSIOLOGIC AND DEVELOPMENTAL PRINCIPLES

To distinguish abnormalities, dysfunctions, and deviations from normal, one must have a basic foundation in normal development. We must also be open to the possibility that some or all of the dysfunctional patterns we see in the growing premature infant are, in fact, "normal" physiologic responses to the insult of prematurity, for we do not yet know the natural history of this "disease."

We will operate on the basis of six developmental principles:

1. Development is a continuous process from conception to maturity.

The significance of a CNS insult can be quite different when it occurs to a very young, immature brain, than when it occurs to a more mature brain. For example, a stroke that occurs in an older person quite frequently may leave rather devastating loss of function. When that same stroke occurs in a newborn as a result of difficulties, there are typically minimal or even no long-term consequences to the young infant. We frequently refer to this quality of the young immature nervous system as "plasticity."

A second example of this plasticity is seen in the 18-month-old child who suffers a near drowning, is not breathing for at least 10 minutes, and once resuscitated, is neurologically quite disrupted, with coma, seizures, neurologic asymmetries, irritability, and agitation for perhaps 12 to 24 hours, then awakens and is normal by all neurologic standards.

It is well known that the immature, premature infant's brain is physically underdeveloped compared with the term infant's brain, and it is not difficult to imagine that early insults might be more easily overcome.

2. The sequence of development is the same for all children, but the rate may vary from child to child.

There may be some mild variations to this principle, but in general, infants learn to roll over before they learn to sit, before they learn to stand, and before they learn to walk. Any given child may skip a step or go back to pick one up out of sequence. In general, it is fair to say that there is an order that allows us to predict what probably comes next in the developmental sequence. One of the things we want to look for from a treatment intervention point of view is whether an infant deviates from that normal sequence, whether the infant is just delayed in that sequence, and if treatment will correct or reorder sequencing.

3. Development is intimately related to maturation of the CNS.

You cannot teach a 4-month-old infant to walk; the nervous system just has not matured enough. You may possibly be able to influence the rate of maturation but not increase it significantly. This principle is important when evaluating and establishing a treatment program in terms of what to realistically expect from a child. When we are dealing with premature infants, we must view them from their corrected developmental ages, not their chronologic ages.

4. **Generalized mass activity is replaced by specific individual responses.**

The newborn infant tends to respond with mass activity to any stimulus; for example, with a startle or a total flexion response. Gradually, with maturation, the responses become more selective. As examples, the 2-month-old infant will activate the hands to a visual stimulus, the 3- to 4-month-old infant will be able to reach, and the 6-month-old infant will grab and begin to manipulate.

5. **Development is in a cephalocaudal direction.**

Eye-hand coordination and upper-extremity skills develop before lower-extremity coordination and skills.

6. **The integration of the primitive reflexes and the appearance of postural mechanisms are intimately related to the acquisition of corresponding volitional movements.**

The term *reflex* refers to those responsive behaviors typically present at birth and capable of influencing movement and neuromotor development during the first several months of life. With maturation, they are gradually integrated and brought under the influence of higher centers of control, and they typically disappear by 4 to 6 months of age.

Reactions or *postural mechanisms* refer to those responsive behaviors that are typically not present at birth (the exception is the placing reaction) but that appear during the first year of life with maturation and remain with the person throughout life.

If there are factors that interfere with the maturation of the nervous system or that affect the integration of the various primitive reflexes, there may be interference with the appearance or influence of the emerging postural mechanisms on the function of the developing infant. If factors interfere with the interaction of these two systems, they can result in a significant effect on the volitional movement pattern of the infant. One of the basic premises of therapeutic intervention is that we can modify and affect the integration and influence of these reflexes and reactions and their effect on volitional movement. Primitive reflexes, although not always demonstrable in any given infant, probably serve an important role in the development of the infant. This is perhaps of phylogenic importance.

RELATIONSHIP BETWEEN TONE AND MOVEMENT

Movement is an extension of tone and posture and vice versa. Posture may be dictated by position and reflex activity, particularly if reflexes are obligatory. Tone may also be influenced by position and primitive reflexes. Tone can also be determined if a variety of areas of the brain are damaged. This occurrence will result in a predominance of certain tonal patterns unrelated to position, movement, or posture. For example, you may have an infant who manifests increased extensor tone in the supine position. This tone could result from tonic labyrinthine input being activated by the supine position. When this infant is turned over into the prone position, you may see tone either disappear or become increased into extension. Or the tone may be the result of a specific lesion and will be essentially unchanged in any position in which the infant is placed. You may also see an infant with basic underlying hypotonia who has increased tone only with attempts at movement. Premature infants who have spent most of their lives lying on their backs and intubated sometimes will develop opisthotonic posturing that may take weeks of therapy and repositioning to reverse. This occurrence may be the result of constant stimulation of the tonic labyrinthine reflex in the supine position.

"Normal" tone varies at different chronologic and gestational ages. The normal newborn is predominantly flexor in tone, and over the first 4 months develops increasingly controlled extensor tone. The increased flexor tone seen in the normal newborn may well be due to the flexion positioning in utero. The preterm infant is basically hypotonic and tends to posture in extension. If we allow this posture to go unopposed, we may see a picture of opisthotonic posturing, as discussed above.

It is important to make a distinction between resting tone and tone that exists with attempts at movement or changes of posture. Oftentimes, an infant will be basically hypotonic but will have increased tone with attempts at volitional movement. This superimposed abnormal tone will then interfere with normal movement patterns. Other times, abnormal tone will only show up in patterns elicited with the primitive reflexes. Both of these are quite different from infants who have abnormal tone even at rest. Their increased tone may be flexor, extensor, or a combination, but it is consistently present independent of posture or movement.

Typically, with premature infants we see a picture of underlying hypotonia with some superimposed increased extensor tone in the lower extremities and flexor tone in the upper extremities. We may also see the effects of various primitive reflexes. These tonal patterns tend to change with age; and it is possible that what we are seeing may, in fact, be recognized as the natural course of the ill premature infant. The more classic fixed abnormal tone patterns do not seem to show up until later; for example: (1) the hypertonia does not go away; (2) the increased extensor tone, believed to be due to posturing, in the unopposed supine position does not break up as expected; or (3) primitive reflexes do not become integrated, and they begin to dominate posture and tonal patterns as well as movement patterns. There is certainly a period of many months when the premature infant may demonstrate significant neurologic aberrations, but these stand a good chance of disappearing with time or intervention.

Earlier, a distinction was made between true abnormalities and neurologic dysfunction. It was noted that it is not easy to distinguish which infants will ultimately fall into these categories. We now see that as a frequent picture in the sick premature infant, and it may even be seen in the term infant who is stressed in the perinatal period. It may well be that the increased tone, the increased DTRs, and the delays in maturation are simply manifestations of a highly stressed, overstimulated, immature nervous system. It is obviously important to make a distinction between dysfunction and abnormality as soon as possible, for prognostic as well as diagnostic reasons. At the present time, we do not have reliable criteria for this distinction. Because of this difficulty in making an accurate early diagnosis, early treatment, using the diagnosis of neurologic dysfunction, should be encouraged. The diagnosis can be adjusted later as required.

EVALUATION PROCESS

The purpose of collecting data is to obtain a data base from which to draw conclusions; it is a means of assessing clinical problems and establishing whether there is a need for treatment and ongoing modification of a comprehensive treatment plan. There are, in my mind, four basic categories in which to collect data:

History: This should include existing medical records, previous evaluations, and an interview with the patient and/or family. What do you want to know? What records do you absolutely need? Who do you talk to? What is important information? How do you summarize and make sense out of the history?

Observation: This should include informal as well as formal evaluative tools. Observation should not only be of the patient but of the family as well, and interactions should occur with various persons in the environment. What is important to observe? How do you elicit the information needed? What tools do you use to facilitate observation? How do you sort out what is important?

Examination/Hands-on: This should include physical interaction with the patient. How do you get the data needed from an infant or young child? Is there anything special you expect to find?

Special tests/Other evaluations: This should include accessory but meaningful supplementary data. What do you want to know that is not available to you at the completion of your evaluation? How can you get it? From whom can you get these data? How do you obtain needed resources?

Having some format for each of these data collection areas is important. I use an outline for history taking that reminds me what to ask and whether it seems important at the time. I also use a format for observing and examining the infant. It does not matter what format you use as long as it allows you to gather the data you need to make your complete assessment of the patient. More data will need to be collected than will necessarily be used, but collect it all so that no important information is overlooked.

The history may sometimes be overwhelming. One should not get bogged down in details but rather should come away with a feel for the past and present medical pictures and an understanding of how the parents perceive the situation.

Observation of an infant is the most useful means of gathering objective data. Often, infants will not cooperate well during the hands-on evaluation. One can fine tune observation skills to the point of hardly needing to touch the infant to gather most data. By combining good observation skills with a knowledge of what data to obtain, including the interrelationships of reflexes, reactions, tone, posture, and movement, much can be accomplished in a short time. The use of age-appropriate toys and activities to facilitate movement and responses from the infant will further promote data collection. Infants may not always be cooperative, so it is wise to have a large repertoire of activities and techniques. Flexibility and adaptability are most helpful. If you are rigidly locked to a format of data collection, your ability to collect needed information may be limited accordingly.

One of the difficulties with observation is that it borders on being subjective, or at least tacit. I can look at an infant and make a comment about something I see, and a student will ask me how I know. I am often hard put to answer that question. Part of it is experience—an ability to integrate and intercept bits of data into a unified whole. It relates to knowing how to pick and choose what is important among a huge volume of data.

Hands-on evaluation is important because you can feel things you cannot see: subtle tensions, tonal patterns. Remember though, the mere act of touching the infant may put the infant into a state of stress and thus influence resting tone and movement patterns. Through handling, you can promote various movements or postures and begin to see the infant's response to being handled. In this sense, the evaluation can also be a treatment period.

The last area of data collection is special tests and evaluations. With the aid of these tests, you can fill in some of the missing areas of information. Are vision and hearing normal? What is the intellectual or language potential? What is the social situation? What is the infant's general health? All of these questions produce answers that may influence the infant's response to your treatment program.

In addition to knowing how to acquire needed information, one should be able to obtain it in the community. Is there a developmental clinic that can more fully evaluate the infant? Does the physician need to make the specific referral? What other options are available?

ASSESSMENT

This task is perhaps one of the most difficult in the evaluation process: interpreting and making some sense of all the data that has been collected. Thinking of assessment in terms of three objectives helps. One is to *identify the specific diagnostic issues* worthy of addressing. For you, this may already be done; and you can organize your findings accordingly, perhaps detailing or subcategorizing under broader, more general, diagnostic areas. The second objective is *to identify the specific problem areas* worthy of addressing in treatment. The third is to *identify areas requiring more information*—those unanswered questions.

Even using these guidelines, coping with large amounts of data can still be a problem and requires a certain amount of experience. It may be useful to relate the data to developmental theories, but here we must be careful. Others may not share our theories or agree with our categories. We must not be too rigid or locked into our own theories and interpretations. We must be willing to entertain new options as new data or theories come to our attention. We have looked at part of the basic theoretical framework that can be useful in interpreting data. There are more in-depth theories, and there are conflicting theories. It may not matter so much what framework you use as long as you understand it and can explain it to others so that they can also understand the basis of your interpretations. Remember, many of our evaluations and treatments are based on theory and are not necessarily agreed upon by all.

In examining the collected data, it is important to look for common threads. By sorting data into common problem areas, it may be easier to interpret and make sense of them. This process also enables you to see what additional information might be useful to complete your assessment and to define goals for a treatment program. Do you know all you need to know about the etiology of the problem, the appropriate diagnosis, and related problems, including family and social issues? Do you know how and where to get the missing information?

TREATMENT PLAN

Working from my problem list is an easy way to set up a treatment plan. Some of you will have many problems (splitters), others only a few (lumpers). Your approach is important as long as it makes sense to you, and you can develop treatment approaches around your various problem areas. Remember too, with infants, treatment is really an extension of evaluation, and it is imperative to continually re-evaluate your treatment and to modify it accordingly.

Your problem areas can be rewritten as goals. Then specific objectives can be identified for each, with the treatment procedure selected accordingly.

CASE PRESENTATION

The infant underwent a 28-week gestation period and is now 6 months old. The infant was treated for hyaline membrane disease, with respirator therapy for 6 weeks and oxygen for another 2 months for bronchopulmonary dysplasia. The infant had a grade III intraventricular hemorrhage. The infant was discharged at 3 months. Physical therapy was initiated at 6 weeks for opisthotonic posturing, which responded rapidly to therapy except for some lingering increased extensor tone unrelated to reflex postures or position.

EXAMPLE OF ASSESSMENT AND TREATMENT GOALS AND OBJECTIVES

Findings:

- lack of head control
- lack of flexion
- clonus
- shoulder retraction
- paucity of movement
- asymmetry (asymmetrical tonic neck reflex)
- disorganization of movement

Diagnosis: Neuromotor dysfunction manifesting as increased extensor tone, asymmetries, and delayed motor development.

Interpretive Comments: Development is overall delayed and disorganized even for her corrected age of 3 months. There are no specific hard-core neurologic abnormalities, but concern exists about the persistence of increased extensor tone and asymmetry in spite of 3 months of treatment. The oral-motor problems may lead to later articulation problems. This infant's overall intellectual potential is good.

Treatment Goals and Objectives

1. Decrease overall abnormal extensor tone. Promote flexor tone and more normal extensor tone both as a basis for maintaining posture and to provide a stable base on which to superimpose movement.
2. Decrease asymmetry with subsequent facilitation of midline activities.
   a. Maintain protraction of shoulders for several minutes while engaging in midline play in supported sitting—4 weeks.
   b. Maintain shoulder protraction in assisted rolling—4 weeks.

Be careful about getting locked into a static treatment program. Part of what we are promoting is changes of posture, as well as stability and function within a posture. Most young infants are not going to tolerate a static treatment program anyway because they become bored or stressed quickly. It may be necessary to provide the posture and stability for the infant and then work on promoting movement.

Remember that with infants, unlike older children and adults, you will see rapid changes and responses to treatment, and your treatment program is an ongoing evaluation and updating. The general overall goals will remain the same over fairly long periods of time, but the more specific objectives may change rapidly. What you choose to work on next is partly determined by the progress the infant is making in each goal area, as well as by maturation and developmental sequence.

When you are not making expected headway on an objective, it is important to examine why. Is it an inappropriate objective or unrealistic expectation? Have you selected the wrong treatment technique? Are there extenuating circumstances? One explanation often rendered is that therapy does not work. To me, the main thing that justifies therapy is having a rationale—a theoretical framework from which to operate. By selecting goals and objectives that fit into this framework and by applying treatment techniques that make sense within this same rationale, we can begin to objectively measure our successes and failures.

It is inadvisable to draw conclusions that the specific treatment technique directly caused the accomplishment of the objective; however, with input, we can influence tone, promote the integration of primitive reflexes, and facilitate the emergence of the various postural mechanisms. There is absolutely no proof for these beliefs, but it is sensible within the theoretical rationale we have presented. As long as we operate within this rationale, we can justify what we do and can monitor whatever results we see. The day may well come when we will change the rationale because we see a new piece of information that tells us that the way we have been operating is not working, and in fact, we make subtle changes all the time. We should not become so attached to our rationale that we use it whether or not it works. Nor is it wise to have a treatment approach that we either do not understand or for which we have no rationale.

SUMMARY

Some of the etiologic and diagnostic considerations relating to neurologic dysfunction in infancy were reviewed. I have made a careful distinction between dysfunction and true abnormality. The patterns seen in the typical ill premature infant as the infant develops are initially those of dysfunction. We do not have an accurate means of predicting those infants who will continue to have problems that can later be labeled static encephalopathy.

I have developed a rationale of neuromotor development in the infant that relates maturation of the various reflex behaviors and postural mechanisms, tone, and posture, to the acquisition of normal volitional movement patterns and postural control. A case was analyzed and a treatment program was developed relating to the rationale of neuromotor development. The importance of having a rationale for evaluation and treatment was emphasized.

Chapter 14

CLINICAL DECISION MAKING: SPORTS PHYSICAL THERAPY

PHILLIP B. DONLEY, M.S., P.T., A.T., C.
RONALD G. PEYTON, M.S., P.T., A.T., C.

To be comfortable with and most productive in the decision-making process in sports physical therapy, it is essential that clinicians have the areas of responsibility clearly defined and that all of the individuals with whom they interact be aware of their capabilities.

Working circumstances for the sports physical therapist may fall into any one of the following settings:

1. educational institutions
   a. college settings
   b. high school settings
2. professional sports
3. sports medicine clinics and/or centers
4. private practice as a sports physical therapist
5. physician's office—serving independently or in conjunction with other sports-related health care specialists.

In each of these settings, there must be well-defined areas of responsibility for the sports physical therapist. It is best if there is a written contractual arrangement that identifies the scope of the responsibilities. In most states, a physician will serve as the respondent superior for the actions of the sports physical therapist. It is, therefore, vital that a written agreement between these two be arranged.

Sports physical therapy has many characteristics that are quite different from the usual physical therapy setting. It requires independent action and many skills not usually taught in the physical therapy curriculum. There must be a clear definition of the independent actions and skills, and they must be agreed upon by the physician and the sports physical therapist.

The competencies for sports physical therapy have been identified, and a national board test will be forthcoming.[1] In the future, it will be imperative that those who purport to be sports physical therapists do, in fact, possess these competencies. The sports medicine physician can only be comfortable as the respondent superior if the skills are present.

Standard operating procedures for emergency care, return to play, referral to other physical therapists or other health care specialists, disqualifying conditions, injury screening, and other additional circumstances as they arise will all need to be developed. These standard operating procedures will facilitate the decision-making process and encourage independent action, such as applying casts, aspirating cauliflower ears, reducing dislocations, dispensing medications, and so forth. The standard operating procedures and/or contract must be reviewed.

Several areas of responsibility have already been identified and are being performed by athletic trainers and sports physical therapists who work in close contact with athletes.[2] One of these areas is the prevention of athletic injuries and includes: (1) conditioning, (2) the safety of both the practice and competition areas, and (3) diet. Emergency care procedures is another area, and the sports physical therapist must become certified in both first aid and cardiopulmonary resuscitation. An area to which physical therapists have had very little exposure is the first evaluation for an acute problem, where the severity of the injury or illness is evaluated during an initial screening process. To facilitate the early return of the athlete to competition, the initial treatment will often be initiated without a physician evaluation. This means that the sports physical therapist must make judgments about the seriousness of the injury and must determine whether the injury can be treated without physician evaluation or referral. In addition, the sports physical therapist may be responsible for changing treatment without consulting the physician. The optimal arrangement for the therapist is to have the sports medicine physician available when needed but not constantly present. Rehabilitation progression must be the responsibility of the sports physical therapist.

The physician takes care of the acute care and turns the athlete over to the sports physical therapist when it is time to start sports physical therapy. It is then the responsibility of the sports physical therapist to prepare the athlete for full return to competitive practice. When these clearly defined lines are drawn, all of the members of the sports medicine team—the physician, the sports physical therapist, and the coach—will better understand their roles, and the athletes will have less confusion as they move toward full competition.[3]

One of the unique characteristics of sports physical therapy, which is a by-product of the evolution of the athletic training profession, is the athletes' broad-based knowledge before they become patients. In the past, this component was an unorganized process in which the knowledge was obtained through informal daily contact and incidental conversation. The athletes' medical histories became common knowledge to the trainers as they became more familiar with the athletes. As a result of this interchange, the athletes learned to trust, respect, and look to the trainers for all of their health care needs. The team physicians were not physically present on a daily basis. They were, however, available when the trainers needed them. It was the trainers' responsibility to screen all injuries and illnesses and to refer those needing medical assistance to the physicians. The athletes became very comfortable in this environment because there was someone who knew them and their medical histories, knew and understood their athletic stressors, and was available at almost any hour.

Today, if sports physical therapists are to gain the same trust and confidence from the athletes, the athletes' pasts must be known, and an appreciation of how the past impacts on their present and future athletic participation must be rendered.

Presently, formalized preseason screening is being performed to obtain a more complete health information base for each athlete. It is not a substitute for personal contact but is intended to enhance it. There is still a need for an in-depth knowledge of each sport's characteristics and for the physical presence of a clinical practitioner (sports physical therapist).

CASE HISTORY 1

The only unique characteristic of this particular case history is that considerable time was taken to prepare it for public consumption. The same kind of decision-making process is taking place each day by athletic trainers and sports physical therapists in their respective work areas. It is performed on several athletes at a time from a variety of sports. It becomes part of the daily norm of "business as usual." Very little is formalized with regard to the collection of the data, and most of it is collected informally and stored almost subconsciously by the practitioner for future reference. It is used much like the intuition that an experienced athlete draws upon during competition. This hidden "bag of tricks" is possessed by a good, experienced clinical practitioner in sports physical therapy.

A sample medical history form is shown in Appendix 1 at the end of this chapter. Keep in mind that once the information has been supplied by the athlete, the sports physical therapist is then responsible for reviewing this history with the athlete. The medical history form in this chapter is not intended to be a model but is the result of many continuing revisions. The case study athlete's responses follow. It represents the first assessment of the patient and was performed in September 1980.

Jack S., a 20-year-old white male wrestler who was 5 feet 11 inches tall and weighed 180 pounds, answered items number 3, 23, 24, 25, 35, and 36 positively. What are the implications? What decisions need to be made?

Item 3: At age 13, he had pneumonia in the left lower lobe, with no serious consequences; however, because wrestling is an endurance sport, this element within the medical history could present problems. Endurance training in the form of outdoor running in cold weather could create respiratory difficulty. The indoor endurance work is often conducted in dusty, dry air during winter months and could present respiratory problems.

Item 23: The back is a frequently abused area in wrestling. The strength training programs wrestlers undertake often involve heavy lifting, which can strain a healthy back. An interview with the athlete to explore this is necessary.

Item 24: We should defer this to questioning later for more details in the medical management.

Item 25: If vigorous exercise and/or heavy lifting cause pain in the back, a detailed evaluation of the back by the therapist is necessary.

Item 35: An interview revealed the following history: Jack hyperextended his back in a wrestling meet in June 1979. He had less pain as he got warmed up in subsequent workouts. Roentgenograms were negative. By August 1, 1979, he had pain radiating down his left leg and into his foot. On August 19, 1979, he had a laminectomy with removal of the L4-5 disk. He was discharged from the hospital on August 24, 1979, with few or no directions for back care. He entered college in September and was wrestling by November 15, 1979. He continued to have soreness after workouts. However, different joints were also sore after workouts, for a variety of reasons.

Item 36: Tetanus shots are usually given to athletes when wounds require stitches. It is wise to know the date of the last booster so that excessive shots are not given.

What plans must the sports physical therapist now make to ensure that this medical history information becomes a valuable part of the athlete's conditioning for wrestling? The following plan was instituted:

> *Examine the Low Back.* The findings of the examination showed limited active motion in both right and left lateral flexion. Flexion, extension, right and left rotation, and passive spring testing of the lumbar vertebrae revealed hypomobility at all levels. Sacroiliac testing was negative. Reflexes were normal, with no unilateral differences. He had tight hamstrings bilaterally and tight hip flexors and lumbar extensors. There was no leg length difference and no scoliosis.

What actions should have been taken by the sports physical therapist? In light of the above data, the action taken was to provide flexibility exercises for the hamstrings, hip flexors, and the lumbar spine in all planes. The exercises were a combination of static stretching techniques and PNF exercises using the buddy system.

In addition to the medical history, a physical examination has always been a part of pre–sports participation for some sports. This has been improving in content, scope, and skills of application with the advent of mass physical examinations with a variety of health care specialists administering the examination. With such a mechanism, participants in all sports, both men and women in a particular school or professional team, can be screened in a short period of time. This provides a rich data base for the sports physical therapist to further plan for and administer to the health needs of the athlete. It is, however, not a substitute for frequent personal contact and private interviews.

Jack's physical examination (Appendix 2 at the end of this chapter) was performed several days after the medical history questionnaire was completed but was prior to the start of wrestling practice on October 15. Wrestlers usually work out on their own most of the year, but the official NCAA date for beginning formal coaching is October 15. The assessment at this particular time again revealed that Jack was 5 feet 11 inches tall, weighed 180 pounds, and was a white male wrestler who had 13-percent body fat. This may have presented a problem because he wanted to continue to wrestle in the 158-pound class. He had to lose 8 percent of his body fat to achieve a more reasonable 4- or 5-percent body fat by his first match in December

1980.[4] A loss of 8 percent fat would have lowered his weight to 166 pounds. He would then have needed to lose 8 pounds of water to reach 158 pounds, not an unreasonable task. He therefore had until December to lose 14 pounds of fat, allowing him an 8-pound drift for water. He was very comfortable with and careful in maintaining reasonable eating habits, fluid balance, and electrolyte balance. His blood pressure was 113/80, with a pulse rate of 56 beats per minute. His urinalysis, eyes, teeth, gums, neck, chest, back, heart, lungs, axillary nodes, abdomen hernias, inguinal nodes, skin, and genitalia were all within normal limits. His nose had a left deviation of the septum, which forced him to breathe through his mouth most of the time. His left ear was more cauliflowered than his right, which almost occluded his external acoustic meatus and caused frequent external ear impactions of wax and subsequent infections. This last item will present some problems and needs to be dealt with by the sports physical therapist. What should the plan of action be?

The action taken was to add him to the list of wrestlers who might have to be seen by the sports physical therapist for ear aspiration and packing. He also was sent to the infirmary on a monthly basis for an ear irrigation to prevent wax accumulation. In both cases, there was no need for a physician referral or for a physician to examine the patient. The team physician had already given permission to the sports physical therapist to manage cauliflower ear problems as they occurred.

The posture examination revealed a mild genu varum bilaterally and pes planus bilaterally as seen in the front view. The back view revealed ankle valgus on the right. The side view revealed a total weight shift forward on the foot, placing all segments in front of the line of gravity. In addition, he had decreased thoracic and lumbar curves and an increased cervical curve, forward head, and flexed knees. His gait was a toe-out, flat-footed pattern, with little or no thrust at push off. What did this posture examination reveal that required subsequent action?

The action taken was to conduct a test of Feiss' line to the medial longitudinal arches to determine if pes planus was structural or functional.[5] It was functional, with the right navicular bone dropping lower than the left. Because of ankle valgus, the subtalar motions were measured as follows: inversion on the right was 25 degrees and on the left, 15 degrees; eversion on the right was –5 degrees and on the left, –10 degrees. These findings indicated not only a decrease of motion but also a marked imbalance, since usual inversion and eversion ratio is 2 to 1, or 20 degrees inversion to 10 degrees eversion.[6] Should this wrestler be referred to a sports podiatrist? The rationale for asking this question is that a functional flat foot frequently causes shin splints,[7] and the intensity of running for endurance work, as well as for weight loss, of wrestlers is very high. The decision made, in this case, was not to refer him to a sports podiatrist because he had no acute symptoms.

Orthopaedic stability testing revealed decreased joint play in the shoulders, knees, and ankles. These are the only joints tested routinely in this physical examination format. The implications of such findings are that we would not expect this athlete to be susceptible to dislocations or sprains in these joints because of their high degree of stability. In fact, they were restricted in motion as opposed to being hypermobile.

Flexibility tests of all movements were evaluated with active motions only. However, because this athlete had so many limitations, almost every

TABLE 14-1. Results of Flexibility Tests

The neck had 15 degrees of right lateral flexion, and 10 degrees of left lateral flexion; 60 degrees of flexion, and 50 degrees of extension; 65 degrees of right rotation, and 80 degrees of left rotation. The trunk had 30 degrees of right lateral flexion, and 20 degrees of left lateral flexion; 45 degrees of right rotation, and 60 degrees of left rotation; 50 degrees of flexion, and 20 degrees of extension. The shoulder had 20 degrees of hyperextension; 140 degrees of flexion; 25 degrees of right internal rotation, and 20 degrees of left internal rotation; 35 degrees of right external rotation, and 25 degrees of left external rotation. The elbow extended to 0 degrees, with 120 degrees of flexion and no hyperextension. In addition, the carrying angle was negative bilaterally. The forearm had 80 degrees of supination and 90 degrees of pronation bilaterally. Wrist flexion on the right was 30 degrees, and on the left, 60 degrees; extension was 65 degrees bilaterally. Hip flexion was 115 degrees and extension 0 degrees bilaterally. Hip medial rotation on the right was 20 degrees, and on the left, 15 degrees; lateral rotation was 25 degrees on the right, and 30 degrees on the left; abduction was 45 degrees bilaterally; adduction was 15 degrees bilaterally. The hamstrings on both sides lacked 30 degrees of motion. Knee extension was 0 degrees bilaterally. Knee flexion was 120 degrees on the right, and 115 degrees on the left; external rotation was 30 degrees on the right, and 25 degrees on the left; internal rotation was 30 degrees bilaterally. Ankle dorsiflexion was 0 degrees bilaterally. Ankle plantar flexion was 30 degrees on the right, and 40 degrees on the left. Strength test revealed no weaknesses and no unilateral differences.

joint was restricted. His motion was measured with a goniometer.[8] The results are shown in Table 14-1.

The next decision for the sports physical therapist was to determine what had to be done, based on these findings, relative to the conditioning and preparation of this athlete for wrestling. The plan of action taken was to institute a general flexibility exercise program for the whole body, which was to be performed before and after strength training sessions and also on all other days of the week. These were general types of exercises, and there were no unusual, specific techniques.

The fitness assessment on Jack provided the following information:

1. The *12-minute walk/run test,* or *Cooper test* (a standard for wrestlers at West Chester): The distance that must be covered is 2 miles, which predicts roughly 60 ml/Kg/min of oxygen uptake and is excellent for endurance.[9] Jack ran 2.25 miles, far in excess of the minimum required for the preseason assessment.
2. The *vertical jump,* also known as the *sergeant jump test:* This test is given because it appears to be the single best indicator of general motor ability.[10] It is based on considerable unpublished data from West Chester State College testing as well as on unpublished opinions of professional sports scouts. A 24-inch jump ranks in the 80th percentile of all college-aged men[11] and is considered as minimal for West Chester wrestlers. Jack jumped 16 inches.
3. *Parallel bar dips:* These dips estimate shoulder girdle strength and endurance.[12] The standard for preseason testing is 20 repetitions. Jack did 30 repetitions.
4. *Pull-ups:* This task tests shoulder girdle and elbow strength and endurance.[13] The standard is 15 repetitions. Jack did 23 repetitions. Both the dips and pull-up scores are important for comparison to subsequent scores if the shoulder or upper extremity is injured in

the future. A return to the standard or 80 percent of actual scores is necessary to return to full wrestling practice.

5. *Sit-ups:* This exercise measures abdominal strength and endurance.[14] The standard is 80 repetitions in 2 minutes. Jack did 100 repetitions.

The overall orthopaedic assessment revealed that Jack was a strong and well athlete with excellent endurance. He had severe flexibility problems requiring intensive work and additional preventive exercises for his low back.

The following related medical history should be available to the sports physical therapist. The right ankle injury occurred in March 1981. Prior to the ankle injury, seven different injuries occurred that resulted in the loss of wrestling time for 12 days and required 96 treatments, 37 of which were for low back pain. This is an average injury rate and treatment frequency for wrestlers, who as a group, average 14-percent time loss for injury during the course of a season. Wrestling has been the most hazardous sport at West Chester for the past 17 years. Only football comes close in terms of time loss, which is 7 to 8 percent per year.[15]

Additional information of importance in Jack's sports-participation history. Jack had 4 years of high school wrestling, with a record of 88 wins, 14 losses, and 2 draws. He had 2 years of college wrestling, with a record of 65 wins and 7 losses. He ran cross-country in the 9th and 10th grades but gave it up because of shin splints. He was a transfer student whose primary interest in wrestling, aside from the pleasure and notoriety it gave him, was the impact it could have on helping him locate a good coaching and teaching job after graduation. He was a B+ student. He had average pain tolerance. His personality was one of a friendly, mild, outgoing person, and he was fairly confident about his abilities both in and out of sports. He was strongly motivated to wrestle and was considered to be mentally tough—a term that implies the ability to persist during difficult times. He had been competing in wrestling at the top of the collegiate levels for the past two seasons. He had no drug habit and did not smoke. He consumed mild amounts of alcoholic beverages during the off season. Knowledge of this information is important for the sports physical therapist to effectively deal with future medical problems. Once filed away in the subconscious, it becomes readily available during a crisis and is necessary for proper planning to prevent health problems and to respond to a crisis situation.

A description of the case injury follows. On March 13, 1981, during Jack's second match in the NCAA, Division I, wrestling tournament (he won his first bout earlier in the day), within seconds of the end of the first period and while kneeling on his right knee, his right ankle was forced into plantar flexion inversion as his buttock was forced against his heel. He continued to wrestle and finished the period but then called for an injury time-out. It should be noted at this point that a maximum of 2 minutes is allowed for injury management during a wrestling bout.[16] If, at the end of 2 minutes, the athlete is unable to continue, he is disqualified. The first decision the sports physical therapist had to make was how to best evaluate this injury, and what to do if it was decided to allow him to continue. The 2 minutes is the total permitted time-out for an entire match. The therapist would not want to use more time than was necessary in case it would be needed later in the match, providing the therapist allows the athlete to continue.

Appendix 3 at the end of this chapter is a checklist of important items to evaluate in ankle injuries. The sports physical therapist had to determine which of the items on the checklist should be evaluated in this particular case, given the 2-minute time constraint. Keep in mind that much of the information requested in this checklist is already mentally filed away because of previous evaluation by observing the match.

The first decision rendered was to examine the ankle with the shoe and sock on because there was insufficient time to remove them, evaluate, and replace them if needed before the injury time ran out.

Each of the items evaluated is indicated with an A or B. If the item has a letter A, it means that it was chosen to be evaluated first, in this case because of the time constraint and the previous history. The letter B is used to indicate those additional items that were evaluated later, such as on the sidelines or in the locker room, when time was not a factor.

The results of the physical examination revealed that:

> The lateral malleolus had a 1+ tenderness. The anterior tibiofibular ligament had a 3+ tenderness. The anterior talofibular ligament had a 1+ tenderness, and the capsule had a 1+ tenderness. Active motion of plantar flexion and inversion revealed 2+ pain in both motions. Passive motion in dorsiflexion had a 1+ pain, and passive plantar flexion 2+ with passive inversion 3+. It is significant to note that there was no support on the ankle and that stability tests and fracture tests were negative. Muscle tests for dorsiflexion, plantar flexion, inversion, and eversion were all 1+ for pain. Functional tests were performed. Heel raisers were normal. Jack was able to hop with a mild decrease in height on one foot. He was able to walk without any problem. However, to be able to make sharp change in direction or to take two or three running steps presented some problem.

Based on this information, the next decisions to be made were to determine the degree of this injury and what was to be the next plan of action. It was decided that this injury was a first-degree sprain of the anterior tibiofibular and talofibular ligaments with minor physical impairment. The plan of action was to tape the ankle over the wrestling shoe and allow him to continue if he so desired. He said that he wished to continue and the coach agreed. The match went on with 15 seconds left for injury time.

Jack lost the match but had no further problem with his ankle and required no additional injury time. He now had an opportunity to wrestle again if his victor won his next match. Under these circumstances, he would then enter the consolation bracket, or the so-called "wrestle-back bracket," to determine third and fourth and lower places in the final standings. In essence, this tournament was a form of double elimination for places after first and second.

The next decisions that had to be made were as follows: (1) What additional evaluation measures were necessary? (2) What emergency care was necessary? (3) Should a physician be consulted? and (4) What treatment was necessary? The action taken was to undress the ankle. Those items on the ankle injury checklist that were marked with a letter B were then evaluated. We were now ready to use the SOAP format.[17] *S:* There were no new symptoms. *O:* There was no new information. *A:* This was considered to be a first-degree sprain of the anterior tibiofibular ligament. *P:* Consult with a tournament physician to reassure the sports physical therapist and the wrestler. Treatment was instituted with ice for 30 minutes on and 30 minutes off. Since walking was not painful, no crutches were necessary, but the ankle was taped and directions were given to stay off of his feet until it was known whether or not he had to wrestle the next day.

Jack's victor won his next bout, so Jack had to make weight by 11 PM to qualify to wrestle the next day. He needed to lose 5 pounds. The next decision facing the sports physical therapist was: What was the best way for him to lose 5 pounds without aggravating his ankle? Should he run, skip rope, or do form wrestling (which is also known as "rolling around" with his partner)? The action taken was to allow him to "roll around" because there was less stress on the ankle and more general body movement to encourage water loss under the plastic suit. The ankle was taped. He made weight. He was then instructed to continue his ice applications over the tape. He was given no medication.

March 14, 1981, 10:30 AM: *S:* Jack had mild general pain and moderate point tenderness over the anterior tibiofibular ligament. He could not push off hard; in other words, he was unable to plantar flex forcibly against resistance, that is, against another wrestler. *O:* There was no change. *A:* This was considered to be a first-degree sprain of the anterior tibiofibular ligament with general soreness due to the inflammation. *P:* What decisions now had to be made? Which physical agent should be used for pain relief? What would be the best method of support during the match? The decision was to use electroacupuncture for the relief of pain because: (1) a machine was available to treat another wrestler who had a 2-week-old undisplaced fracture of his right eighth rib and had been able to practice without limitation following treatments; (2) the half life of beta-endorphin is longer than the endogenous opiates activated with the TENS portion of the same unit. Also, the hyperstimulation analgesia activates ACTH—an anti-inflammatory agent;[18] and (3) ice applied for 20 minutes provides a limited analgesic effect.

He was taped with a Gibney pattern using heel locks, reinforced with moleskin stirrups and Elastikon to check-strap both inversion and eversion. Function was then checked with the tape in place and presented no problem.

He lost the match, but the ankle did not seem to be a major factor. It was, in fact, a mild irritant. He was able to jog, hop, make quick lateral moves, but not "drive off" when pushing against his opponent.

His season was now over. At the post-match evaluation, *S, O,* and *A* showed no change. *P:* Jack's ankle was to remain taped for 1 week, and he was to continue his ice treatment one to two times per day. He would be re-evaluated in 1 week.

On March 23, 1981, he reported to the training room with the following information. *S:* He reinjured his ankle while wrestling in preparation for an AAU match. Wrestlers never have a true off season. There are all kinds of post-season tournaments, and they enjoy working out with one another from time to time to break up the monotony of off-season conditioning programs. It also serves as an opportunity to learn new skills. *O:* There was no change except for increased point tenderness over the anterior tibiofibular ligament. *A:* This appeared to be an aggravation of his unhealed first-degree sprain. *P:* Which physical agents are now most indicated? The action taken was to use contrast baths, which would more effectively utilize the Gate theory of reducing pain, and to use electroacupuncture for the reasons stated earlier.[18] Ultrasound in combination with cortisone cream was also utilized to decrease the local inflammation.[19]

On April 6, 1981, the following was observed: *S:* There was no improvement. *O:* There was no change. *A:* Although running backward is not a usual activity for wrestling, this patient was so tested, and the result was pain similar to that felt with a hard "push off." A rupture of the ankle capsule causes such a symptom. Our experience with such cases (three football players and one basketball player) was that they all had this one common symptom; however, they had no pain with any other movement. The older literature and the experience of Dr. M.L. Levy[20] of the New York Nets professional basketball team suggest that such a rupture is likely with repeated ankle sprains. Jack did not have a history of ankle sprains; however, it seemed possible that he had a tear of the ankle capsule. Was this the time to refer him to an orthopaedic surgeon for roentgenograms and/or an arthrogram to look for possible chondral fracture of the dome of the talus and/or a rupture of the capsule? The action taken was to refer him to our team orthopaedist, who has had experience with both types of problems among our athletes. Jack was instructed to use contrast baths if he had persistent pain.

On April 10, 1981, the following was observed: *S:* There was no change in symptoms. *O:* Plain roentgenograms and the arthrogram were negative. *A:* The physician and the sports physical therapist agreed that the condition was an unhealed first-degree sprain of the anterior tibiofibular ligament. *P:* Should Jack be placed in a walking cast, or could he be trusted to limit his activities and be held firm with tape? In general, my experience dictates that athletes respond better in these cases if they are casted. However, in this case, the physician decided to use taping. Jack's ankle was taped for 3 weeks, providing 24-hour-a-day support. The tape was changed every 3 days, and no athletic activity was permitted.

On May 5, 1981, the following was observed: Summer vacation time was near, and an off-season conditioning program had to be designed. *S:* There was no change in his symptoms. He tried to "roll around," with some pain in the usual "push off" positions. *O:* There was no change. *A:* Jack's ankle should have been healed; but the question remained: why did he still have pain? *P:* Decisions had to be made regarding the direction of the summer conditioning program and how much wrestling Jack could undertake. The action taken was to institute the regular conditioning program given to the other wrestlers. Jack was advised to perform wrestling drills but not to engage in live, competitive wrestling. He was also sent to a sports medicine podiatrist. The podiatrist's opinion was that Jack's restricted subtalar motion was not directly related to his present symptoms. It was decided that there was no necessity for sport-thotics at this time.

As of September 8, 1981, Jack had been treated eight times over the summer. Each time he had been given cortisone, ultrasound, and electroacupuncture. He tried to wrestle four or five times during the summer and had the same symptoms each time. He was discouraged and scared that this situation might not improve and that it could have a very negative influence on the upcoming season. *S:* There appeared to be no change. *O:* There was no change. *A:* There must be something we had overlooked. *P:* What next?

Jack had not had a significant change since the original injury occurred. What were the options? The action taken was to seek a second opinion. Our team orthopaedist had no problem with this decision, so there was no need to ask him. The wrestler was sent to a second orthopaedist, who was located at a sports medicine center and had done a lot of arthroscopic surgery on knees and ankles.

On September 10, 1981, arthroscopic surgery was performed on Jack's right ankle. A small, dime-sized chondral defect on the anterolateral aspect of the talar dome was observed. Curettage and drilling were performed on the defect through a new incision. A portion of the adjacent synovium was removed. Jack was casted for 2 weeks with a short leg walking cast. What new plan of action should the sports physical therapist have taken? He was to instruct Jack in the weight training of all his well parts and also to ride a bicycle dynamometer with the cast in place, at 600 KPM for 10 minutes daily.

On September 25, 1981, the following was observed. *S:* The cast had been removed and Jack had a general sensation of stiffness but no pain. *O:* He lacked 10 degrees of plantar flexion and 5 degrees of dorsiflexion and had 5 degrees of both inversion and eversion. There was no swelling, and there was mild point tenderness over the incision. *A:* This was a common post-cast ankle with the usual amount of strength and range of motion restrictions. *P:* What kind of rehabilitation program was needed? The action taken was to use contrast baths to stimulate his circulation and decrease his discomfort. The Elgin ankle exercise machine was used to gain range of motion and to strengthen the ankle. We continued to use weight training for all of the well parts. He was taped when walking to heighten his sense of security. He was placed on a bicycle ergometer at 600 KPM for 15 minutes daily, which raised his exercise heart rate to 160 beats per minute.

On October 8, 1981, the following was observed: There were only 7 days until the official start of wrestling practice, and Jack was becoming a little edgy because of his desire to get back to competitive wrestling practice. *S:* There was no discomfort. There were good confidence and high expectations. *O:* The motion was back to presurgical levels. *A:* This had been excellent progress, and we continued on the same level. *P:* What decisions needed to be made? The action taken was to start proprioceptive training on the biomechanical disk for range of motion and strength, in addition to the Elgin ankle exercise program. Weight training for all the well parts was continued, and the intensity of the bicycle work was increased to 750 KPM for 15 minutes, with a target heart rate of 180 beats per minute. Orthotron exercises were given for the ankle, in both plantar flexion and dorsiflexion, with a setting of 3 on the speed control for 10 repetitions of 3 sets. Heel raisers and Achilles' stretch were also added.

On October 13, 1981, the following was observed. *S:* Very positive attitude and no pain. *O:* Complete range of motion. *A:* It was time to increase the work load. *P:* What decisions needed to be made? The action taken was to bicycle for 20 minutes at 750 KPM with a heart rate target of 180 beats per minute. Increase the disk height to 3 inches. Rope skip on both the injured foot and on both feet. Continue the weight training for the well parts. No wrestling was permitted until functional testing on October 20.

On October 20, 1981, the following was observed: *S:* Jack could not wait to wrestle. *O:* Jack passed all functional tests, which included hopping, jogging, sprinting, and carioca drills, without tape. Cybex tests were performed at 30 degrees per second. Scores were: dorsiflexion—right 14, left 12; plantar flexion—right 60, left 42. At 180 degrees per second, dorsiflexion—right 4, left 2; plantar flexion—right 14, left 5. Assessment was that Jack was ready for full wrestling practice. *P:* Return to wrestling full speed with tape on the ankle.

On November 3, 1981, the following was observed: *S:* Jack had no pain with any movement or activity. *O:* Cybex tests were performed at 30 degrees per second: dorsiflexion—right 16, left 15; plantar flexion—right 64, left 72. At 180 degrees per second: dorsiflexion—right 4, left 4; plantar flexion—right 28, left 20. *A:* Complete recovery from successful surgery. *P:* Tape the ankle for practice and competition for 6 to 8 months. This was the probable time required for complete healing and strength of ligamentous and capsular tissues.[20]

The total number of treatment visits after the cast was removed was 4 in September, 22 in October, 24 in November, 18 in December, and 9 in January. He had no recurrence of ankle pain all season. Cybex tests at the end of the season were not significant because he injured his left ankle in much the same fashion and had the same symptoms and signs as the right ankle injury.

CLINICAL PROGNOSIS

It is the general impression of orthopaedic surgeons and sports physical therapists that the ankles and adjacent joints allow no freedom for slack motion or excursion to take up the impingement forces of bones when the joints are torqued at high speeds. The result is chondral damage and synovial pinching resulting in disabling pain. The joints have ligamentous stability. Jack will probably be bothered by this type of problem as long as he proceeds with the intensity of his training and competition. The long-range plan is to limit Jack's training activities to less traumatic activities for his ankles, such as bicycling instead of running for endurance; mat drills instead of wrestling in the off-season; weight training for strength; flexibility exercises to gain and maintain some degree of flexibility; swimming for endurance, including running in waist-deep water; and trampoline-type exercises for gaining strength and balance in the ankles. It is important to note at this point that Jack has not only acquired a similar type of injury and disability in the left ankle, which occurred in late February 1982, but that he also has acquired arthritic changes due to frequent injuries of his left acromioclavicular joint, possibly necessitating surgery when his competitive days in wrestling are finished.

Jack's summer program for 1982 included strength work with overhead presses, bench presses, dips, pull-ups, arm curls, wrist curls, half squats, universal knee flexion and extension, ankle exercises, sit-ups, neck exercises with a head harness, trunk rotation, trunk extension to 0 degrees, hip flexion and extension, and adduction and abduction exercises. His flexibility program included Achilles' stretch in three different positions, hamstring stretch, adductor stretch of the hip and hip flexors, trunk rotation flexibility both with and without a partner, and stretching of the shoulder rotators, both internal and external. His endurance program included rope skipping and mat drills. Mat drills included the activities of running in place, falling forward; running in place, left shoulder roll; running in place, right shoulder roll; running in place, backward roll. The mat drills are performed for 1 minute at a time with 1 minute of rest between sets.

Jack had also been instructed to perform suicides on the mat, which means that he ran to one seam in the mat and then returned to the starting position, then ran to the next seam and returned to the starting position, and so forth. He was to sprint at full speed on each of these runs. At the seams, he did a forward roll or, for variation, he did a backward roll. The suicides were also performed by sprinting backward while doing forward and/or backward rolls at each seam. The suicides were also done with a carioca-type step in which he did either a backward roll or a forward roll at each seam. All of the exercises were performed on the wrestling mat to lessen the shock of heel strike, which would be somewhat disabling to Jack and would certainly create a lot of excessive wear and tear on his joints. A new type of exercise was being used this year with Jack that involved the use of a Nordic Ski Trainer. This trainer is a cross-country skiing device that does not provide any kind of heel strike and still provides a great deal of upper- and lower-extremity motion and extremely high heart rates when resistance is applied to the machine. Jack was to continue to work on the bicycle ergometer as well as to do a great deal of swimming. He was discouraged from running any farther than 2 miles a day, a distance that seemed to allow pain-free training. Most importantly, he was instructed to do no wrestling until October 15, 1982. This restriction included not only free wrestling but also wrestling drills and was a very difficult assignment for Jack; but he complied with these directions.

EPILOGUE

At least 70 percent of this case report had to be reconstructed during prolonged interviews with Jack. I am indebted to him for taking the time to not only recount the experiences, but also to pose for the 140 slides that were taken to be used in the presentation of this case to a live audience. Roentgenograms and physician reports are a matter of record, as are his training room visits for treatment, evaluation, and taping; however, the rest is routine business for an athletic trainer or sports physical therapist who is working closely with athletic teams. There is never enough time to record all of these events because of the large numbers of athletes involved.

CASE HISTORY 2

D.S., a 23-year-old white man, injured his right knee on July 26, 1980, while playing semiprofessional football. The weather was mild in the evening, and some dew was present. The playing surface consisted of grass with bare spots, and the grass needed to be cut. D.S. was wearing long cleats, and his ankle was taped. He was not wearing knee protection, and he had had no previous knee injury. The injury occurred during the third quarter, while he was performing a sweep play to the right. He moved laterally, planted his foot, externally rotated his lower leg, and internally rotated his upper leg. A player rolled into the lateral portion of his right knee while it was in a flexed position. D.S.'s cleats hung in the turf, and he experienced immediate pain with position and no further activity. His right knee immediately locked.

He was taken to the hospital on the evening of July 26, where roentgenograms showed normal bony architecture. He was first seen by an emergency room physician, who, in turn, referred him to an orthopaedic surgeon. The knee was lacking 5 degrees of extension, with flexion to 120 degrees showing an opening on the medial aspect of the knee with a valgus stress. An anterior drawer sign of +1 on the left and +2 on the right was noted. There was minimal effusion and marked tenderness over the medial collateral ligament and the anterior joint line just over the tibial plateau. Impressions at that time were: (1) internal derangement of the right knee, (2) possible unholy triad, (3) possible torn medial collateral ligament, and (4) a stretched anterior cruciate ligament.

ACTION OF THE MEDICAL TEAM PRESENT

At the time of this injury, none of the personnel present were physicians, athletic trainers, sports physical therapists, or emergency medical technicians. In summary, there were no qualified personnel to manage this particular type of injury. The immediate management consisted of an ice bag, with no specific instructions. D.S. was transported to the hospital after the game by a girl friend.

SURGERY

On July 27, 1980, the medial collateral ligament was repaired with the use of a staple. The anterior cruciate ligament was not repaired; the medial meniscus was removed; and D.S. was placed in a long leg cast flexed to approximately 40 degrees. He was in a cast for approximately 7 weeks. The cast was removed on September 25, 1980.

PHYSICAL THERAPY EVALUATION AND TREATMENT

After the cast was removed, the knee range of motion was measured. At this time, he lacked 25 degrees of full extension and was able to flex to 90 degrees. D.S. began physical therapy with the following goals: (1) to increase his range of motion, (2) to strengthen all muscle groups, (3) to decrease atrophy as well as pain, and (4) to condition all other parts of the body while he was receiving his rehabilitation therapy. The patient received 4 weeks of physical therapy, and the following treatments were selected:

1. *Therapeutic Pool:* The therapeutic pool provides an atmosphere of relaxation as well as an opportunity to derive the benefits from hydrotherapy; that is, the athlete can concentrate on gaining strength and range of motion without undue stress being placed upon the joint. The therapeutic pool is the best means of treatment for the patient with an anterior cruciate insufficiency.
2. *Mobilization Exercises:* Mobilization exercises consisted of the athlete's grinding maneuver as well as patella fibril shifting. Gentle mobilizing exercises are excellent for trying to gain an increase in range of motion without stressing the ligaments about the knee joint too much.

3. *Progressive Resistive Exercises:* These exercises consisted of ankle weights and pool jogging to help increase the strength prior to gaining maximum range of motion.

The main emphasis of the program was to gain strength before motion for this particular pathology. The results of this rehabilitation program were less than favorable. D.S. had a slight gain in extension (5 degrees) and was still only able to flex to 90 degrees, the range he had attained coming out of his cast.

The physician was extremely concerned about his progress and elected to perform an arthroscopy on October 29, 1980, to remove scar tissue and manipulate the knee. There was significant scar tissue formation, and the manipulative procedure resulted in a gain to 110 degrees of flexion; however, D.S. still lacked 20 degrees of full extension. Once again, he was put on 2 months of physical therapy. The same type of therapy was selected for the same reasons, and after 2 months, he was re-evaluated. At this time, he still lacked 10 degrees of full extension and was flexing to 101 degrees. The patient was unable to maintain the range of motion following his manipulation and arthroscopy.

The physician and therapist felt that the knee again needed to be manipulated, and on April 18, 1981, arthroscopic surgery and manipulation were performed. The results after this procedure were more favorable. D.S. was able to extend to –5 degrees and flex to 110 degrees. Again, scar tissue had formed in the knee since the last arthroscopy.

The same selected therapy procedure was again followed. On May 20, 1981, D.S. became disenchanted, and on May 30, 1981, he saw another physician in a different city. This physician recommended surgery to remove the staple, which might have been contributing to impaired motion. The surgery was performed on June 12, 1981, to remove the staple and excise more scar tissue.

On June 14, 1981, D.S. started active, aggressive treatments in the therapeutic pool for 3 hours per day to keep the tissues stretched out and to prevent adhesion formation. He tolerated this therapy very well and almost immediately began to gain range at –5 degrees of extension to 125 degrees of flexion. His strength was excellent. His Cybex report showed normal ranges. By June 20, the range was to –3 degrees of extension and 128 degrees of flexion.

An intensified program began on June 21, 1981, consisting of therapy both in the pool and in the exercise gym. He performed high-speed repetitions on the Cybex unit (8 sets of 10 repetitions) and hamstring and quadriceps stretching (15 times for 3 sets). He was also able to tolerate the universal knee flexion and extension units, and with assistance, he could do 5 sets of 10 repetitions.

By July 14, 1981, D.S. had almost gained full range of motion; he showed excellent strength; and the rehabilitation results were considered superb. Upon gaining full range of motion and strength, he was then placed on a functional exercise program of running, cutting to the right and to the left, figure eights, carioca drills, running backward, and jumping rope. He did not require the use of a knee brace or any type of support, and he was able to tolerate his functional testing very well.

PHASE EVALUATIONS

Every sports physical therapist will be making critical decisions when evaluating the athlete from the time of the injury to the time of his return to sports. Each evaluation is slightly different and is performed in various locations. The phase evaluation is as follows:

Phase I —on the field
Phase II —on the sideline
Phase III—in a treatment facility (which may be the athletes' training room)
Phase IV—in a treatment facility (or the physical therapy facility)
Phase V —in a functional testing facility.

In *Phase I,* the primary decision process is to determine if the athlete is injured seriously enough to be transported to a hospital as an emergency case. It is imperative that an organized, sequential process be followed to keep the thinking process organized as each of these steps is followed. In Phase I, the sports physical therapist's evaluation should be made while the athlete is actually on the field, immediately after the injury is sustained. Initial observations will tell you whether the athlete is conscious or unconscious; holding an extremity will give you a clue about which anatomic structure is actually hurt and whether the athlete is coherent or not.

The next process is the emergency evaluation, at which time you determine whether the athlete is in a serious predicament and will require transportation to a hospital for further evaluation. An immediate evaluation will determine the extent of this injury.

The next process involves taking a short history to determine the extent of the injury. Because of the time element, questions should be short, concise, and relative to the injury itself. A more detailed history can be taken on the sideline. The primary concern here is to determine the seriousness of the injury prior to transporting the athlete.

The next process involves performing a structural evaluation, wherein a quick scan of the gross anatomy will indicate if any bones or joints are obviously broken or malaligned. This component would then be followed by an evaluation to determine whether the athlete has both sensation and motor capability. The athlete is simply asked, "Can you feel the part? Now, can you move the part?" The response to the second question is first undertaken *actively,* with the athlete initiating the move; a passive check then follows, during which time the sports physical therapist would stress the joint in a passive manner to evaluate its integrity. After all these on the field tests are completed, you should determine how the athlete will be transported to the sideline. The thought process here involves the use of a stretcher, the assistance of other athletes, the assistance of splinting devices, or the determination if the athlete can move under his own power.

Once the athlete has come to the sideline, *Phase II* of the evaluation begins. In this particular instance, usually the part of the anatomy is exposed and compared to the opposite side for standardization. A more thorough history is taken at this time to give more definitive findings prior to making a diagnosis of the injury. Also, first aid should be initiated to minimize the injury.

After this phase has been completed, the athlete is then transported to initiate *Phase III*, within the treatment facility, athletes' dressing room, locker room, or whatever facility is designated for injury evaluation. The decision that is to be made here is one based on the end results of the previous findings, and it determines the treatment and/or splinting techniques to be applied. This decision depends on the situation and rapport with the physician. The athlete may then be transported to either a hospital or a physician's office for roentgenograms to rule out any serious fracture. Once the physician eliminates a serious injury, a treatment plan is outlined, with the goal of returning the athlete to activity as soon as possible, but not at the expense of further injury.

Phase IV primarily involves the treatment regimens and selective programs for rehabilitation. Once the athlete has returned to a satisfactory level of performance, with full range of motion, pain-free activity, and adequate strength, he is put through a testing procedure considered to be *Phase V.*

Phase V is the functional component involving actual testing of the athlete prior to returning to activity. Most athletes will return immediately to that activity and will perform the same maneuvers and exercises that caused the injury. It is therefore important that the determination of the athlete's return be based on sound kinesiologic principles to prevent the same accident from recurring. The functional testing must also be designed on an individual basis. Every athlete is different, and every position within each sport is different. Therefore, there are no "general types" of functional testing programs. When the athlete has successfully performed the functional test for the sports physical therapist, the therapist makes a recommendation to the physician, and a final resolution regarding the athlete's capabilities is reached.

SUMMARY

The process of preparing and presenting this case history, as well as the editorial process of putting it into a written format for publication, has given us considerable time to reflect on the clinical decision-making process in sports physical therapy. So much of what the athletic trainer/sports physical therapist does is intuitive. It is the result of scraps and bits of information collected as one deals with athletes on a daily basis, as well as the accumulation of ideas that occur as the result of contacts with coaches and others involved in both the athlete's academic and athletic performance.

The full flavor of all of this cannot adequately be presented in textbooks or in live presentations. It has to be experienced to be both appreciated and learned.

There is no substitute for experience in the field. There has been considerable criticism by physical therapists of the National Athletic Trainers Associations' requirement that physical therapists have an additional 800 hours or more of clinical experience in an athletic training setting supervised by a certified athletic trainer. It should be very clear that there is far more to dealing with athletes' health care than has been taught in a standard physical therapy program. It is, therefore, our contention that the additional hours in a clinical setting are important if the physical therapist wishes to be certified as an athletic trainer or if, in the future, the physical therapist wishes to be certified as a sports physical therapist. Those who wish to deal with athletic injuries effectively should then either: (1) become qualified through the process that is established for that kind of certification; or (2) admit their ignorance and be willing to work, collectively, with those who deal most directly with the athlete, namely, the coaches and/or athletic trainers and/or parents or any other experts in the area so that they can most effectively understand the mechanisms of injury and, perhaps, more importantly, understand what the athlete has to contend with in the way of stressors. For physical therapists to open a sports medicine clinic or to be involved in a sports medicine center without adequate training is probably unethical. In addition, for physical therapists to proclaim to be sports physical therapists or to feel that they can advertise as being qualified to treat athletic injuries without the proper qualifications of either certification in athletic training or boarding in sports physical therapy is probably unethical. It is our hope that, through these particular case presentations, more people will become aware of their limitations and their need to be honest in dealing with the public regarding such a commercial issue as the treatment of sports injuries.

REFERENCES

1. Skovly, RC: *Results of the Task Analysis Study Sports Physical Therapy Section American Physical Therapy Association.* Journal of Orthopedic and Sports Physical Therapy Spring:229–238, 1980.
2. National Athletic Trainers Association, Professional Education Committee: *Guidelines for the development of an undergraduate athletic training education program.* NATA, pp 15–30.
3. Donely, PB: Presentation: *Functional Testing for Return to Activity in a Wide Variety of Sports.* Dogwood Conference, Atlanta, 1981.
4. Gale and Flynn: *Max O_2 and relative baby fat of wrestlers.* Med Sci Sports 6(4):232–234, 1974.
5. Leivin, PE: *The Foot and Ankle: Their Injuries, Diseases, Deformities and Disabilities,* ed 3. Lea & Febiger, Philadelphia, 1947, p 169.
6. Subotnick, SI: *Podiatric Sports Medicine.* Futura Publishing, Mount Kisco, NY, 1975, p 24.
7. Ibid, p 49.
8. American Orthopaedic Association: *Manual of orthopaedic surgery.* AOA, Chicago, 1972, pp 185–186.
9. Cooper, KH: *A means of assessing maximal oxygen uptake.* JAMA 203(3):135–138, 1968.
10. Clarke, HH: *Encyclopedia of Sports Sciences and Medicine.* Macmillan, New York, 1971, pp 290–292.
11. Johnson, BL and Nelson, JK: *Practical Measurements for Evaluation in Physical Education,* ed 3. Burgess Publishing, Minneapolis, 1979, pp 201–202, 274.
12. Ibid, pp 131–132.
13. Ibid, pp 124–125.
14. Ibid, pp 120–121.
15. Donley, PB: Unpublished material, West Chester State College 1969-1981 Athletic Training Annual Reports Man Days Lost Per Sport.
16. NCAA 1980–1981 College Wrestling Rule Books. NCAA, 1980, p 16.
17. Feitelberg, SB: Problem Oriented Record System in Physical Therapy. S.B. Feitelberg, Burlington, Vt, 1975, pp 34–36.
18. Bishop, BP: *Pain: Its physiology and rationale for management.* Phys Ther 60:13–27, 1980.
19. Kleinkort, JA and Wood, F: *Phonophoresis with one percent versus ten percent hydrocortisone.* Phys Ther 55:1320–1326, 1975.
20. Levy, ML: Personal communication, January, 1973.

APPENDIX 1

Date ____________________

WEST CHESTER STATE COLLEGE
ATHLETIC TRAINING

MEDICAL HISTORY QUESTIONNAIRE

NAME ____
Last First M

BIRTHDATE __________ AGE __________ HEIGHT __________ WEIGHT __________

PARENT OR GUARDIAN ______________________ PHONE __________

HOME ADDRESS ______________________________________

CITY ______________ STATE ______________ ZIP ______________

SCHOOL ADDRESS ____________________________________

CITY ______________ STATE ______________ ZIP ______________

SCHOOL PHONE ______________________________________

HIGH SCHOOL VARSITY LETTERS WON __________________________
(Indicate number of letters won in each sport)

I AM A CANDIDATE FOR THE ______________________ (SPORT TEAM)

THIS INFORMATION WILL BE KEPT CONFIDENTIAL

INSTRUCTIONS: When reply is yes, give date of injury or treatment. Please indicate as near as possible anatomic site of injury, left or right, plus any data you consider important.

Circle the appropriate answer:

DISEASES AND ILLNESSES

Yes No 1. Have you ever experienced an epileptic seizure or been informed that you might have epilepsy?

Yes No 2. Have you had hepatitis?

Yes No 3. Have you been treated for infectious mononucleosis, virus, pneumonia, or any other infectious disease?

Yes No 4. Have you ever been treated for diabetes?

Yes No 5. Have you ever been treated or informed by a medical doctor that you have had scarlet fever?

Yes No 6. Have you ever been treated or informed by a medical doctor that you have had rheumatic fever?

Yes No 7. Have you ever been told you have a heart murmur?

Yes No 8. Have you had any illness requiring bedrest of one week or longer during the past year? If so, give date and nature of illness.

Yes No 9. Have you ever been treated or informed by a medical doctor that you have asthma?

HEAD AND NECK INJURIES

Yes No 10. Have you been "knocked out" or experienced a concussion during the past 3 years? If yes, give dates.

Yes No 11. If answer to Question 10 is yes, did the attending physician have you stay overnight in a hospital? If yes, give dates and details.

Yes No 12. Have you ever had any injury to the neck involving nerves, vertebrae (bones), or vertebral disks that incapacitated you for a week or longer? If answer is yes, give dates.

EYES AND DENTAL

Yes No 13. Do you wear eyeglasses or contact lenses?
Yes No 14. If answer to Question 13 is yes, do you wear them during athletic participation?
Yes No 15. Do you wear any dental appliance? If answer is yes, underscore appropriate appliance: permanent bridge, permanent crown or jacket, removable partial or full plate.

BONES AND JOINTS

INSTRUCTIONS: Please give dates and indicate left or right for any injuries or procedures listed below that you received during the past 3 years.

Yes No 16. Have you ever been treated for Osgood-Schlatter disease?
Yes No 17. Have you ever been treated for osteomyelitis?
Yes No 18. Have you had a fracture? If answer is yes, indicate site of fracture and date.
Yes No 19. Have you had a shoulder dislocation, separation, or other shoulder injury?
Yes No 20. Have you ever been advised to have surgery to correct a shoulder condition?
Yes No 21. If answer to Question 20 is yes, has the surgery been completed? Give date.
Yes No 22. Have you experienced a severe sprain, dislocation, or fracture to either elbow? If answer is yes, give date.
Yes No 23. Have you ever had an injury to your back?
Yes No 24. If answer to Question 23 is yes, did you seek the advice or care of a medical doctor?
Yes No 25. Do you experience pain in the back? If answer is yes, indicate frequency with which you experience pain by underscoring answer: very seldom, occasionally, frequently, only with vigorous exercise, or heavy lifting.
Yes No 26. Have you experienced a sprain of either knee with severe swelling accompanying the injury?
Yes No 27. Have you ever been told that you injured the ligaments of either knee joint?
Yes No 28. Have you ever been told that you injured the cartilage of either knee joint?
Yes No 29. Have you ever been advised to have surgery to a knee to correct a condition?
Yes No 30. If answer to Question 29 is yes, has the surgery been completed? Give date.
Yes No 31. Have you ever experienced a severe sprain of either ankle?
Yes No 32. Do you have a pin, screw, or plate somewhere in your body as a result of bone or joint surgery? If answer is yes, indicate anatomic site and date of surgery.
Yes No 33. Have you ever had a bone graft or spinal fusion? If answer is yes, indicate anatomic site and date of surgery.

GENERAL

Yes No 34. Have you ever been told that you have a hernia? If yes, has the hernia been surgically repaired? Give date.
Yes No 35. Have you had any operations? If answer is yes, indicate anatomic site of operation and date.
Yes No 36. Have you ever been inoculated for tetanus? Give date.
Yes No 37. Are you currently on prescribed medications or drugs on a permanent or semipermanent basis? If so, indicate name of drug and indicate why it was prescribed. (E.g., birth control, epilepsy, high blood pressure, etc.)
Yes No 38. Are you allergic to any medication? (E.g., aspirin, penicillin, etc.)

Give full name and address of your family physician. ______________________

____

All of the above questions have been answered completely and truthfully to the best of my knowledge.

Signature ______________________________

APPENDIX 2

WEST CHESTER STATE COLLEGE
ATHLETIC TRAINING

Name ________________

Date ________________

MUSCULOSKELETAL EXAMINATION

A. POSTURE EVALUATION:

	OK	NOT OK (with remarks if necessary)
I. Front view:		
1) Nipple levels		
2) Muscle symmetry		
3) Level of hips		
4) Level of patellae		
5) Genu varus or valgus		
6) Pes cavus/pes planus		
7) Q angle		
II. Back view:		
1) Scoliosis (Adams position)		
2) Shoulder levels		
3) Scapulae		
4) Level of hips		
5) Ankle alignment		
III. Side view:		
1) Spinal curves (lordosis/kyphosis)		
2) Genu recurvatum (OK if absent)		
3) Head alignment		
IV. Gait evaluation		

B. ORTHOPEDIC STABILITY:

	OK	NOT OK (with remarks if necessary)
I. Knee		
II. Ankle		
III. Shoulder		

C. RANGE OF MOTION (FLEXIBILITY) EVALUATION:

	OK	TIGHT	LOOSE	REMARKS
I. Neck				
II. Trunk (pain, difficulty moving, etc.)				
III. Shoulders:				
1) Arms over head				
2) Hands behind back				
3) Hands clasped behind neck				
IV. Elbows:				
1) Flexion				
2) Hyperextension (10° OK in girls)				
3) Carrying angle (girls more than boys)				
V. Forearms: (pronation/supination)				
VI. Wrists & Hands: (flexion/extension)				
VII. Lower extremities:				
1) Hamstrings (supine)				
2) Heel cords (supine or standing)				
3) Quadriceps (prone: palpate for VMO)				

D. GROSS STRENGTH EVALUATION:

	OK	WEAKNESS	INEQUITY	REMARKS
I. Neck:				
II. Shoulders (elbows at sides, bent 90°)				
III. Quadriceps (sitting)				
IV. Hamstrings (prone)				

APPENDIX 2—*continued*

E. FITNESS TEST—Sport—*WRESTLING:*

	Standard	Actual
I. Endurance (12-min run)	2 mi	
II. Vertical jump	24 inches	
III. P bar dips	20	
IV. Pull-ups	15	
V. Sit-ups (2 min)	80	

F. PERSONAL HISTORY

I. Sports history ____

II. Success ____

III. Variety ____

IV. Frequency of injury ____

V. Personality ____

VI. Motivation ____

VII. Level of competition ____

APPENDIX 3

WEST CHESTER STATE COLLEGE
ATHLETIC TRAINING

Name ______________________________

Date: ______________________________

ANKLE EVALUATION

Case History: Lateral ankle pain in a wrestler.

Ankle: R-L; Examiner ______________

Key: A—Check at time of injury on the activity area.
B—Check after match in locker room or on sideline.
C—All items could be checked in the clinic or training room.

I. History (how, what, why, where, when)
   A. Weather
   B. Playing Surface—A, B
   C. Shoe—A, B
   D. Sole—B
   E. Ankle protection—A, B
   F. Protection for knee—B
   G. Protection for foot—A, B
   H. Shoe correction
   I. Part of practice
   J. Part of game—A, B
   K. Activity when injured—A, B
   L. Direct blow—A, B
   M. Indirect blow—A, B
   N. Audible sound at time—A, B
   O. Previous injury to area—B
   P. Time of swelling—B
   Q. Previous R_x incl. F. Aid—B
   R. X-ray
   S. Physical—B
   T. Medication

II. Physical Examination
   A. Observe
      1. Swelling—A, B
      2. Deformity—A, B
      3. Discoloration—B
      4. Ankle valgus
      5. Ankle varus
      6. Toe in, toe out
      7. Feiss' line
      8. Abducted foot
      9. Adducted foot
      10. Callus
      11. Tibial torsion
      12. Hammer toes
      13. Cavus
      14. Equinus
      15. Hallux valgus
      16. Pump bump
      17. Shoe wear
      18. Gait shoes—B
      19. Gait barefooted—B
      20. Scars
   B. Active motion
      1. Dorsiflexion—A, B
      2. Plantar flexion—A, B
      3. Inversion—A, B
      4. Eversion—A, B
      5. Toe flexion—B
      6. Toe extension—B
   C. Passive motion (Mobility tests for hypermobility and for pain in ligaments.)
      1. Dorsiflexion—A, B
      2. Plantar flexion—A, B
      3. Inversion—A, B
      4. Eversion—A, B
      5. Midtarsal motion—B
      6. Drawer sign—A, B
      7. Metatarsal arch
      8. Mortise spring—A, B
      9. Fibular spring—A, B
      10. Talar tilt—A, B
      11. Thompson test
      12. Calcaneal percussion—B
      13. Tendon stretch (pain)
         a. Dorsiflexion (knee flexed and knee extended)
            1) inversion—B
            2) eversion—B
         b. Plantar flexion
            1) inversion—B
            2) eversion—B
   D. Palpate
      1. Defects, tenderness, crepitus
         a. Medial malleolus—B
         b. Lateral malleolus—A, B
         c. Shaft of tibia—B
         d. Shaft of fibula—A, B

e. Calcaneus—B
f. Tarsals—B
g. Sinus tarsi—B
h. Vital ligaments
1) anterior tibiofibular—A, B
2) posterior tibiofibular—A, B
3) ant. & post. talofibular—A, B
4) calcaneofibular—A, B
5) naviculotibial—B
6) ant. & post. talotibial—B
7) calcaneotibial—B
8) distal tibiofibular syndesmosis—A, B
9) proximal tibiofibular syndesmosis—A, B
10) calcaneonavicular—B
11) calcaneocuboid—B
i. Pulse P. Tib.
D. Pedis
j. Temperature—B
k. Sensation—A, B

E. Manual muscle tests
1. 15 heel raisers (gross plantar flex) 2 feet, 1 foot—A, B
2. Dorsiflexion (gross)—A, B
3. Inversion (neutral) (gross)—A, B
4. Plantar flexion (inversion & eversion)—A, B
5. Dorsiflexion (inversion & eversion)—A, B
6. Great toe flexion—B
7. Great toe extension—B
8. Lateral toes extension—B
9. Lateral toes flexion—B

F. Goniometer measurement
1. Plantar flexion 50°
2. Dorsiflexion 20°
3. Subtalar & midtarsal joint—combination
4. Subtalar inversion 20°
5. Subtalar eversion 10°

G. Neurologic
1. Sensation L_4 medial, L_5 dorsum, S_1 lateral—B
2. Achilles reflex S_1—B

H. Functional tests
1. Heel raisers (1 foot)—A, B
2. Hop (1 foot)—A, B
3. Walk—A, B
4. Run—A, B
5. Change directions or figure "8"—A, B
6. Sprint & stop—A, B

	°/sec.	°/sec.	Endurance
R dorsiflexion			
L dorsiflexion			
R plantar flexion			
L plantar flexion			
R inversion			
L inversion			
R eversion			
L eversion			

Chapter 15

QUESTION AND ANSWER FORUM

The following information is excerpted from an exchange among contributors to this text and physical therapists attending a conference on clinical decision analysis. This forum took place *after* the presentations that subsequently formed the basis of this text. Components of the exchange have been reordered in some instances to maintain continuity of thought or content.

ON EDUCATION

Paris: Dr. Geneva Johnson was talking about the need for us to earn doctoral degrees. I'd like to ask if she envisions all physical therapists needing to do this and if she has considered the costs in terms of patient care if, indeed, that was to result.

Johnson: I suggested that everyone should have a doctorate, but not necessarily a PhD. The PhD study really is fairly costly; however, there are ways to offset that cost. If we press ourselves, we can probably find several ways to support the cost of doctoral study, or what I would call a professional degree of a doctorate in physical therapy. The cost to the patient, I don't believe, is going to be that much increased. For one thing, what I see in the clinical specialist and those people whom I consider to be master clinicians is a great deal less time spent in trying to figure out what to do. A program of doctoral study for the initial professional preparation probably would take a minimum of 3 years, and that would give us approximately 4 academic years. That's 1 more year than we are thinking about now. I don't think it's an exorbitant cost. Does that help you at all?

Paris: You're thinking of a physical therapy doctorate.

Johnson: Yes, for the initial professional preparation, and then the PhD as the scholarly degree for research and for teaching.

Paris: What I have noticed is that many physical therapists who obtain PhDs may have done so after being master clinicians, to use that term, but they finish up doing something else entirely. Their efforts are lost to patient care.

Johnson: We don't want that to happen. I'm emphasizing that we need such people with both expertise and knowledge in the clinical or treatment setting.

Audience: My question to Geneva Johnson is: Isn't it a commentary on our profession that there are so few people known? All of you, our distinguished faculty, have advanced degrees in other fields. There are so few people and so few opportunities to pursue purely within physical therapy that we always have to rely on other professions to obtain further formal education. We are not self-sufficient, and our best-known physical therapists are identified first as doctors, physiologists, or educators. The RPT gets lost with all the other initials. I would just ask how you would feel about that.

Johnson: For now, you are right. We have the pathokinesiology doctoral program at the University of Southern California, and we have an interdisciplinary program at Boston University. Iowa has an exercise physiology program, and NYU has a doctoral program. It does seem a sad commentary that as yet we haven't developed graduate study for ourselves. We are really just getting underway with some pretty solid master's degree programs, and we have been reluctant to admit that we even have anything worth graduate education, let alone worth doctoral study. I do not belong to that camp, but there are people who do; so that's one of the reasons we really need to move quickly to get advanced degrees. We all draw from the same well of knowledge. We just need to take from all the areas that have something applicable for us. The unique way in which we can apply that knowledge is what makes us different. I think that, in time, we will have doctorates.

Ramsden: I think that you've raised a question that is common in the minds of many people, and my reaction to it is almost inevitably to look at history. Harry Truman said many years ago that there isn't any new history except the history you haven't read. I think that we can learn from history; and if you look at the evolution of medicine over the years, I think you will find an interesting pattern and some interesting analogues as you compare the evolution of physical therapy with that of medicine. This is not to say that we will follow the same ultimate track in the long run, but I think the growth of the professions so far has been very similar. So I would say it is timely now for us to develop a generic doctorate and to encourage our physical therapists to pursue the advanced degrees for research and teaching responsibilities. Ours is a relatively young profession.

Sahrmann: I cannot help but comment here because I approach that problem in a different way. I concur with Dr. Johnson that the problem with not having our PhD in physical therapy is because we did not have a body of knowledge within a content area identifiable among physical therapists. So that history does not have to wait until all of you are as aged as we are, I think it becomes important that we begin to identify a treatment area unique to physical therapy. I am a strong advocate of considering physical therapists as movement specialists. And I equate this notion to my experience in neuroscience. When I began my degree in neurobiology, the field of neuroscience had really been identified for only 2 years, meaning that all of those people who studied the nervous system were either in the pharmacology, anatomy, physiology, or another basic science department; but once they pulled those people interested in the nervous system together, one of the largest scientific groups rapidly emerged.

I relate this occurrence to the whole concept of the doctorate that has been brought up here. I strongly believe that down the road, we will have a clinical doctorate; and I equate this belief to the idea that if the eye and the tooth and the foot dictate separate doctorates, then all human movement really does. My other rationale for this belief is that my colleagues in neurology and in medicine are now biochemists. In addition to pursuing the anatomic location of a problem, they worry about the biochemistry and immunology associated with that problem, because these are elements of a disease. When my neurologist colleagues identify sickness in my area of expertise, what they really care about is finding the location of the stroke and the part of the brain that is damaged, or how, in the future, stroke can be prevented. They do not know all that much about the disturbed motor behavior. I think that that applies to almost any area of the practice of medicine. We have a unique system that desperately needs us both in prevention and remediation. We ought to get on with putting that body of knowledge together so that, like neuroscience, we can get to where we need to go both for academic study, which is the PhD, and for clinical practice, which is the clinical doctorate.

Audience: What can we do to maintain or increase our professional status and yet, at the same time, make it physically and financially feasible to serve a population dependent on long-term, constant care? If we increase our status, what will be our requirements of the paraprofessionals who work with us?

Hislop: I think the issue of what will happen to the support personnel for physical therapy if we move into the clinical doctorate is very clear. In my perception at present, in day-to-day clinical life, if I visit a physical therapy department I am very hard put to distinguish the roles of the professional physical therapist, the physical therapist assistant, and less frequently, the aide. Perhaps costume delineates the aide more from the others. If we move to the clinical doctorate, I do not perceive any need at the moment to change the educational role in the preparation of the physical therapist assistant; nor do I see the role and the on-the-job training for the aide changing. But certainly there will be a marked and very distinct difference in the functions and roles of the professional physical therapist.

Campbell: It is not necessarily to get a better product. You have to invest an initial outlay of capital, and I do see what's being suggested here as costing a lot initially. We will have to research factors that will tell us whether what we do works. I hope that such research endeavors will help us to become more efficient in knowing that what we do is going to have a predictable outcome.

Unfortunately, on the negative side, I think that we are also in a time when very harsh realities are facing us in universities as well as in other institutions in our country. We are going to need strong alumni support if we are going to try to move in different directions. My university, and others, have moratoriums on new degrees, much less raising existing ones to a higher level.

Hislop: Dr. Campbell brought up something that I think is worth responding to with respect to the cost of adding new degrees. I happen to be in one of those universities that now has the doctorate in physical therapy—the PhD. It has not cost us substantially in terms of university funding to add this degree to our program, with the exception that we now have been able to justify equivalent and higher salaries for the kinds of faculty we are now able to employ and will have to employ in the future. But that has come along with the recognition of a legitimate degree. Secondly, when you look at cost, we are facing the demise of physical therapy educational programs within universities because they do not meet the coin of the realm. Having the PhD in physical therapy is financially economical because you now have the coin of the realm of the university, and a PhD faculty must meet the same academic requirements for tenure and promotion within the university as members of any other department. Thus, the economic savings, perhaps, come through in part by the assurance of the continuity of that program in the university, where without it such programs would be in a much more tenuous situation.

Paris: Helen, would a doctorate in physical therapy meet the coin of the realm—the standard of physical therapy?

Hislop: Yes, I think it would. Without any question, it would be highly respected and looked at much more favorably by higher university administrators.

Watts: Let me comment from a different standpoint. What matters is not the letters that come after your name, but what you can do. So if we say that the problem we are trying to solve is how to improve our capacity, our ability to do good things at a reasonable price in an accessible way, then I guess I like to look at different options. It is possible that the clinical doctorate or the PhD represents an option. It is certainly one that I would want to examine. But let me just describe very briefly an option that at the moment tempts me even more, and that is an option of realizing that the start is not the finish. Entry level is not an ending level. Competence does not have to be learned entirely in school and does not at all have to be totally recognized by an academic degree, which serves a very particular purpose in our society.

There are many other, perhaps more real, forms of recognition of competence than academic degrees. It seems tempting to me to think of our having real careers for clinicians beginning at an entry-level preparation that is adequate for starting a career. I am impressed that we appear to have such an adequate entry point now. This point is not adequate, as it has had to be in the past, for a total career. We will need to build on it. Yet, I am not personally ready to reject the starting point that we have. I am only ready to reject it as a stopping point for the individual. My impression, from sessions such as the one in which we have participated for the past couple of days, is that many of my colleagues have gone very far beyond their beginnings; they have developed careers that have not only gone in different directions, but have also developed an imposing, exciting, and useful level of clinical competence beyond anything that I think is necessary to teach at the entry level. And I find that attractive because it seems to me that we then have opportunities for people to begin at one level and to move on to other levels. I would like to see those levels include as many options as possible for different ways to accomplish progression. A degree-labeled path might be one; but many of you have the clinical competence at an advanced level, which I admire, and have done it through a very different route. I am not ready to discard some of those other alternative routes, including learning through experience, through independent study, through continuing education, and through contact with colleagues who can teach, whether it is one on one or in groups.

I guess my hope is that as we keep our eye on the ball, which is developing competence, accessibility, price control, and the things that will let us do that, we do not put all our eggs in one basket, nor reject anything that is working, but try to get as many routes to the goal as possible, because some things work for some people and some for other people. This notion is not in disagreement with what some of these folks are proposing. It is just to say that we ought to also keep some other avenues open.

ON SPECIALIZATION

Blessey: I wonder how the faculty see the relationship between the drive toward specialization and certification in a specialty area, and the clinical doctoral degree? Do you see one supplementing the other, or do you see it as two options? I would be interested in hearing responses from some of the educators on the process of specialization and how it may interrelate or help stimulate people to consider the clinical doctoral degree.

Paris: I think that before one becomes a physical therapist, that person would have already reached competence for one of the boards as a requirement. So one could become a doctor of physical therapy in the clinical area and become certified at the same time.

Audience: Where will physical therapists receiving their PhD degrees go?

Sahrmann: First of all, I really strongly believe that those of our students who are receiving a baccalaureate education are taking many more hours than required for a standard baccalaureate degree. In most programs, they are also taking courses with graduate students and medical students at a level well beyond what most other professions require for a master's degree. Social work, speech pathology, and other health-related baccalaureate programs do not have the same kind of academic standards in their educational programs. Furthermore, a limitation on the development of future faculty is that people often join faculties to become schoolteachers and not to become academicians. We are subject to tenure requirements, which means that we've got to do research, we've got to publish, and we've got to have an area of expertise open to public scrutiny. The hard thing for people to do is to join faculties not knowing that they have to be academicians, and it was hard for them to come on not having appropriate training. I think it is critical that people understand what the requirements are and that they possess the background on which they can build and then meet those university requirements.

Young: I want to go back for just a moment to some of Dr. Watts's comments. I might also just remind everybody that I was a physical therapist and wanted to go on for a further degree. I did not want to go into academia, so I went to medical school instead. This opportunity allowed me to remain in a clinical setting. With that in mind, I'd like to return to the statement of taking yourself seriously. I've been very impressed in my encounters with physical therapists about how much you do know, particularly in comparison with medical students and physicians. You are movement specialists, and you know more about that than any physician will ever know. The gap that needs to be bridged is for you to know that you are specialists, to take yourselves seriously about that, and to put it out there to the world of physicians. You do know something about what you are doing, who you are, and what you are all about.

One of the thoughts that has occurred to me as we were sitting here talking is that perhaps physical therapy needs a longer internship. As physicians, we have a required 1 year of internship, and for most people, I think, to get out of residency in less than 3 years is almost unheard of. After being in a classroom for 1, 2, 3, or 4 years, you must then have some time to really practice and develop those skills in a supervised learning situation that would allow intuitiveness to develop more competence. You people already know this. It really bothers me to see that awareness being kept under wraps. So that is my challenge to you.

ON CLINICAL PRACTICE

Hislop: I'd like to throw a challenge out to clinicians. I've done this in many places and at many times in the past in terms of your own recognition of yourselves, and it is in full support of what Dr. Watts said a few moments ago about options. In the clinic, by and large, we have staff physical therapists. The staff physical therapists, in place for 1 or 2 years, need an increase in income. In order to get the increase in income, the staff physical therapists either go into private practice or, if they stay in institutional practice, move upward. In moving upward, they move laterally away from patient care. They become seniors or instructors or supervisors or chiefs, and the more they move up, the further they move away from the patient. I would challenge you to make a system of incentives for remaining in patient care that includes salary incentives, time away for study incentives, and so forth. You must move up from a staff clinician, just as in academia we move from instructor to full professor. So consider the incentives of moving from staff physical therapist to a recognized title of master clinician. You have heard that title over and over this week—the master clinician. You have a group of master clinicians sitting at this front table. I dare say, none of them has ever been given the opportunity and the accolades to use that as a title of respect in the clinic. This is another option, and there could be requirements, experiences, self-learning, or formal learning to achieve that goal.

Personius: I would like to pick up on that and say that I wholeheartedly agree. I think that we need to get on with specialization and recognition of master clinicians. I have a very specific mechanism for that recognition and attainment of competences.

We have master clinicians. I have no problem personally awarding a doctorate if a person attains enough capabilities to be labeled as a master clinician. So there is a challenge, on the purely clinical side, to have levels of competence and to make them really mean something. However, there is also a challenge within the university. We have also talked about movement specialists; and to really borrow from several things that have been said here, we have a discipline, identified by Dr. Hislop several years ago—the study of normal and abnormal movement. We can justify the development of that discipline in the academic setting. On the other hand, do we have clinical specialists? I, for one, think that we do. What we need is a mechanism to move on and recognize that. But what is needed to relate clinical expertise to academic excellence is not occurring in the university.

I would like to go back to the comments that were made just a minute ago. What we need are people within universities who can provide very strong clinical role models in concert with very strong role models working in the clinic; in other words, academic faculty and clinical faculty who work very closely together. Therefore, within education, one must have clinical and academic components as well as research experts who are working very closely together. How many universities with physical therapy programs and clinics can be identified in which the clinicians are looked upon and feel like people working strictly on an 8-hour day? How much interaction is there between academic research and clinical groups? How many incredible wedges are driven between the two so that there is very little high-quality teaching going on with patients who are in the hands of academic faculty? To put it another way, how often is the real responsibility for judging whether people are competent to practice handed over to clinicians? I think that we are looking at a problem of people getting together—the academic part of it, the research part of it, and the clinical part of it, with recognition and high standards on both sides.

Coogler: I am a person in a doctoral program who plans to go back to the clinic—who wants to—but it seems no one believes I can. My fellow clinicians are totally appalled by that idea. They feel that I will pursue a teaching career. The academic faculty feel they need doctorate people and try to enlist them. However, there are clinical educational programs designed to put master's level people back in the clinic. I think that as a profession, both the academic and the clinical components will have to change their thinking a little bit so that advanced-degree students are geared toward improving the quality of patient care.

Johnson: I want to speak from a practical standpoint. I have a PhD, and I am in a clinical setting. On my staff, I have a PhD in physiology, and until recently, I had another person with a

PhD in physiology. My goal for the past 8 years has been to develop a staff with a minimum of a master's degree and to develop the clinical specialist, a title we use instead of master clinician. We developed an opportunity for people to stay in clinical practice and to be rewarded for developing clinical skills and to be recognized by the title of clinical specialist. It is not easy to develop this concept, and I am telling you that I have been at this now for 8 years. We also have a program of clinical research, and at the last national conference, we presented papers. I think young people are serious about wanting to contribute and learn to be better clinicians. I agree with what everybody is saying about the need to develop those clinical skills, but I want us to use them in appropriate clinical environments.

Hislop: We expect our faculty to work in the clinic.

Johnson: We do have those opportunities available, and maybe you just are not looking in the right place. Another thing that we have done is to develop fellowships for new graduates from master's degree programs, so that they have an environment in which to work and to be treated as professional practitioners while being required to do some clinical research. Some of them stay on the staff; some of them go on to other things. So one can create environments that encourage the development of comprehensive professional competence.

Audience: We talked about academic people who teach not being aware of what their expectations were. I think that one of the problems with prospective physical therapists is that they are individuals who want to help people. I see a problem in that people are entering into physical therapy school not knowing what our expectations are for them. I am wondering if, besides the long-range suggestions that Dr. Johnson mentioned, there are characteristics that I can look for in student applicants that would help foster the direction that we are trying to take here?

Paris: I think that entering and exiting expectations are obviously going to be different. I don't know of any medical students who entered medical school wanting to become proctologists.

ON CONSULTATION

Watts: Could we add a question to those we have been considering? Let us suppose that we have managed to get past this first layer of the problem, and we have more master clinicians. I think that many, but not all, of these clinicians will have specialized to develop that level of mastery. For the moment, let us put aside whether they have done that in the degree program or through subsequent training. As I have had the privilege of going from session to session during the last few days, I have been struck by the very advanced level of much of what is going on, by some of the unanswered, very primitive questions that are either being ignored or that we are not prepared to answer yet, and by the fact that frequently I would see a case problem in one session that really needed attention from another session as well. For example, I finished up this morning in pediatrics and saw Dr. Young's very interesting film about an infant with a very striking breathing problem and wished that Scot Irwin and Ray Blessey (cardiopulmonary) could have seen the film. It would have been fascinating to see if we could have merged those two groups so that two kinds of specialists looked at the problem (pediatrics and cardiopulmonary). While I was with the sports physical therapy group, I was wishing that Shirley Sahrmann (neurology) could have looked at the posture of a young man with an ankle problem that limited his wrestling ability. When we develop clinical masters, is it going to be necessary for new therapists to, in many cases, be specialized? If so, what kind of communication system can we use within our profession to see to it that we do not fragment the patient in the way that some other professions have? Is the only solution for everyone to be a master clinician in all areas, or can we find ways to consult with one another?

Wolf: As you think about responding to that question, perhaps Dr. Watts's thoughts could be tempered by the knowledge that in many jurisdictions throughout the country, physical therapists are striving for more autonomous practice; and inherent in that thought is the entire concept of responsibility and professional maturity, of knowing when to ask for help and when to act as independent medical agents. That concern was one of the themes of this conference. I hope that as the clinical faculty respond to Dr. Watts's question, they keep this thought in mind.

Ramsden: I would like to suggest that we have been serving as consultants for quite some time, but we seem to have some resistance to accepting that title for ourselves. This probably relates to our not taking ourselves seriously enough. I suspect that most of you talk with a physician every now and then about a patient. What you have discovered about the patient's condition and your excitement about the patient's potential, I would call a consultation. I suspect that you have consulted with other health professionals, whether nurse, social worker, or occupational therapist, about a patient's condition and your understanding of the patient from your perspective, and that is a consultation also. I think that those bonds need to be strengthened in response to Dr. Watts's very teasing kind of question. I think fundamental to strengthen those bonds between and among us is to accept the role that we have already taken.

ON GENERAL PRACTICE SPECIALIZATION

Paris: I think that Dr. Watts has raised a very important point. The task force on clinical specialization has been active in setting out specialty boards and has recommended that there be a specialty area of general practice. The House of Delegates of the American Physical Therapy Association (APTA) abandoned that idea. I personally felt that that was a big mistake. Medicine made that mistake, so I will relate it to medicine in this regard: it overspecialized the human body into components. To address Dr. Watts's concerns, one way of tying the system together is to elevate the specialist in general clinical practice to the same level as the specialist in any other area. I think it is very important that the general practitioner specialist be put into the board certification process.

Young: Medicine has done it now with the Family Practice specialty.

Paris: Medicine has made a mistake and has corrected it. Let us take a lesson from medicine.

Audience: A problem that concerns me, as a clinical faculty member who has been training students over the years, is that I have noticed educational systems developing added curricula as each new specialty emerges. If we are going to have a general specialty, as opposed to specialists in particular areas, we will be in school forever. I would like to know from the educators what we will eventually do if the program becomes lengthened to 4 or even 6 years. There is no way we can learn every aspect to be a very good generalist in 4 to 6 years. I think that Dr. Young's idea to get the basics and then to spend from 1 to 4 years in an internship while learning a specialty is excellent. Then you can also be more of a generalist. I just do not know how we can keep adding more courses in physical therapy schools.

Sahrmann: I have some information relevant to that concern. I want to elaborate on two points because I hate to leave things unclear. When I was talking about academic physical therapists, I was referring to people who do exactly what Mr. Personius is talking about—clinical practice, research, and teaching. These people do not have many other hours to do other things. This is just as the clinical medicine departments do. I refer to physical therapists who have expertise in different areas; we have people who really know a lot about the knee, the ankle, and the back. I do not know a lot about the knee and the ankle and the back, so I use those people. I trust that all of you do. Informally, if not formally, I hope you refer to others who have additional expertise.

We convened a session in Missouri because I had the same concern that a lot of you do about overloading our physical therapy educational programs. We asked all of the specialty sections of the APTA to send a representative to present position papers on what they think ought to be taught at the entry level. This experience turned out to be exciting to me because in group sessions we identified what was common and different about our practice among these specialists. What was common was all about movement. We did not end up with that many different things, because people were essentially practicing almost the same thing with a few extra areas. Somehow, we get locked into a notion that if information doesn't come in a course called Sports Physical Therapy, you cannot possibly apply it to Orthopaedics. So much of what we have done is to put false labels on things that are actually common to almost everything we do. The sooner we get on with the business of what it is we are focused on, the faster all of us will recognize that that is exactly what we are doing.

ON THE ROLE OF FACULTY

Campbell: I would like to follow up on that a little bit. I think that other people have a different vision of a clinical doctorate than I do, but I would like to share mine. We should not add more academic courses; we should add more clinical practice. I have a neighbor, for example, who is a dental student, and she has hundreds of hours required in her dental curriculum. That is very important because she is working beside faculty members. I think that there are a lot of reasons why faculty members in our institutions do not undertake clinical practice. Some of them probably became academians because they really did not like clinical practice. Some of them are teaching 30 hours a week, and it is unrealistic to expect them to do research and clinical practice as well. But there are also some hard institutional realities. We have not been involved in clinical practice facilities, as have physicians and dentists. We have not had access to clinical income that has made it possible for us to have the time to do clinical practice. A lot comes down to economics in the long run. My division recently attended a meeting in Washington with a number of school directors and found out that over half of our schools were establishing clinical faculty practices within which faculty will be treating patients and achieving clinical incomes. I think that that has to happen in the future as a basis for allowing faculty members to undertake clinical practice.

Personius: I believe that most faculty members should be practicing and should be master clinicians. I think that we should place our students into the clinic to work with patients and to be guided by master clinicians in the first semester of education. We need academic faculty treating patients with the students. Further, we need to tremendously upgrade clinical preceptors so that these people will not train students out of the goodness of their hearts while getting practically nothing from it and, in the process, be forced to make ultimate decisions about whether students pass or fail.

Stockmeyer: Over the many years that I have been in the field, new graduates or people about to graduate always come to the faculty and ask where they should work to obtain really good learning experiences. I think that one of the really good things that we could do for ourselves would be to initiate some kind of a register of places in the country where we could take advantage of not just what a faculty person could teach a student, but of what people who are already master clinicians could teach a new colleague.

ON REGIONAL PRACTICE

Audience: As a continuation of the schooling process, we are talking about independent practice, and yet we are talking about all this education occurring in groups or in facilities. One of the problems medicine and dentistry have had is in encouraging their graduates to go out to where the patients are, which is out in general practice. Physical therapy right now is failing to meet the challenge of solo practice.

Watts: It seems to me that there are several ways in which we can particularly deal with the problem of patients in the remote areas and the therapist who goes there almost alone to help them. One option is, perhaps, to provide a preceptorship that allows the clinician a chance to learn how to do that from clinicians who have already experienced this. Another option is to try within our profession to develop more circuit riding services—group services that serve a geographically distributed population. I do not know if our educational programs are educating people to deliver in some of the new patterns that we have been able to design. So it seems to me that really we have both a matter for the clinicians to develop ways to deliver services and then a need for our educational programs to provide opportunities for students to do extended practical work with people within those delivery systems. The University of Vermont has developed a prototype that includes both testing and using a new delivery service.

ON EDUCATIONAL COSTS

Audience: Quite honestly, the reason we cannot train students well is because it is extremely expensive. It costs a lot of money—not in the time factor, but in logistics and gasoline, because we have to go to the patient. Otherwise, we are charging the patient for education.

Hislop: Let me just comment that the costs are as great for educating the student in the hospital, but they are not as visible. I think that we have managed to ignore them because it is convenient to; but the costs of clinical education, no matter where it takes place, are enormous. This is why it needs to be undertaken with great care and why I think we look at proposals to extend the internship and establish a residency program while always asking what it will cost and who will pay that cost. Most of us know that third-party payers for patient care are less and less willing to subsidize education.

Paris: As a private practitioner, it is very expensive to have students in our clinic, just as it is in the hospital. We can estimate what it costs because we have a direct budget, and it is expensive.

Hislop: Both the educational programs and the clinics have to take some onus for the lack of trust and lack of responsibility that we invest in students. Some years ago we did, I think, what may be a prototype for some outreach physical therapy services today. We established a program in Shiprock for the Navaho Indian Reservation, and because of lack of money, we could not send students over with a preceptor. We had no preceptors to send, so we took a chance and sent students without the preceptor. They did marvelously well.

From a clinical perspective, the problem with the cost of clinical education is that clinicians won't trust our students to go one on one with a patient without a preceptor. Every student has to have a preceptor, and yet I know of remarkable institutions that will take high-school students in off the street as candy stripers and allow them to do mat classes, gait training, and a variety of things without a preceptor. Somehow, physical therapy students have to have a preceptor with them every minute of the day, and there comes cost. So how do we get over trust and responsibility?

Audience: I really wanted to make a comment. I feel that I was fortunate to have had my physical therapy training in England, because we did have a clinical internship. Our program was 3 years. It was not a degree program, and that really did not bother me one little bit because I think I came out just as good a physical therapist as anybody else--maybe a little bit better. The reason I say that is because over the years in America, I have taken a lot of students from bachelor's degree programs, and the one thing I find lacking in them is the competence in dealing with any type of patient. I think that in England, in the 3 years we rotated through all of the specialties, we had time to practice, and we had time to absorb. I find that lacking here. I find the American students that I am dealing with come out with wonderful didactic knowledge and very little practical skills. I think that is not necessarily the fault of the faculties that teach them, but it is just a matter of the time that they have not had to absorb the skills.

To Helen Hislop I would say, you have a point, because my preceptor was a senior student when I was a junior. I learned from senior students, and we had one preceptor in each department who was a member of our faculty. Senior students supervised the junior students, and we learned a great deal from them. In my own clinical practice, I have students from different programs, and I sometimes use that method.

Hislop: And I think if you will recall what I said in the first plenary session, a physical therapy student cannot learn to be a physical therapist without a patient. I would be the first to agree with you that in this country, we need more of the English system, and I wasn't trying to put all of the blame for clinical education on the clinician. I agree that the universities must change, and I thought we had really addressed that by saying that we needed more time. In our institution, just as an example, we have an entry-level master's degree that requires 79 units of university credit. Our university says 24 is the minimum for the master's degree and 36 is the maximum. Sixty post-baccalaureate units are required for the PhD. We're almost 20 units more than what is required for a PhD degree.

ON PROBLEM SOLVING AND EVALUATION

Wolf: I have an obligation to try to make sure that there are several aspects of what was encompassed in this conference that are going to be addressed today. We have emphasized primarily education and qualifications. There is another component to this meeting that deals with problem solving at the clinical level. And it seems that we have lost sight of that. In the light of the experiences of the last several days, are there any changes in your thinking that you might be able to incorporate in your practice?

Audience: When I went to school 10 years ago, we were told by our teachers not to tell the doctors what we can do but simply to show them. Now, 10 years later, we are showing them what we can do, and they know we can do it. This meeting is teaching us about decision analysis and research to demonstrate why it works. If we see something that we can analyze, should we chart this? As a clinician, this is my only record.

Stockmeyer: Well, I do not know whether you should necessarily chart it. I think that is going to depend on a lot of factors. At one point, I was both the teacher and the clinical instructor of a group of students, and I required them to develop treatment plans that included the rationale for everything they did on a patient. In essence, that became part of the chart; so we all knew that they understood why they were making a decision. When I first began as a staff therapist, I often had to do that. I had to justify, in front of a team, the rationale for everything that I wanted to do. Some of that can be mental; you may not put it all down on paper. I think it falls into the same category as decision analysis in that you often identify a rationale word for word in writing. But it seems to me that we do have an obligation to at least do it in our heads, even if we can't do it with every patient.

Irwin: I would just like to comment on what Dr. Hislop had to say about trust and responsibility. I think that she sort of threw the onus at us, and I would like to throw a little bit back to her. I think a lot of the times when I am in a clinical setting with a student, the student needs a preceptor because somewhere in our educational programs, whether it be at the undergraduate-physical-therapy-school level or back in the sixth grade, our educational system creates individuals who learn by being spoon-fed and spitting things back. Students do not necessarily learn by the methodology used here in the last 4 days to problem solve and then decide a rationale for treatment. I think that that is part of the reason clinicians have trouble turning the trust or responsibility for a patient over to those students. I think that a lot of times, students are not challenged in the educational setting to problem solve, and I know I am as guilty as many educators for not doing that enough.

Audience: I'd like to express a concern on the part of the clinicians. I had conversations with some therapists this morning asking them how they felt about the sessions. They all felt that they were wonderful. We can think and solve problems only to return to the clinic and try to go through problem-solving approaches until a physician tells us to treat a patient in a specific manner. We are also faced with the fact that in a few settings, we have to treat over 16 to 20 patients a day while being crammed into rooms where there are 15 other clinicians treating patients. All of these factors tend to hamper problem solving.

Paris: I would like to address the issue of doing what the physician says. We are all professionals. We have an obligation to do evaluations and to make decisions. It is then up to us to decide how that patient should be treated. We have no business treating a patient in the manner that does not fit the results of our evaluation. We must stand up and tell the physician that we do not agree with the prescription for treatment. We should accept only referrals. Those of you who are happy to accept prescriptions (and I hope there are none in this room) and to perform as you are told are doing us a disservice. I have never, after my first year as a clinician, treated by prescription. On the rare occasions that doctors, after hearing about my evaluations and findings, have insisted that patients be treated by their prescriptions, they are informed that an aide will comply but that there are no therapists who will.

Wolf: Several issues were brought up here regarding the practicality of the number of patients that are being treated versus the time to do evaluations.

Irwin: That is a reality. The reality of the situation is that it is all well and good for master clinicians to defend themselves in their areas of specialization against physicians. It is much more difficult to have a generalized specialist do so. I would not begin to speak to an orthopaedic surgeon about someone's low back pain in the way that Stan Paris can and with his level of confidence. I think that as we become a larger group of master clinicians, it is going to be very difficult to be a generalist master clinician. We will always confront the physician who has a problem ego, or a problem with not wanting to agree, and the only way we are going to get through is to inform the physician that either the patient will be treated by an aide or will not be treated at all.

Coogler: I just wanted to say something about the time factor. I think that time was stressed over and over again at this meeting. We've got to make sure that the information we gather is only what is needed to make our decisions. I think possibly some of the clinical sessions stressed that the method by which you gather the information can be done rather quickly to make early decisions. Some of our evaluations give us information that may be nice to know but is not always necessary. I think that we do have to begin to look at what we are evaluating because time is of the essence in a clinic. I do agree with you on that. We are limited with time, and we do have to see how we can reduce time usage to obtain just the clinical data we need.

ON PROFESSIONALISM AND PRODUCTIVITY

Young: Until you are willing to stand up for what it is that you know you are doing and how you are reasoning things through, decision analysis will not become a part of you but rather an extra little task that you do just to satisfy somebody or something. Until it becomes part of who and what you are and part of your evaluation process, you will not have the respect of the physicians who ask what you are doing and why. They are not going to listen to you until they hear you really using analysis and rationale as part of your treatment. As long as you are willing to sit back and be told what to do, you will gather limited respect.

Audience: I just want to respond to some of the questions that arose about the clinical setting and discussing issues with physicians. I have to agree with the responses of Paris and Young. I think that it is imperative for physical therapists to stand up for themselves under any and all circumstances. I, personally, have sat on medical tribunals in which the primary lawsuit was against the physical therapist. The medical society in Massachusetts had requested the presence of a physical therapist in order to judge a case. I think that with that kind of activity, you cannot ever hide behind a physician telling you what to do, because you would be the person who would be liable if you did not act upon what you firmly thought to be right. In response to the case load, I think it does behoove the clinicians to be able to speak up and define what constitutes these patient treatments. I hear a lot of argument and discussion about productivity. Productivity is income-producing activity and what the third-party payers will reimburse. If you are talking about applying the experiences from this conference to what constitutes patient care, discussions with a physician or other health care professional should be defined as a component of physical therapy productivity. It has to be. If we define productivity as only our income-producing time, then we will have to turn over 16 patients a day.

Donley: I think that the problem with excessive case loads is that everybody is standing around wringing their hands because they see a lot of patients and are uncertain about what to do with them. This probably results from never having learned how to analyze the patients' problems. Therefore, you have never dealt with them efficiently. Sixteen patients is not a lot of people if you know what to look for.

Audience: How do I explain what I do to a resident physician when we don't agree ourselves, especially with respect to evaluations? We are very delineated in what we are doing. I think we have that problem.

Paris: I just quickly turned to Dr. Young and asked if all physicians agree. She said no. I think the answer to that is, "Well, doctor, I have evaluated this patient using a system that I know works for me with this type of case, and I'm quite confident that what I recommend is the best way for this problem. I know that there are other ways of treating it, but for me, I have found this way to be effective. Just as you have differences in your disciplines, as we see on your rounds, we have them in ours. But I'm sure that if you'll let me do this, you will get good results."

Irwin: I think that we could take that thought one step further. How many of you have physicians who practice together, and how many of them treat patients the same way? None that I know of. I tell physicians that I use a specific methodology for a patient because I am capable of providing it well and it is effective.

RETROSPECTIVES

Donley: Regarding the process that we have tried to go through here, case history approaches to problem solving, I think it has at least a minor problem. Learning a decision-making process is very dependent on what you know. If you do not know very much, then you are not looking for very much. If you have specific knowledge regarding a particular problem, it is easier to make meaningful and rational decisions.

Irwin: I think that it was very interesting trying to prepare for this meeting. I don't know whether the other clinical faculty had problems similar to mine, but it is very easy to fall back into a mode of expressing content. It is very difficult to know when you have expressed enough content before you present a patient case. What is the group going to come back with, and are you prepared to answer some of their questions? After a while, I thought that the responses and the processes were phenomenal. I thought that the group was able to interact and to recognize one another's abilities and to just utilize the faculty as resources. To me, it is the model that we should have in the future.

Coogler: We said that one of the major themes for this meeting was consultation, or using other people, and I think that is one thing that became apparent. I certainly know that it wasn't really alluded to in the sessions that I gave, but everyone was doing it; they were consulting with each other in their decision-making processes, and that is what we are talking about.

Paris: I learned a great deal from this experience. I have done a lot of teaching. I usually teach, but I found in this way I will constantly remind myself to involve the group, ask them questions, and get them to see how I was thinking. In the process, I believe that the group received a lot more from it.

Irwin: I think, as I referred to earlier, that the process utilized here is what I would like to see happen in the schools.

Wolf: Perhaps we can each admit to our own frailties and shortcomings and emphasize the importance of a basic human trait—communication. All of us have certain skills that can make us unique and exceptional as professionals and that can give us a basis upon which to build.

Chapter 16

SUMMATION: IDENTIFICATION OF PRINCIPLES UNDERLYING CLINICAL DECISIONS

STEVEN L. WOLF, Ph.D., R.P.T.

To the reader who has attempted to absorb most, if not all, of the preceding chapters, the content must appear interesting and, hopefully, relevant. At the same time, it would not be surprising if the volume and complexity of the information left one with a sense of being overwhelmed. Part of this feeling might be attributed to personal reflections of inadequacy or incompleteness with respect to clinical competence. Recall that the information contained herein is provided to you by some of our most profound professional stalwarts and master clinicians. A more constructive introspection, therefore, might revolve about a sense of challenge to enhance one's future productivity and performance.

Toward this end, it would be worthwhile to reassess the content of this text with a primary intent of identifying principles that span all aspects of clinical decision making. Such principles are derived from the presentations in this text and are not intended to be viewed as all inclusive. On the other hand, an assessment of whether certain aspects of the decision process are unique to a specific field of specialization within physical therapy will also be rendered.

A review of all presentations within this book yields a series of opinions. These opinions are repeated so often within the context of a treatment plan or a philosophic conceptualization that they may be deemed principles. These principles would appear to characterize the essentials for comprehensive and autonomous practice. To deny their existence is to perpetuate and promote a technologic approach whose demise is long overdue.

PRINCIPLES

1. Effective treatment must be based upon a plan.

A plan is derived from the acquisition of *quantified* data (for example, active range of motion, integrated electromyogram, vital capacity, oxygen consumption). These data must be essential, relevant, and meaningful. We tend to want more information than is essential to formulate a treatment sequence. While excessive and extraneous information provides us with a sense of security, it is not cost-effective and dilutes efforts toward professionalism. The truly masterful clinician learns through experience and *thought* how to gather the minimal yet most relevant data in a *systematic* manner. Too much data may cloud the paths to decision.

2. Effective treatment forsakes empiricism as a primary guide.

For too long, physical therapists have based treatments or explanations of outcomes upon empiricism. The "I do it because it works" philosophy promotes technicians and retards professional growth. A reasonable blend of intuition and experience certainly contributes to the unique character of every physical therapist. Reliance upon these attributes, however, tends to facilitate a lackadaisical attitude toward concrete data acquisition and denies the active pursuit of new knowledge. Superb clinicians appear to be in an unending information-seeking venture through explorations that find empiricism unacceptable.

3. The cornerstone of effective clinical decisions is the ongoing acquisition of knowledge.

Most clinicians seek knowledge through lecture, workshop, or continuing education formats. While these vehicles toward more meaningful clinical analysis capabilities often supplement practice, they are insufficient. Additional contemporary information can be gained from ongoing library searches and literature reviews. The unavailability of these resources to practitioners in rural or "deprived" areas can be overcome through relatively inexpensive subscriptions to such publications as *Current Contents* (Life Sciences or Clinical Sciences weekly volumes) or to abstracting services. These resources list contemporary articles and journals with mechanisms for directly contacting authors for reprints.

4. Effective treatment is based upon integrative and often multiple treatment approaches.

Expert clinicians express treatment plans in terms of multiple options and several integrative techniques (e.g., the use of electromyographic feedback during therapeutic exercise for the spinal cord injured patient, to direct both patient and therapist toward activity in key muscles). The notion of one and only one treatment approach to ameliorate a movement limitation is archaic and retards the use of comprehensive approaches to effect maximal improvement.

5. Re-evaluation of treatment efficacy must be an ongoing process.

The re-evaluation process is built into each treatment plan within decision-analysis models. Quantified data obtained within the re-evaluation phase help to guide future decisions and to promote cost-effective treatment. This phase of patient management spans all clinical specialties.

6. The body of knowledge that characterizes physical therapy practice is growing exponentially and promotes specialization.

This principle has evolved from the further education obtained within physical therapy and elsewhere by many of our clinical specialists and researchers. Like professions that emerged years ago, the rapid increase in knowledge fosters special-interest groups. Within the American Physical Therapy Association, the number of specialty clinical sections has increased substantially within the past decade. Clearly, as new techniques emerge and information to corroborate or explain existing procedures develops, the amount of knowledge required of new therapists will be correspondingly greater. In time, it will be virtually impossible to be an effective clinician in all areas of physical therapy. Undoubtedly, subspecialties will emerge from specialties to lend further diversity to our knowledge base. Witness the multiple educational courses in orthopaedic physical therapy that are now capable of devoting days or weeks to clinical management and treatment rationale for virtually any musculoskeletal component (elbow, knee, lumbar spine, shoulder, and so forth). From this principle, another emerges.

7. Enhanced clinical expertise comes from knowing when you do not know; clinical wisdom is born from knowing with whom to consult and when to effect the best treatment.

A theme that ran through most presentations is that not knowing information or not having answers with which to clinically decide is certainly acceptable provided every reasonable effort has been made to seek the appropriate information or answer. This recognition of one's knowledge limitations can only enhance professional status and integrity and promote inquiry processes. Given time constraints and growing specialization, it is perfectly legitimate, and perhaps morally obligatory (see below), to seek consultation by requesting that others who possess more appropriate or superior clinical skills treat the patient or attend to a certain aspect of patient management.

8. The more chronic a patient's condition, the more time will be required to effectively make decisions and treat.

Many practitioners within clinical and private practice environments have generated remarkable revenue for their institutions or themselves through "assembly line" or "volume" oriented approaches. Quantity may facilitate cash flow, but it does not assure quality treatment. In no circumstance is this more true than for chronic patients, who probably have proportionately greater disruptions of more physiologic systems leading toward more profound limitations of movement capabilities than their acute counterparts.

This realization is apparent in all specialty areas of physical therapy. Clearly, new conceptualizations are necessary with respect to time, cost-effectiveness, and reimbursement (see below). For chronic patient populations, "quick" treatments to treat more patients and produce greater revenue are counterproductive and retard professional growth and responsibility.

THE UNIQUENESS OF SPECIALTY AREAS

These eight principles are not unique and, indeed, are probably applicable to any phase of physical therapy patient management. There are, however, several features within the five specialties represented in this text that are different. These differences may be more apparent rather than real because of the manner in which the contributors offered their respective problem-solving approaches; however, there is good cause to believe that these unique features are acceptable to the physical therapy community.

It would appear that no group makes use of clinical laboratory data more effectively than those clinicians responsible for rehabilitating cardiac or pulmonary patients. Changes in regularly gathered laboratory results or fitness testing serve as a primary basis for making decisions on treatment progression or modification.

The need to make rapid clinical decisions that may be altered or modified within subsequent hours and, ultimately, days, weeks, or months is most readily seen in sports physical therapy. Assessments of sudden injuries require immediate decisions that often are rendered by physical therapists because they are the most senior medical specialists available. Often, these decisions transcend physical therapeutics, but the application of a rational approach, governed by thorough experience and knowledge, will influence subsequent treatment for what become primarily musculoskeletal disorders. Sports physical therapists also find themselves dealing with a unique personal interaction—the psyche and motivational drive of the competitive athlete. These interactions are often as difficult to manage as are those interactions with chronic pain patients so often seen in orthopaedic and neurologic physical therapy. In both cases, clinicians must confront patients with attitudinal sets and behaviors that are influenced by multiple psychosocial and cultural factors, each of which can affect decision making.

Perhaps the most dynamic and changing patient is the newborn or pediatric patient. Clearly, pediatric physical therapists are faced with a constantly developing nervous system already thrown into a non-homeostatic state by virtue of the underlying pathology. This situation requires much flexibility on the part of the clinician. Therefore, the development of a fixed treatment plan becomes most difficult, and decision analysis may necessitate the creation of an entirely new avenue of approach. This reality is further complicated by the comparatively limited knowledge base available to the pediatric physical therapist. So little is known about the developing human nervous system and its potential for plasticity under normal circumstances, let alone plastic changes in the presence of pathology.

Chronic problems are most likely encountered with greatest frequency among neurologic and geriatric physical therapists. As can be gleaned from the neurologic presentations within this text, treatment of such patients is time consuming and comprehensive and necessitates rendering diverse decisions. Such patients cannot be treated in short order within one session or within limited time. Like orthopaedic physical therapy, treatment decisions for neurologic patients necessitate numerous options that must be systematically assessed, integrated, and implemented based upon knowledge and demonstrable effectiveness and not upon habit or favoritism.

EMERGING CHANGES

If we can believe that the principles outlined above are acceptable and that clinical specialties have common as well as unique features, then several changes in practice must emerge. Chronic or complex patients often provide the clinician with an overwhelming challenge by virtue of the multiple physiologic systems that may be disrupted. To best effect optimal treatment for these patients, we are obligated to actively seek consultation from physical therapists most qualified to treat or provide suggestions for the treatment of specific symptoms. Too often, physical therapists have been reluctant to pursue this course of action for fear of being viewed as inadequate or incompetent. In reality, while consultation might imply to some a loss of revenue, such a procedure is a symbol of strength and promotes professionalism.

Given our rapidly growing body of knowledge and our emerging specialty areas, the position that a failure to consult when such consultation can best benefit the patient is morally unsound (and may even conflict with ethical principles) is easily defensible. In the same vein, referring a patient to another therapist who is more qualified to treat a specific problem is a behavior that must be exercised with greater frequency.

Most physical therapy services are structured to be ancillary and "money makers." This philosophy is often espoused by administrators and catered to by clinicians. Justifiable reimbursement to physical therapists who have unique skills is not considered in such an approach. For at least the chronic patient, treatment must be comprehensive and, by necessity, time-consuming if it *is* to be cost-effective. Therapists and their clinics or practices must be reimbursed accordingly, even at the expense of numbers of patients treated per day. The complex surgical case is not rushed. The intricate medical complication is assessed and treated over time with multiple diagnostic procedures. So it must become with the complicated patient in rehabilitation. Physical therapists and their immediate supervisors must promote policy changes that offer adequate reimbursement and time. Treating for numbers can only be justified for acute or relatively simple conditions. A failure to provide quality treatment because of inadequate time is a disservice to the promulgation of professionalism within physical therapy practice.

Given the escalating costs of all medical services, physical therapists must consider branching their skills and interests beyond reparation of injury. Promotion of wellness and prevention of movement limitations are emerging concerns that require the attention and intervention of many health professionals, including physical therapists. It is not unreasonable to suggest that significant financial reimbursement will emerge from premorbid interventions because they will ultimately be cost-effective. Therefore, the winds of change dictate expansion of patient services beyond the "repair" phase.

These are a few notions. To some extent, they may be thought-provoking. They challenge the physical therapist to *actively* seek change rather than to stereotypically follow the dictates of others. They imply recognition of what is needed to gain the respect due to professional rank. They digress from the blind adherence and passivity so characteristic of technicians. To a large degree, they are the bases for respect and professional status within the medical community. Their implementation is limited only by self-imposed restrictions on dedication, creativity, and imagination.

Chapter 17

IMPLICATIONS FOR THE FUTURE AS OUR IMAGE CHANGES

Geneva Richard Johnson, Ph.D., F.A.P.T.A.

Change in physical therapy is as inevitable as change in every area of our lives. That change can be a forward step or a backward one, for better or worse, a challenge or a defeat. In the years immediately ahead, our image as physical therapists will undergo some major alterations. Because we, the physical therapists, are the profession, the image of physical therapy will be modified, too—for better or for worse—by us. The outcome depends on all of us but mostly on the young ones among us.

As I try to make my vision of physical therapy sharp and clear, the vision seems to ebb and flow like the tide. Instead of a stable, distinct image, I see a kaleidoscope of images, each one clear and identifiable for a moment, then blending and merging with the next so smoothly that I am awed by what I see in that panoramic view of the future that flashes on my own private screen. What will our tomorrow be like? What will make our tomorrow different? Let us briefly examine some of the factors that will make both our immediate and distant futures different as our image changes.

FACTORS CONTRIBUTING TO IMAGE CHANGES

EDUCATION

First in the minds of many these days is the effect that changes in education will have on our practice and on current practitioners. The responsibilities in patient care are staggering in their import for clinicians and faculty alike. Consequently, our educational preparation must be extensive—broad enough to prepare a generalist for practice and of sufficient depth to provide a firm foundation for that practice.

As our leaders in education are meditating on the future, I hope that they are allowing themselves the luxury of dreaming the *impossible dream,* because whatever we dream, we can make a *reality.* Hislop[1] discoursed eloquently on that subject a few years ago in her McMillan lecture.

I hope that the natural consequence of our dream will be the establishment of our educational programs at the doctoral level, with the award of a professional degree like those given in medicine, dentistry, and law. I do not mind if you think I am crazy. For more than 20 years, plenty of people have thought that I was a bit strange—that I walked with my head in the clouds—because I strongly advocated graduate education as the appropriate preparation for the practice of physical therapy. But in 1979, we passed a resolution in the House of Delegates that mandates us to move our educational programs to the post-baccalaureate degree level by 1990. Why not the doctorate in physical therapy?

If I had held the slightest reservation about the urgency of moving our educational programs to the post-baccalaureate degree level, the content of this book has dispelled my doubts. Reading the words of the contributors has confirmed my belief that we do not know enough about the effects of our interventions. We may not even know enough to intervene, and I am overwhelmed by what we need to know.

Education cannot stop with the completion of the initial professional preparation no matter where we set the degree level. The habit of independent study for continued professional and personal development must be instilled in, and expected of, the student from the very beginning.

To fulfill the promise of our future, our curricula must be dynamic. The curriculum in any institution will be a reflection of the resources available within the institution and in the community, especially in the treatment environments such as hospitals, agencies, schools, private practices, and any other environment in which patient care is provided. Because each institution has its own characteristics and resources, programs can and will vary markedly in the future, just as they do now. Some elements will be common to all.

Faculties must include new and different approaches to management of patient care, and those must be founded on sound scientific principles resulting from research. We must eliminate the teaching of certain procedures just because some physician might order them sometime. Fortunately, we are less hampered by the physician's orders today because many physicians do not know the variety of procedures we can offer a patient. That obliges us to be discriminating in our evaluation and treatment procedures, to be competent to make the necessary choices about patient care, and to be knowledgeable about the options available and the probable outcomes of their use.

I believe that we have an extremely important obligation as a profession to plan now for ways to give our currently practicing physical therapists opportunities to acquire new knowledge and skills in the anticipation of the changes we all face in the near future. More programs of advanced study in physical therapy must be developed soon to meet the needs and interests of clinicians.

STUDENTS

I do not want to dwell solely on education, although I consider education to be the key to change in our image. In the selection of students, we will be dealing with individuals who are older and more mature; whose career choice is based on an exploration of several comparable options. Students who are committed to extensive preparation for practice will expect to be held accountable for a large part of their education, and then to be rewarded with "prestige, power, position, and possessions"[2] for those years of preparation. That does not mean that we will become a "careless" profession because we seek those rewards. Rather, our concern and care will deepen as we clarify who we are and what we are about.

I do not believe that we will have more intelligent or intellectually able people in our field in the future. We have plenty of those now. But we will attract more people who could choose other careers.

FACULTY

To participate in the future as our image changes, faculties must make major changes. The number of physical therapists who are eligible for faculty appointments must increase several-fold and very quickly. Our acceptance of the expectations of a faculty member must move nearer to those of any other university faculty member. To make ourselves true members of a university faculty, all physical therapists who hold positions as educational administrators, all those who presently hold positions as members of a faculty, and all those who aspire to such positions must learn what being a faculty member means.

Let me say first some of the things that being on a university faculty do *not* mean:

- time clocks—punching in; punching out
  A student may need to see a faculty member at an unscheduled, odd hour; an emergency may call for the presence of a faculty member at an early or a late hour. Those occasions will be rare. Each faculty member must have freedom to schedule regular office hours instead of being available at all hours.
- 20 to 40 contact hours weekly in the classroom or laboratory and additional hours in counseling or advising students
- 12-month contracts
- different rules for appointments, promotions, or tenure from those applied to faculty in other departments or schools
- remaining aloof from colleagues in other departments or schools
- the option to participate in the affairs of the academic community, such as committees, faculty meetings, special events, and graduation ceremonies.

Being a faculty member *does* mean that:

- candidates selected for appointments will meet the qualifications imposed on all faculty candidates in the university
- assignment of a teaching load will be based on the same criteria used in other departments and schools; for example, consideration will be given to the number of classroom and laboratory hours; the number of students assigned for advising; the number of students assigned for supervision of research; the expectations of the faculty member

for productive research, attendance at professional meetings, and presentation of papers; and the expectations that a faculty member will maintain a clinical practice, when that is practical and desirable.

Although the model we want to use for our faculty probably does not exist yet, I suggest that we dream hard about that, for the future is upon us. When education changes, our practice inevitably changes. When physical therapists with doctorates, either a professional degree or a PhD, are in treatment settings working with patients, I believe that many of the problems that currently interfere with our ability to provide services to patients will disappear.

PRACTICE

As a result of expanded educational opportunities, we will have the knowledge (the science) and the skill (the art) on which to base our practice. We will seek the freedom to function and will earn the respect of our colleagues in other health professions. Then, to function independently, physical therapists will need to make contractual arrangements with treatment facilities, such as hospitals, to provide services. In essence, most physical therapists will be in private practice, in a group practice, or will be employed by physical therapists who are in independent practice.

STATUTES

The struggle for independence in practice is in progress in several states. Autonomous practice is a legal reality in 4 states (California, Maryland, Massachusetts, and Nebraska), and evaluation without physician referral is legal in 17 more states.[3] An inescapable and immediate obligation of every physical therapist is to devote time, energy, and financial resources to the passage of legislation that will permit autonomous practice for qualified physical therapists in all states.

Autonomous practice carries with it serious obligations as well as professional, financial, and personal rewards. Those obligations should not frighten us, but we must be prepared to accept the consequences of being the entry point into the health care system. The variety and intensity of the demands that that will place on us are unknown, but we can anticipate that they will be enormous when we consider the opportunity to practice in all four components of physical therapy—development, prevention, maintenance, and restoration.

As professional practitioners, we acknowledge our obligation to the public to be qualified through education and experience to provide excellence in patient care. That means a continuing commitment to increasing our knowledge and enhancing our skills. We are obliged, then, to participate in research that will: (1) uncover new knowledge that will give direction to the expansion or modification of our services and (2) substantiate the bases of our practices at any given time.

The knowledge acquired through research must reach the practitioner and the student through the process of education. Clearly linked, then, to the move to independence in practice will be changes in the methods used to provide opportunities for learning new or different approaches to patient care. The teaching/learning process must focus on preparing practitioners who are capable of dealing with the present while participating fully in the creation of autonomous practice for a near future.

Other obligations imposed by autonomous practice, and the legal mechanisms that support it, may be less evident. One implication that deserves consideration is what the license to practice will require and allow. Control of specialization in clinical care currently rests with properly constituted bodies within the American Physical Therapy Association. In the future, licensure laws may dictate requirements for receipt of a license that permits or limits the practice of a physical therapist to areas of proven competence through examination.

COMPONENTS

All of the things that I have said so far may have caused you to feel uneasy. I hope so. Because I have meant to alert you to the obligations we have if we intend to reach true professional status and to serve the public accordingly.

Serving the public means more than restoration of an individual to a functional state. As our image changes, we should look carefully at four components of physical therapy:

- *development* of normal motor behavior at all ages
- *prevention* of damage to the body systems through fitness programs and education for protection against injury
- *maintenance* of health or of functional status achieved following illness or injury
- *restoration* of function when injury or disease has interrupted function in one or more body systems.

Our services have focused almost exclusively on restoration of function. Few physical therapists have had the time or the inclination to participate in the other three components of physical therapy. In the future, our services must encompass all four components with equal emphasis—development, prevention, maintenance, and restoration.

DEMANDS FROM OTHER SOURCES

PATIENTS

Demands from our consumers (patients, clients), our sponsors who support our services, and our colleagues will require us to change our image. Our consumers, patients and others, will expect expert, caring service. They will want services that help them to meet their goals, not ours, and services that are reliable, dependable, and reasonably priced.

They will want to choose who will deliver the service. We seldom allow a patient to select the physical therapist who will deliver services. Instead, the physical therapist is assigned to a patient because time is available in that person's schedule.

SPONSORS

The sponsors, our third-party payers, will demand the most service possible for the least expenditure of funds. They will expect precision in the identification of a patient's problems and an estimate of the time required to eliminate or ease those problems. Sponsors will want predictable outcomes.

COLLEAGUES IN OTHER PROFESSIONS

Our colleagues in other professions will expect us to be:

- knowledgeable about physiologic and anatomic functions of the human body in health and following illness or trauma
- skillful in the delivery of physical therapy services
- articulate in expressing ourselves in speech and in writing.

In addition, they will expect us to:

- add to the body of knowledge in physical therapy and to the general body of knowledge that we all share
- share what we learn through publications and presentations at scientific meetings.

COLLEAGUES IN PHYSICAL THERAPY

Our colleagues in physical therapy will expect the same as colleagues in other professions and much more. For example:

- models to emulate in clinical practice, research, and education
- opportunities to use knowledge and skills that they have acquired and to continue learning in their employment settings
- opportunities to prepare for advancement in a variety of ways (e.g., a work/study program that would permit movement from one facet of physical therapy to another without completely sacrificing employment income)
- participation in political action that helps to further a cause on behalf of the public, physical therapy, and physical therapists.

IMPLICATIONS FOR THE FUTURE

First, my message is that if we want to survive as a profession, we must substantiate the basis of our practice through research. The dearth of clinical research, particularly descriptive research, strongly suggests a mandate to all clinicians. Descriptive studies are necessary to identify the important basic and applied research for which we must accept responsibility as a group and in collaboration with our colleagues in other disciplines.

The next implication is that education must change drastically. The curriculum must prepare a physical therapist for a role that is not yet clearly defined, but one that will surely be different, demanding, challenging, and rewarding. We can expect the physical therapist of the future to fill a role that may require functioning in any of the following facets, as well as in others: administrator, care giver (generalist), change agent, clinical specialist, consultant, educator, evaluator, manager, political activist, supervisor, teacher, researcher. When additional facets of the role emerge, as the physical therapist accepts other responsibilities in health care, the educational programs must be prepared to respond to those needs without undue delay.

Another implication is that students will be older and less likely to follow blindly where we might want to lead them. More students in the future will have a breadth and depth of knowledge on which to build the foundation for the practice of physical therapy. They will expect us to make preparation for practice a thrilling, rewarding, and challenging experience instead of a drudgery to complete until they can do what they say they really want to do—work with patients.

Another serious implication as our image changes is that the faculty must be leaders in education, and participants in research and patient care when that is practical and desired. Their credentials must equal those of other faculty in the university. To have an adequate number of qualified faculty to prepare the physical therapists of the near future, many of you will need to hurry back to the ivied halls of learning for advanced degrees, perhaps at great personal sacrifice and considerable expense.

A frequent complaint that I have heard from physical therapists about graduate study is that no program exactly fits their needs. My advice is to take the program that comes closest to fitting your needs and make that work for you and the profession and, consequently, for your patients. Since our need for faculty knows no bounds, you may seek a doctorate in physical therapy, physiology, kinesiology, sociology, psychology, neuro-linguistics, education, curriculum, teaching methodology, administration, financial management, or personnel management. Since that is hardly an exhaustive list of the possibilities, one can hardly say that no graduate program is available that fits a need or an interest.

SUMMARY

As we gain independence in practice, our horizons will be unlimited. Education will be a major force in changing our image in the future through the initial professional preparation and continuing education. Our role will expand to include a greater variety of services that emphasize development and maintenance of health as well as new approaches to the restoration of function.

An implication for major curriculum change is that all physical therapists in the future may have a doctorate, either the professional degree for entry into the field as a practitioner or a scholarly degree, the PhD.

Concern that the physical therapist with an advanced degree will have difficulty in finding desirable employment is unfounded. Physical therapists with master's degrees have paved the way. When a majority of physical therapists are in independent practice, suitable employment opportunities for those with advanced degrees will fade as an issue.

If we want the responsibilities that are inherent in independent practice, we must be willing to accept the consequences:

INDEX

A "t" following a page number indicates a table. A page number in *italics* indicates a figure.